SHOCK TRAUMA/ CRITICAL CARE MANUAL

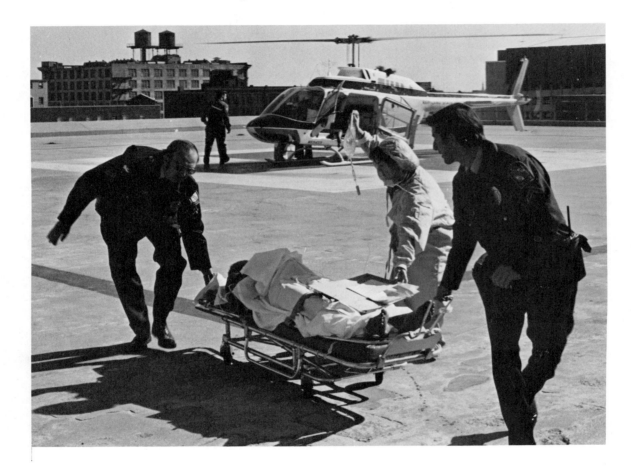

In the race against death, a patient is rapidly transported to the Shock Trauma Center where resuscitation will be continued and definitive management initiated...

SHOCK TRAUMA/ CRITICAL CARE MANUAL

Initial Assessment and Management

Edited by

R Adams Cowley, M.D.
Director

and

C. Michael Dunham, M.D.
Attending Traumatologist

Maryland Institute for Emergency
Medical Services Systems
Baltimore, Maryland

University Park Press
Baltimore

UNIVERSITY PARK PRESS
International Publishers in Medicine and Human Services
300 North Charles Street
Baltimore, Maryland 21201

Copyright © 1982 by University Park Press
Second printing, May 1983

Typeset by University Park Press, Typesetting Division
Manufactured in the United States of America by The Maple Press Company

Cover photograph courtesy of MIEMSS, Public Relations Division.

Library of Congress Cataloging in Publication Data
Main entry under title:

Shock trauma/critical care manual.

Includes index.
1. Emergency medicine—Handbooks, manuals, etc.
2. Shock—Handbooks, manuals, etc.   I. Cowley, R Adams,
1917-   . II. Dunham, C. Michael. [DNLM: 1. Wounds
and injuries. 2. Critical care—Methods. 3. Emergency
medicine—Methods. WO 700 S559]
RC86.7.S463   616'.025
ISBN 0-8391-1712-4   AACR2

Contents

Preface

This book is the culmination of work over a number of years in the development of an evolutionary clinical program on the assessment and management of the critically ill and injured patient. When the shock trauma program was conceived 20 years ago, there was no existing model care system for the acute management of the severely injured and ill patient. From our experience in this program we developed our philosophy and treatment protocols into a teaching manual. As the program developed and our knowledge increased, the manual was expanded, updated, and refined each year. Thus, what is presented here is our current experience on the management of multiple trauma and critical care problems, as seen in the Shock Trauma Center at the Maryland Institute for Emergency Medical Services Systems.

Unlike other publications, this book focuses only on the clinical problems that are seen daily in a large trauma/critical care center. A conscientious effort has been made to include all necessary aspects of successful patient management during the acute phase of illness. We have tried to make the information as clinically relevant as possible, and have purposefully deleted or minimized historic and pathophysiologic information to avail maximum space for the presentation of our experience in the day-to-day management of catastrophic injury and illness.

We strive to provide many answers to questions asked about the acute management of these victims. It is our hope that this manual will provide a practical and ready clinical reference for the surgeon, the anesthesiologist, the critical care specialist, the emergency room physician, the nurse, and the house officer. We have included guidelines on general procedures for various critical problems, immediate resuscitation, stabilization, and diagnosis and treatment. We have developed extensive expertise in the management of multiple system injuries, the ruptured aorta, chest contusion, and abdominal, central nervous system, and extremity injuries; these injuries are presented in depth in this volume. Cross-references to supplemental information are listed in parentheses throughout the book.

Many authors of surgical trauma books deal extensively with penetrating wounds, and most physicians who come into our program already have a generous experience with penetrating wounds from the war in Vietnam and the upsurge in violent crimes. Their experience with blunt trauma, however, is often minimal. Both types of injuries are discussed in this work, with greater emphasis being placed on life-threatening blunt injuries.

In our hands this manual has been of significant assistance in minimizing death and permanent disability. It has also provided a useful educational tool in this clinical arena.

Large community and university hospitals can no longer pretend to be everything to everyone. More comprehensive management systems must evolve to provide the necessary care for survival of the acutely injured and ill patient. Therefore, in the emergency management of these unfortunate victims, the first objective is to *save the life*. The second objective is to prevent disability. The third objective is to provide a rehabilitation system that will return the patient to an active and productive life. The final objective is to make such a dedicated program cost-effective. These objectives require constant surveillance, scrutiny, and creativity if the goal of optimal care is to be met. The concept of holistic care also becomes an important element of our philosophy and demands teamwork at every level, especially in rehabilitative care. A change in thinking about this latter aspect, as it relates to acute care, is required if we are to lessen disability.

Finally, hypoxia, the destroyer of all life, insidiously tears down the biochemical energy-transducing systems so necessary for survival. Therefore, the message throughout this book is to prevent hypoxia: maintain ventilation, control the hemorrhage, and maintain optimal tissue perfusion.

R Adams Cowley, M.D.
C. Michael Dunham, M.D.

Acknowledgments

My deep personal gratitude is expressed to C. Michael Dunham, my co-editor. He, more than anyone, has made the publication of this manual possible.

Both of us are indebted to the many physicians, nurses, and administrative personnel who participated in the 20-year clinical evolution of the MIEMSS shock trauma program. They gave generously of their time in writing up each clinical procedure performed in caring for our patients. I wish I could mention and personally thank each individual; they have not been forgotten for their contribution. Space prevents naming all those who have made a contribution to the program. A special thanks goes to Dr. William S. Stone, former Dean of the University of Maryland Medical School, and Dr. Sam F. Seeley, Brig. Gen. USMC (Ret.), for their constant encouragement and advocacy of the program over the years of its development.

Special appreciation goes to my present clinical staff and consultants, listed below, who gave of their time and expertise in the preparation of this manual.

Mr. John Ashworth	Dr. Dorothy Gordon	Dr. Thomas Phillips
Ms. Sandra Bond-Lillicropp	Mr. Alex Gretes	Dr. Ameen Ramzy
Dr. David Boyd	Dr. J. Alex Haller	Dr. Ken Ransom
Dr. John Britten	Dr. Kirk Hamilton	Dr. Richard Richards
Dr. Sheldon Brotman	Dr. John Hoopes	Dr. Aurelio Rodriguez
Dr. Bruce Browner	Dr. Alexander Kuehl	Dr. Thomas Saul
Dr. Ellis Caplan	Dr. Larry Leonard	Ms. Elizabeth Scanlan
Dr. Peter Chodoff	Dr. Thomas Majerus	Ms. Ann Scanlon
Dr. Alasdair Conn	Dr. Paul McClelland	Dr. Bruce Shack
Dr. Everard Cox	Dr. Frank McCormack	Dr. Clayton Shatney
Dr. Raymond Curtis	Dr. Paul Manson	Dr. Carl Soderstrom
Dr. Ben Dawson	Dr. Peter Margand	Dr. Joseph Sperrazza
Dr. A. Lee Dellon	Dr. Edmund Middleton	Dr. John Stene
Dr. Thomas Ducker	Dr. Philip Militello	Dr. Benjamin F. Trump
Dr. C. Michael Dunham	Dr. Roy Myers	Dr. Stephen Z. Turney
Ms. Marge Epperson	Dr. Ole Otteson	

They drew on the work of predecessors and updated and refined each chapter to reflect our most current techniques in managing catastrophic medical problems. In addition, this work would not have been possible without the patient cooperation and sacrifice of the families who supported the staff during the long hours of manuscript writing.

Our secretarial staff must also be acknowledged for the painstaking care given in typing the many manuscript drafts.

Finally, a special acknowledgment goes to Ruby Richardson of University Park Press. Her personal interest and enthusiasm for the publication of this manual, her broad knowledge and attention to detail, and her support and encouragement to the staff were invaluable.

R Adams Cowley

To Liz, Sandy, and Mike

RAC

Introduction

Trauma is responsible for the deaths of more than 150,000 persons in the United States every year. An additional 10 to 17 million are disabled annually as a result of trauma, 380,000 of them permanently. Trauma ranks as the third greatest killer in the United States, surpassed only by heart disease and cancer. Yet the impact of trauma on American society is not adequately reflected in these statistics, grim as they are. Whereas cancer and heart disease typically strike in middle or late life, the toll of trauma falls disproportionately on the young. More Americans between the ages of 1 and 44 die as a result of trauma than from any disease. Accidents alone kill four times more children (1–14 years) than the next leading cause of death, and motor vehicle accidents by themselves account for 38% of deaths among those aged 15 to 24. Trauma causes three quarters of all mortality among teenagers and young adults. It extinguishes lives that have just entered their productive years, and taxes heavily one of society's most valuable assets—its young people. The cost of trauma goes far beyond what is spent on initial emergency care, although that sum in itself is enormous. The unseen costs of trauma are measured in decades of lost productivity and earnings, in families left without a chief provider, and, frequently for those who survive the injury, in a lifetime of expensive rehabilitation and therapy. The total costs of trauma to society therefore probably exceed those associated with the other major types of illness.

Thus, the crisis in medicine today is in the delivery of emergency care. For the two greatest killers, cancer and heart disease, new discoveries are needed to reduce mortality, and national institutes have been established with federal funding to do the requisite research. For trauma, a systems approach is needed to meet the specific challenges trauma presents.

Such a revolutionary systems approach to the treatment of shock and traumatic injuries began in Maryland in 1960. A clinical shock trauma unit was established in Baltimore through a contract with the U.S. Army Office of the Surgeon General, with the overall goal of ensuring every citizen's right to the best emergency care regardless of type of illness or injury, its severity, the patient's financial circumstances, or geographic location. A simple proposal was made: bring the hospital's resources to the patient by building the hospital around the patient. The patient would not be moved. Every resource would be adjacent and readily available. Everything needed for the patient's care and for the study of the patient's condition would be there. Medical knowledge as well as the patient's well-being would therefore be advanced at the same time. The success of this pilot unit led to the awarding of a NIH Research Facilities grant in 1963 to build a model facility devoted exclusively to the critically ill or injured patient. This model facility, the Shock Trauma Center, after many years of research, trial, and error, was completed in 1969.

During these years of initial organization, it was learned that the first 60 minutes, "the golden hour," after a life-threatening incident dictates whether a patient will live or die. Another factor influencing survival is access to an emergency medical system providing on-site resuscitation, evaluation, triage, and communication and transportation with care en route to a definitive care facility. The Maryland group, therefore, set out with the cooperation of the Maryland State Police Air Med-Evac System and ambulance services statewide to formalize an emergency health care delivery system with the primary goal of saving lives and coordinating emergency health efforts throughout the state (see Appendix section on Trauma/Emergency Medical Services Systems).

In 1971, a plan for the development and organization of a statewide, systematized emergency medical services program for Maryland was written and submitted to the Governor. The plan was based on a regional concept and encompassed communications, transportation, education, training, implementation, and evaluation. On February 26, 1973, the Governor by executive order created a Division of Emergency Medical Services to implement this program and complement the University of Maryland Center for the Study of Trauma.

In 1977, legislation was passed amalgamating the emergency medical services program with the Shock Trauma Center into the Maryland Institute for Emergency Medical Services Systems (MIEMSS), an autonomous institution on the campus of the University of Maryland at Baltimore. This merger combined the educational, research, and professional expertise of the academic and clinical programs with the state emergency medical services system.

Today MIEMSS is the clinical core of the state's emergency medical services system. As a public institution its mission is to make available specialized patient care, develop new concepts of care, and provide educational and research resources to those institutions, agencies, and citizens of the state of Maryland as well as others who wish to study shock and trauma and emergency medical services problems. In addition, MIEMSS provided the impetus to the formation of an eight-state EMS council to raise emergency care in the region to state-of-the-art standards.

MIEMSS' first responsibility is to save life and prevent disability. The overall care of the severely ill or injured patient is beyond the capabilities and experience of any individual physician. Thus a holistic approach to treatment and the cooperative efforts of a multidisciplinary team of specialists at the attending staff level are required.

On admission, all patients are assumed to be dying and much of the "golden hour" for total stabilization has passed. Thus, the fight for survival begins immediately. Treatment begins before diagnosis—a necessary break with tradition. Resuscitation and stabilization have priority as many victims would die awaiting an accurate diagnosis.

MIEMSS' basic philosophy is to provide total preparedness for any life-threatening injury. This requires the immediate availability of seasoned experts to manage the clinical program 24 hours a day, 7 days a week. MIEMSS receives those patients whose only chance for survival is through the aggressive, state-of-the-art care that MIEMSS offers. Criteria for admission include any of the following: severe injuries (two or more body systems), head and spinal cord injuries, cardiac and major vessel injuries, uncontrolled shock from any cause, multiple injuries with complications (e.g., shock, sepsis, organ failure), severe facial and eye injuries, burns, gas gangrene, and carbon monoxide and other poisonings, including attempted suicides.

In managing life-threatening problems, unplanned therapy can be disastrous. Indecision and procrastination with therapy is hazardous. Because of the urgency and the type of patient treated, standardized modes of therapy have been developed and are the substance of this book.

These standard treatment protocols offer the advantages of 1) a single coordinated approach to patient care problems, 2) standardization of training, 3) facilitation of research and evaluation via a standard data base, and 4) a basis for legal standards for trauma care.

The probability of patient survival is greatly improved when time is not wasted by the team determining a possible care plan. Communication between the physician, nurse, and paramedic is simplified. All team members know their roles and tasks. Thus, they function independently, automatically, and efficiently throughout the resuscitation and stabilization phase. In addition, the protocols ensure that essential steps are not inadvertently left out or forgotten, jeopardizing the treatment plan.

Protocols facilitate planning and conducting of an extensive training program. The didactic content of lectures is based on the educational requirements needed to understand and perform the treatment protocols used at MIEMSS. Psychomotor skills are also taught to ensure proper technique.

Standardized protocols provide a concrete basis by which to measure the quality of patient care provided by new treatment protocols undergoing trial. The morbidity and mortality of different treatment modes can also be evaluated, providing a mechanism to change and improve patient care.

This protocol system provides the accepted standard for trauma care in the State of Maryland. Treatment protocols are reviewed yearly by MIEMSS' Protocol Review Committee. Each protocol is updated by the appropriate specialist to reflect the state of the art. Then the committee, consisting of the Director, the Clinical Director, the Chief of Traumatology, the Chief of Anesthesia/Critical Care, and the Director of Nursing, approves the proposed changes.

MIEMSS' clinical operation and philosophy can be better appreciated by following the course of a patient through the various care units.

The Admitting Areas, where the initial resuscitation, evaluation, and stabilization procedures outlined in this book are conducted, are always prepared for the admission of patients with life-threatening injuries. Loaded intravenous lines, surgical packs, monitoring devices, and resuscitation and diagnostic equipment stand ready. Once the estimated time of arrival is known, one of the four trauma teams is immediately mobilized. An anesthesiologist and a nurse are dispatched to the helipad to await the arrival, while the remainder of the team, consisting of the Team Leader (a surgeon), a trauma nurse, an anesthesiologist, and one or more surgical or emergency room residents, stand ready for the patient's arrival in the Admitting Area. There is no waiting. Radiographic equipment, blood, and all other life-saving components are available on the spot. If necessary, the patient can be moved a few steps to the adjacent operating room. All patient admissions are the responsibility of the Team Leader under the immediate supervision of the senior attending physician. The Team Leader directs the resuscitation, stabilization, and triage of all patients.

The surgeon and the anesthesiologist discuss the surgical and anesthetic plan before surgery is started. They act as a team throughout the surgical procedure and during the postoperative phase. Decisions regarding patient care are made according to the protocol system described.

The Team Leader has the responsibility for care throughout the patient's hospital stay. The Team Leader and the primary nurse for each nursing unit, supported by multidisciplinary specialists and therapists, participate in the patient's total care. A consultant writes patient orders in an emergency when the Team Leader or designate is not available. Should a consultant need to write orders, the Team Leader is immediately notified of the action.

Once stabilized in the Admitting Area or operating room, the patient is moved to the 12-bed, sophisticated Critical Care Recovery Unit (CCRU). There the patient is closely monitored, and all orders are reviewed and rewritten. A chest x-ray, EKG, lab profile, and any other pertinent data are ordered at the time of admission to the CCRU. When a patient is ready for transfer from the CCRU to another unit, the team summarizes the patient's course and writes the necessary orders. Routine transfers occur at 4:30 p.m.; transfers may be made at other times according to bed requirements. The shift charge nurse coordinates all non-routine transfers with the Team Leader or designate.

The Team Leader and the primary nurse are responsible for family contact and support. Telephone contact is maintained with the family spokesperson by the primary nurse. All information given to the family about the patient's condition is cleared with the Team Leader; the Team Leader partakes in as many communications as possible with the patient's family. Through participation in patient rounds, the nursing staff is aware of all changes in treatment, prognosis, and clinical plans.

As the patient improves beyond the need for the highly specialized CCRU care, he or she progresses to a special intensive care unit (ICU) similar to those in other hospitals. When the patient enters the ICU, all previous orders are reviewed and revised as necessary. The ICU primary nurse works with the Team Leader and the disposition coordinator in making rehabilitation and discharge plans for the patient.

Intermediate care at MIEMSS is dedicated as a unit to helping the patient adapt to the environment within the confines of any post-trauma disability. As a process this involves dealing with the patient's total needs, including psychosocial and physical needs. The family now becomes an integral part of the patient's care in reorientation, teaching, and discharge planning, and in helping the family and the community to reincorporate the patient as a useful citizen.

The trauma team coordinates with the nursing staff of the intermediate care unit (IMCU) the smooth transition of the patient from other units to this facility. The mix of patients is quite broad and includes those who are stable with limited injuries and who do not require intensive nursing or electronic monitoring, those who are awaiting the completion of discharge disposition arrangements, and those who are staying at MIEMSS for rehabilitation or follow-up surgery. Patients transferred to the IMCU ordinarily do not require monitoring devices, are not on respirators, do not require balanced traction, and have stable vital signs. Occasionally, patients will be electively admitted to this unit for follow-up surgery or for hyperbaric medicine treatment.

The IMCU primary nurse coordinates and expedites the reorientation of the patient and the follow-up arrangements for the patient prior to discharge. The Team Leader is aware of patient needs and makes regular rounds to include nursing requests for medical assistance. Discharge then is to a rehabilitation hospital, a hospital near the patient's home, a nursing home, or the patient's own home. Should complications occur, the patient is returned to a more specialized unit.

The support functions at MIEMSS are also essential for saving lives. Because of the need for immediate and frequent laboratory data, MIEMSS maintains its own Clinical "Stat" Laboratory. Staffed 24 hours a day, the lab can return most test results within 10 minutes.

Radiologic examinations are carried out in the Admitting Area as well as in the CCRU and the step-down units. Special contrast studies are made in the Radiology Department. Uncrossmatched blood and blood components are always available in MIEMSS' mini-blood bank. MIEMSS cooperates with the University of Maryland Hospital blood bank for the larger amounts of blood and blood derivatives required. A multidisciplinary Family Services branch offers psychosocial help both to patients and their families, crisis intervention and counseling during their stay, and assistance with discharge planning. Psychiatric consultation is always available for patients and staff.

To reduce disability, rehabilitation should ideally begin at the time of injury and continue throughout definitive care. Prevention, maintenance, and restoration are major elements in the rehabilitation process; integration of the appropriate elements at the right time and place facilitates recuperation and patient adjustment. The program is based on individual patient assessment. Most patients need intensive rehabilitation following stabilization and during recovery from trauma. Early evaluation by rehabilitation personnel determines when and which specific therapies should be used. Joint patient rounds and discharge planning conferences are held to facilitate continuity of care.

Research is pursued on both basic and clinical laboratory levels. Physicians, nurses, and researchers are constantly seeking ways to improve patient care. No clinical study is made that would endanger the patient, and all studies comply completely with the University's Human Volunteers Committee.

Professional educational opportunities include 1- and 2-year fellowships in traumatology, critical care medicine, and research. MIEMSS also sponsors training programs for physicians, nurses, emergency medical technicians, and paramedic and helicopter crews. In-house and outreach programs as well as state and national seminars and conferences are available in addition to public education programs.

The education and research functions are less dramatic than the life-saving measures of patient care, but just as important. Research efforts have allowed us continually to provide new modes of therapy, thereby reducing mortality and morbidity. The immediate autopsy program (see Chapter 39) has advanced greatly our understanding of cell injury and its relationship to survival. Current research areas receiving greatest attention at MIEMSS include systemic infection, severe head injury, and hepatic dysfunction, as these remain the chief causes of mortality after initial stabilization. Since the shock trauma unit was founded, our mortality rate has dropped from 70% to 16.3%. Our educational programs have trained numerous physicians who are now establishing and managing trauma centers throughout the country, thus allowing the expertise we have developed to be spread and the original purpose of the unit, better patient care, to be practiced elsewhere.

SHOCK TRAUMA/ CRITICAL CARE MANUAL

Section I
INITIAL EVALUATION AND MANAGEMENT OF THE TRAUMA PATIENT

INTRODUCTION

The multiple trauma patient is received by the admitting team on-call. Each member has a predesignated duty. In most cases, it will be necessary to institute resuscitation measures before a complete diagnostic assessment has been performed. The admitting team has adequate time to scrub and change uniforms prior to the arrival of the patient.

I. **First Priorities**

   A. **Rapidly** inspect the patient on arrival for skin color, alertness, chest wall motion, and extremity movement.

   B. Palpate the pulse (slow, rapid, strong, weak) and obtain a blood pressure.

   C. Auscultate the chest for the presence of breath sounds.

   D. Establish an airway and provide adequate ventilation (see p. 15).

   E. Assess whether the patient follows commands.

   F. Assess the extremity posture to noxious sternal compression.

   G. Assess the size of each pupil and determine whether the pupil reacts to light.

   H. Control external hemorrhage.

   I. Establish intravenous lines and begin volume infusion (see p. 7).

   J. Obtain admission blood work.

   K. Initiate EKG monitoring.

   L. Obtain a baseline arterial blood gas sample. The blood gas should be on room air if the patient is not intubated. The acid-base status and PaO_2/FiO_2 ratio can be calculated to estimate the degree of anaerobic metabolism and the pulmonary shunt (see p. 316).

   M. Stabilize the cervical spine with a hard collar and/or sandbags.

Do not become concerned with peripheral injuries until the cardiovascular, pulmonary, and neurologic systems are stabilized. The first priorities are directed at evaluating these systems, since instability poses an immediate threat to the patient's life. The first priorities are concomitantly performed by multiple team members (surgeon, anesthesiologist, and nurse).

In all but a very few situations, time exists for an adequate preparation of skin prior to the insertion of lines. <u>Remember</u>: Infection is the leading cause of death in trauma patients.

Those measures listed under "First Priorities" will normally require only a few minutes. The second and third priorities are more time-consuming.

II. **Second Priorities**

    A. A brief examination of the head, chest, abdomen, pelvis, and extremities is performed.

    B. Brief and pertinent history is obtained.

    C. A lateral cervical spine x-ray is obtained.

    D. An upright chest x-ray is obtained (see p. 32).

    E. An anterior-posterior (AP) x-ray of the pelvis is obtained.

    F. Insert a Foley catheter.

    G. Pass an orogastric tube.

    H. Peritoneal lavage and/or abdominal examination is performed.

    I. A more complete neurologic examination is performed (see pp. 225 and 230).

    J. Splint extremity fractures.

    K. Emergency surgery is performed, if indicated.

    L. An arterial line is inserted, if indicated (see p. 461).

III. **Third Priorities**

    A. Systematic examination

        1. Facial and scalp evaluation

        2. Evaluation of the extremities

        3. Rectal, pelvic, and perineal examinations

        4. Back examination

B. Radiologic studies

    1. Additional x-rays

    2. CAT scan

    3. Contrast studies

    4. Intravenous pyelogram (IVP)-cystogram

C. Specialty consultation

D. EKG

E. Temperature

F. Urgent surgery

G. Swan-Ganz catheter, if indicated

By the time the third priorities are initiated, the patient's general state should be acceptable, unless emergency surgery is indicated. A repeat, detailed assessment with multidiscipline consultation is indicated in order to completely assess and properly manage the patient's problems.

IV. Procedural Comments

A. The anesthesiologist and nurse assess the patient at the helipad and start appropriate emergency therapy. A status report is given to the receiving team immediately prior to the patient's arrival in the Admitting Area.

B. The attending staff and Team Leader direct the sequence of events from this point on.

C. The anesthesiologist manages the airway.

D. Monitoring the central venous pressure is a necessary part of proper patient management in MIEMSS.

E. After the central line is inserted, 70 cc of blood is drawn for type and crossmatch and all routine lab studies.

F. After blood is drawn, plasma protein fraction or blood is administered at a speed dictated by the patient's condition. **Generally, a colloid expander** (1,500 cc) **is used at this stage as the initial resuscitation fluid** (see p. 35).

G. Surgical priorities are decided by the Team Leader in consultation with the specialty staff.

H. A combative patient must be immobilized early in the course of resuscitation; otherwise, the various intravascular catheters may be pulled out. The patient should preferably be sedated with the approval of the neurosurgeon. If it is unsafe to sedate the patient, it may be necessary to securely tie the patient to the table. If this proves inadequate to properly immobilize and resuscitate the patient, an artificial airway is inserted and nitrous oxide/oxygen and short-acting muscle relaxants are administered. In general, one should avoid narcotics in the Admitting Area until injuries have been clearly defined. **Remember: Hypoxemia is a common cause of restlessness or combativeness.**

I. Once a patient is fully evaluated and a **satisfactory neurologic examination** is completed and recorded, the patient may be anesthetized if immediate surgery is required.

J. The patient's family should be called by the clerk for the following reasons:

1. The Team Leader has a responsibility to inform the family of the patient's accident and condition. The nurse in the Admitting Area should be involved with providing information should the physician be unable to discuss the patient with the family.

2. Information from the family should be obtained regarding the patient's past medical history.

1

CARDIOVASCULAR ASSESSMENT AND STABILIZATION

A primary concern in the post-trauma patient is oxygen transport to the tissues. If there is sufficient pulmonary function, the major focus is on assessing the adequacy of the cardiac output and the hemoglobin concentration, i.e., the cardiovascular status.

I. **Etiology** Although cardiovascular instability is usually due to hypovolemia, absolute or relative, causes of cardiogenic shock must be excluded.

  A. **Hypovolemia** is the major cause of shock in the traumatized patient.

   1. Overt blood loss
      a. Major lacerations
      b. Smaller lacerations associated with severed vascular tissue, e.g., the scalp

   2. Concealed blood loss
      a. Chest (hemothorax)
      b. Major fracture (e.g., pelvic or femur)
      c. Peritoneal
      d. Retroperitoneal

  B. **Cardiogenic shock** (pump failure)

   1. Tension pneumothorax

   2. Cardiac tamponade

   3. Cardiac contusion

   4. Cardiac arrhythmias

  C. **Miscellaneous** (relatively uncommon)

   1. Myocardial infarction

   2. Quadriplegia

   3. Head injury (severe and terminal)

   4. Hypothermia

II. **Clinical Manifestations** Cardiovascular instability is manifested by a characteristic physiologic response. Manifestations of cardiovascular instability are:

A. **Symptoms**

  1. Thirst

  2. Weakness

B. **Signs**

  1. Hypotension

  2. Tachycardia

  3. Pallor

  4. Anxiety

  5. Cool extremities

  6. Decreased capillary refill

  7. Diaphoresis

  8. Cyanosis

  9. Decreased urine output

C. **Laboratory data** Falling hematocrit; the rapidity of the fall relates to the severity of the bleeding.

> **Perspective**
> A patient may not be hypotensive until one-fourth to one-third of intravascular volume has been lost. The normotensive patient with other manifestations of circulatory insufficiency should be aggressively treated before profound cardiovascular collapse takes place.

III. **Treatment** Proper treatment depends on a correct diagnosis which, in turn, is dependent on a thorough assessment of the patient. Since hypovolemia is the most common cause of shock, the primary treatment is volume infusion. Since the primary therapy for cardiogenic shock is not volume infusion, its subtle manifestations should be actively sought.

A. **Central venous pressure** The central venous pressure (CVP) helps to differentiate hypovolemic and cardiogenic shock. In general, extremes of the CVP and the trend of the CVP in response to a fluid challenge are the most helpful guides in regulating volume infusion. More succinctly, very low central venous pressures (less than 8 cm) suggest hypovolemia and very high central venous pressures (greater than 18 cm) imply cardiogenic shock. A rise in CVP in response to volume infusion implies adequate filling of the intravascular space. Minimal to absent rise in CVP in response to fluid infusion implies the presence of hypovolemia.

B. **Vascular access**

1. The initial treatment of cardiovascular instability, in general, in conjunction with securing an adequate airway and ventilation, is directed at volume infusion. The first step in volume infusion pertains to securing adequate venous access. The number and size of venous lines will be dictated by the magnitude of cardiovascular instability. If the blood pressure is stable, the heart rate is less than 100, and there are no manifestations of shock, a long line is inserted in the antecubital fossa and is directed centrally. Through this line, initial blood work is obtained, a central venous pressure is recorded, and volume infusion is begun.

2. If signs and symptoms of severe cardiovascular instability are present, an antecubital long line is inserted in conjunction with a saphenous line. This will allow infusion above and below the diaphragm to ensure that at least one line is infusing a nondisrupted venous system. If hypovolemia is severe, vascular collapse will not allow percutaneous insertion via a peripheral vein. In this state, lines must be inserted via peripheral cutdown and/or central percutaneous venipuncture (subclavian or internal jugular routes). There are potential complications associated with subclavian venipuncture (discussed on p. 470). If the subclavian venipuncture is unsuccessful upon one or two attempts, it should be abandoned, and venous access should be obtained by peripheral cutdowns. Cutdown sites of choice are: antecubital fossa, cephalic vein at wrist or shoulder, and greater saphenous vein in the groin or ankle. Size 10 or 12 French feeding tubes are used for large volume infusion. Massive volume infusion may be performed by inserting a Swan-Ganz introducer by the Seldinger technique.

C. **Infusion rate**   Rate of infusion is dictated by the return of cardiovascular stability and/or a significant rise in the CVP. The rate of infusion should be as rapid as possible and monitored by the CVP, the systemic arterial pressure, and the clinical manifestations of adequate tissue perfusion. Reversal of cardiovascular instability is suggested by the following:

1. Stable blood pressure

2. Slowing of the heart rate

3. Increased level of consciousness

4. Decreased anxiety

5. Improved color of mucous membranes, toes and fingers, and capillary refill

6. Warming of the extremities

7. Increased urinary output (equal to or greater than 30 cc/hr)

D. **Infusate**   Initially, the patient is administered plasmanate. If 1,500 cc of plasmanate is administered, and the patient remains unstable, red blood cell infusion is begun in order to maintain acceptable oxygen capacity of the circulating blood.

Judgment must be made regarding the use of uncrossmatched blood in unstable patients. O-negative blood is an ideal universal donor, but it is frequently difficult to obtain. Uncrossmatched O-positive red blood cells may be used in emergency cases, since major transfusion reactions are rare and maintenance of oxygen-carrying capacity is essential for maintaining patient viability. There is a major concern in administering O-positive blood to women of childbearing age who may develop antibodies to the Rh antigen if they are Rh-negative. The immediate welfare of the potential mother, however, is the primary concern in a hemodynamically unstable situation. (See p. 36.)

E. **Surgical intervention**

1. In conjunction with volume infusion, it is necessary to evaluate sites of probable blood loss and to halt the hemorrhagic process. Most **external hemorrhage** can be controlled with pressure. **Femoral fractures** should be immobilized by traction (Buck's traction or Thomas's splints) or by use of an air splint to reduce bleeding. A patient may lose 500–2,000 cc of blood if the fracture is comminuted and/or in a large thigh. A patient with a **pelvic fracture** usually loses a minimum of 500–2,000 cc of blood. Blood loss will be greater if there is instability, comminution, or associated major vascular injury. Considerations for hemorrhagic control should include Military Anti-Shock Trousers (MAST), application of a Hoffman device, and/or angiography with embolic tamponade, as described on p. 197.

2. Consideration must be made for the presence of **hemothorax** in the post-trauma patient in shock. In general, if the patient is hypotensive and has decreased breath sounds, a chest tube should be inserted into the pleural space immediately and the flow rate monitored. If the flow rate is significant, thoracotomy must be considered (see p. 111).

3. Peritoneal lavage should be performed in the hypotensive patient in order to assess the **peritoneal cavity** as a source of hemorrhage. Splenic, hepatic, and mesenteric injuries are frequent sources of major hemorrhage and must be excluded. If the lavage is positive, the abdomen must be explored (see p. 146).

4. Another area of concealed blood loss is the **retroperitoneal compartment.** Hemorrhage in this compartment is suggested by
   a. Hematuria
   b. Flank ecchymosis
   c. Expanding flank mass
   d. Lumbar spine fracture

   (See pp. 175, 181, and 183.)

F. **Cardiogenic shock** As previously stated, signs and symptoms of cardiogenic shock must be aggressively sought. If the CVP is very high or rapidly rising with volume infusion, cardiogenic shock must be strongly considered. A high CVP presents clinically as neck vein distention.

1. **Tension pneumothorax**   If there are absent breath sounds in the face of hypotension, a chest tube should be inserted into the pleural space. If a tension pneumothorax is present, a gush of air will be expelled; the hemodynamic instability will be alleviated, if hemorrhagic shock is not present concomitantly (see p. 113).

2. **Cardiac tamponade or contusion**   Hypotension in the presence of a high CVP and/or neck vein distention should arouse concern for the presence of cardiac tamponade or cardiac contusion (see p. 120). Frequently, cardiogenic shock is difficult to diagnose, especially if there is associated hypovolemia. The hemodynamic manifestations of cardiac contusion or tamponade may not become apparent until the hypovolemia is corrected. Cardiac valvular and septal tears are rare causes of pump failure.

G. **Miscellaneous considerations**   Other considerations in the hemodynamically unstable patient are: myocardial infarction, quadriplegia, hypothermia, and head injury. A patient may have had an auto accident secondary to a myocardial infarction and, hence, may present in cardiogenic shock. A quadriplegic patient may be hypotensive secondary to sympathectomy. The quadriplegic-hypotensive patient has a bradycardia as opposed to tachycardia which is seen in hypovolemic shock. In this setting, poor perfusion is treated with dopamine (Intropin) to maintain a urinary output equal to 30 cc/hr (see p. 237). A head-injured patient is rarely hypotensive from the central nervous system (CNS) injury, except as a manifestation of a terminal brain stem insult. In other words, hypotension in the head-injured patient should usually be considered secondary to hypovolemia or cardiogenic shock, until proven otherwise. Hypothermia may cause hypotension by myocardial depression, vasodilation, and by creating arrhythmias. As with all trauma patients, the shock patient's temperature should be noted carefully in cold weather.

H. **Monitoring**   In shock, venous access is the initial priority. If the patient has improved, but has multiple injuries, an **arterial line** should be inserted to continually assess hemodynamic function. In the hemodynamically unstable patient, continuous arterial monitoring is indicated. If the femoral pulse is palpable, a femoral arterial catheter is inserted. If the pulses are poorly palpable, a radial arterial cutdown is performed. The radial artery, if pulseless, may be easily located by anatomical landmarks (see p. 462).

A **Foley catheter** should be inserted in the hemodynamically unstable patient to follow urinary output, a reflector of visceral perfusion. Thus, urinary output, vital signs, and physical manifestations of the patient will reflect the adequacy of treatment and guide subsequent therapy.

 Anytime shock recurs in the convalescing patient, intense resuscitation and monitoring should be reestablished.

IV. **Posttraumatic Cardiac Arrest**   Most patients who arrest following blunt trauma do so secondary to profound intravascular volume depletion. The majority of these patients are young. It is an impression that once the youthful myocardium has arrested, it has **usually** received an insult that is irreversible, i.e., recalcitrant to cardiac resuscitation. Usually, the heart that arrests in this situation has incurred such a hypoxic insult that, should cardiac activity resume, the brain is usually nonfunctional because of hypoxia.

Flaccidity and apnea usually imply irreversible brain stem damage, but these findings may be secondary to hypothermia or central nervous system depressants.

In the face of intravascular volume depletion, an effective stroke volume cannot be generated with external cardiopulmonary resuscitation. An arrest that has lasted longer than a few minutes without massive volume infusion and manual compression of the ventricles is most likely to result in hypoxic brain damage, should cardiac activity resume. The patient has a "reasonable" chance at resuscitation if he or she arrests within a few minutes from, or within, the Admitting Area, and if open massage, aortic compression, volume infusion, and ventilatory support are concomitantly and rapidly performed. Short of this aggressive and expeditious form of resuscitation, the patient has a negligible chance of useful cerebral function. The arrest should be monitored by EKG since some perfusion may be maintained by a slow rhythm despite a "nonpalpable" pulse.

Our success rate has been very poor in the postcardiac arrest patient following blunt trauma. The success rate for useful cerebral function following open thoracotomy for the patient who has arrested following penetrating thoracic trauma is better than that following blunt trauma, although only 10–15%. Open thoracotomy following penetrating trauma permits the control of intrathoracic hemorrhage, compression of the aorta, massage of the ventricles, and relief of tamponade.

A. **Manifestations**

1. Absent pulse or blood pressure

2. Absent heart sounds by auscultation

3. Mottling and cyanosis

4. Electrocardiogram
   a. Ventricular fibrillation
   b. Asystole
   c. Electromechanical dissociation (QRS complex without peripheral pulsation)
   d. Idioventricular rhythm.

B. **Treatment** An aggressive approach regarding resuscitation would be indicated in the following:

1. Young patient

2. Arrest less than 5 min in duration

3. Spontaneous movement of the extremities

4. Pupils reactive to light

5. Attempt at spontaneous respiration

6. Uncertainty regarding the effect of drugs, hypothermia, or timing of the arrest

7. History of an arrest greater than 5 min but a situation in which a palpable pulse is obtainable with external cardiopulmonary resuscitation, i.e., effective stroke volume.

These factors should be considered in each case. However, the ultimate decision regarding aggressive resuscitation lies with the physician in charge.

The following is a list of guidelines for the management of posttraumatic cardiac arrest:

—Translaryngeal intubation and positive pressure ventilation performed immediately
—Rapid vascular access
—Massive volume infusion, preferably with red blood cells
—A thoracotomy through the left fourth or fifth interspace
—Manual ventricular compression
—Compression of the thoracic aorta above the diaphragm
—Opening of the pericardium to relieve possible tamponade
—Control of the associated intrathoracic hemorrhage
—Administer sodium bicarbonate, 1 mEq/kg intravenously; follow with arterial blood gases.
—**Ventricular fibrillation** Apply 20–60 watt/sec of direct current to the left ventricle; if the heart does not defibrillate, administer additional bicarbonate, a bolus of lidocaine (Xylocaine) (50–100 mg), and 0.5–1.0 mg of epinephrine if the fibrillation is fine. The epinephrine should be administered by a central venous or intracardiac route. If the patient is hypothermic, the heart should be bathed in warm saline.
—**Asystole** Administer epinephrine and/or calcium chloride (10 cc; 10%).
—**Electromechanical dissociation** Administer calcium chloride, dopamine (Intropin), and/or epinephrine.
—If there is profound bradycardia, but hypotension, administer dopamine and/or atropine.

Perspective
There is a controversy regarding emergency room versus operating room thoracotomy. Our feeling is that it is not the place where the thoracotomy is performed that is important, but whether it is appropriate to perform a thoracotomy in a given patient. If a thoracotomy is indicated for a **recent** arrest or marked hemodynamic deterioration, it should be performed immediately in the emergency room, if that is where the deterioration occurs. If an "overaggressive" thoracotomy is performed and cardiac activity returns, yet the patient has suffered irreversible hypoxic encephalopathy, neither society nor the patient benefits.

V. **Summary of Cardiovascular Assessment and Stabilization**

A. Rapid appraisal of **hemodynamic status**—pulse (present or absent), heart rate, blood pressure, skin color and temperature, auscultation of chest for absence of breath sounds

B. **Venous access**—number and site determined by site of injuries and hemodynamic instability of patient

   1. CVP line is a minimum
      a. Hypovolemia versus cardiogenic shock
      b. Withdrawal of admission lab
      c. Volume infusion

   2. Cutdowns and/or central percutaneous lines, when appropriate

C. **Volume infusion**

   1. First 1,500 cc of plasmanate

   2. After first 1,500 cc of plasmanate, administer red blood cells (RBC).

D. **Arterial line**—continuous assessment of cardiovascular status

E. **Diagnosis and treatment of hypotension**

   1. Absent breath sounds—chest tube (treatment for tension pneumothorax and hemothorax); to OR, if indicated

   2. Compression of external bleeding points

   3. Stabilize major fracture site (e.g., femur or pelvis)

   4. Peritoneal lavage; to OR, if positive

   5. Retroperitoneal hemorrhage; to OR, if major hemodynamic instability (consider MAST trousers or angiography and embolic tamponade)

   6. Cardiac tamponade—pericardial tap; decompress at thoracotomy

   7. Cardiac contusion—treat pump failure and/or arrhythmias

   8. Exclude:
      a. Quadriplegia
      b. Brain stem herniation
      c. Myocardial infarction
      d. Hypothermia

2

RESPIRATORY ASSESSMENT
AND STABILIZATION

Seventy percent of the patients admitted to MIEMSS are intubated and mechanically ventilated within the first hour. Intubation and ventilation are frequently necessary to maintain pulmonary parenchymal expansion, secure the airway, and remove tracheobronchial secretions. By achieving these objectives, oxygenation, which is especially important in the patient in shock, is maintained. Normal pulmonary physiology depends on:

—An intact pulmonary parenchyma
—Alveolar-to-pulmonary capillary hemoglobin gas exchange (blood flow $\times$ Hb)
—An intact pleura
—An intact thoracic wall
—A patent laryngotracheobronchial tree
—Neural innervation

The pulmonary system may be physiologically divided into two major categories:

—Ventilation: gas flow in and out of lungs
—Gas exchange: oxygen and carbon dioxide exchange between the alveolus and blood

Ventilatory dysfunction results from pathology involving the "conduits" extending from the nares and lips to the respiratory bronchioles as well as chest wall components that provide the work of ventilation. Gas exchange dysfunction occurs secondary to pathology involving the alveolar sacs and pulmonary capillaries. Impairment of function at any level may result in the rapid demise of the patient. Pulmonary function, along with cardiovascular function, remains the highest priority for consideration in the immediate post-injury period.

I. **Etiology**   Injuries to certain areas can be associated with early respiratory obstruction and pulmonary insufficiency. Cerebral, maxillofacial, laryngotracheal, and thoracic injuries commonly result in difficulty with maintaining a patent airway and/or adequate ventilation.

   Acute anemia, usually dilutional as intravascular volume is restored with red cell-free solutions after hemorrhage, is a cause of gas exchange failure. Anemia reduces the maximal O_2-carrying capacity of the blood so that the cardiac output needs to be elevated to meet the body's oxygen demand. Since the severely traumatized patient may not be able to raise cardiac output enough to totally compensate for the anemia, the mixed venous O_2 content drops. This lowered mixed venous O_2 content coupled with a reduced pulmonary end capillary O_2 content magnifies the effect of any pulmonary right-to-left shunting on the PaO_2.

The head-injured patient may lose consciousness and be prone to **aspiration.** The soft tissue structures of the pharynx may prolapse into the supraglottic region and cause **partial airway obstruction.**

There may be **massive facial trauma.** The resulting swelling may interfere with patency of the upper airway. Fractures of the maxilla and/or mandible may cause obstruction of the airway due to prolapse of soft tissue into the airway. There may be severe hemorrhage associated with maxillofacial trauma, thus causing the patient to aspirate blood.

Laryngotracheal trauma is not common, but may result in upper airway obstruction if there is a fracture of the larynx or a disruption of the trachea.

Foreign bodies, such as dentures or food present in the mouth at the time of injury, may become lodged in the glottis and lead to partial or complete obstruction. Blunt chest trauma may result in **pulmonary contusion, tracheal** or **bronchial injuries,** a **pneumothorax, hemopneumothorax,** or a **flail chest. Sucking wounds of the chest** may result in profound respiratory embarrassment. A **quadriplegic patient** may have inadequate innervation of the chest wall to maintain adequate ventilation. **Pulmonary edema** is a common sequel to pulmonary contusion, shock, and aspiration. Lung edema causes an increase in the pulmonary shunt with resultant hypoxia.

II. Manifestations of an Inadequate Airway

A. Supraclavicular and intercostal retractions

B. Noisy respiration

C. Flaring of the ala nasi

D. Labored use of accessory muscles of respiration

E. Stridor

III. Manifestations of Inadequate Ventilation

A. Decreased breath sounds (unilateral or bilateral)

B. Cyanosis

C. Associated airway obstruction

D. Minimal or absent chest wall motion

E. Absence of air exchange from the nose or mouth

F. Restlessness, anxiety, and confusion

G. Decreased PaO_2

H. Increased $PaCO_2$ and decreased pH

IV. Manifestations of Inadequate Gas Exchange

A. Tachypnea

B. Cyanosis

C. Infiltrates on chest x-ray

D. Decreased PaO_2

E. Increased dead space

V. Methods of Securing an Airway

A. **Removal of foreign bodies** The removal of foreign materials such as blood, dentures, food, loose teeth, and bone fragments may rapidly clear an obstructed airway.

B. **Jaw thrust** Forward pressure at the angle of the mandible may transiently relieve pharyngeal airway obstruction.

C. **Oral airway** The oral pharyngeal airway is helpful in spontaneous breathing patients by preventing posterior displacement of the tongue. This airway is not well tolerated in the patient who is minimally depressed, and laryngospasm may result.

D. **Nasal airway** A nasopharyngeal airway may be used in a patient who has spontaneous respiratory efforts, but has partial upper airway obstruction. This airway is better tolerated than an oral pharyngeal airway if the patient has minimal CNS depression. A nasopharyngeal airway should not be used in a patient with facial trauma, because the airway may enter the cranial vault if the cribriform plate is fractured.

E. **Esophageal obturator airway** This technique is primarily used in the prehospital setting in which techniques **A–D** have been inadequate to maintain an airway or provide adequate ventilation (see p. 475).

F. **Translaryngeal tube** In competent hands, the passage of an endotracheal tube through the larynx is usually the most expeditious route for maintaining a patent airway (see p. 483).

G. **Transtracheal tube** Occasionally, the airway is unable to be secured using the above procedures; therefore, transtracheal intubation or needle jet ventilation may be required. This is especially likely with severe disruption of the oropharynx, larynx, or cervical trachea (see pp. 45 and 481).

VI. **Ventilatory Management**

A. **Head injury** The head-injured patient is usually intubated with a translaryngeal tube immediately after admission. The primary reason for insertion of a translaryngeal tube is to secure the airway and to provide hyperventilation. Ventilation with a respirator and endotracheal tube minimizes the occurrence of hypoxia and hypercarbia, both contributors to cerebral edema. It is optimal to evaluate the cervical spine with an x-ray prior to manipulating the patient for intubation. Prior to intubation, the following techniques may be used to provide a patent airway:

1. Traction on the tongue

2. Jaw thrust

3. Removal of foreign bodies and secretions from the pharynx

4. Insertion of a nasal or oral airway

5. If intubation is necessary, paralyze the patient to provide optimum conditions, and stabilize the neck in a neutral position during intubation. If the cords cannot be easily visualized, fiberoptic laryngoscope intubation or transtracheal intubation may be necessary to minimize neck movement (see p. 482).

B. **Facial injury** With minimal maxillofacial trauma, the less invasive techniques of airway maintenance are usually successful:

1. Jaw thrust

2. Suction pharynx

3. Removal of foreign bodies from the pharynx

4. Insertion of an oral airway

If the upper airway is more tenuous, translaryngeal intubation should be performed. A patient may develop such massive facial swelling, and/or intraoral hemorrhage, that transtracheal intubation is required. The patient's jaw may swell so much after fluid resuscitation that mobility prevents oral breathing or intubation. When in doubt about the future status of the patient's airway, intubate early. Extubation can always be done if the tube is not needed, but edema formation and swelling can jeopardize the patient's life by creating a difficult intubation later. The same reasoning holds for potential upper airway burns in smoke inhalation patients (see p. 481).

C. **Laryngotracheal injury** Cervical swelling secondary to blunt or penetrating trauma may cause extrinsic compression of the upper airway and require endotracheal intubation. A fractured larynx should preferably be managed by transtracheal intubation because translaryngeal intubation may further damage the larynx. An injury to the cervical trachea is usually best managed with transtracheal intubation; however, translaryngeal intubation may be successful.

D. **Thoracic trauma** Open wounds of the chest are usually best managed by applying a sterile dressing and inserting a chest tube in the pleural space. If the patient has a hemothorax and/or a pneumothorax, this is best managed by decompression of the pleural space with a chest tube. Patients with a flail chest frequently have associated pulmonary contusion with disruption of gas exchange physiology and hypoxia, which is best managed by endotracheal intubation and a ventilator. **Positive end-expiratory pressure** (PEEP) is useful in restoring alveolar volume, which normalizes gas exchange mechanisms. PEEP applied to the spontaneously breathing patient, or continuous positive airway pressure (CPAP), is often all that is required to normalize gas exchange following lung contusion or aspiration (see p. 316).

E. **Quadriplegia** The quadriplegic patient has decreased intercostal muscular function, which may result in hypoventilation. It is not uncommon for a C_5 spinal-injured patient to ascend one or two neural segments, which would also compromise phrenic nerve function. The quadriplegic patient must be closely evaluated for evidence of hypoxia and/or hypercarbia. If oral translaryngeal intubation cannot be easily performed for an emergency intubation, transtracheal intubation may be indicated to minimize neck movement. Fiberoptic intubation should be considered in a difficult elective intubation which involves the quadriplegic. Awake nasotracheal intubation is an alternative method for elective intubation, but requires excellent topical anesthesia to prevent spontaneous neck movement.

VII. **Summary**

A. **Manifestations of airway obstruction**

1. Stridor

2. Labored use of accessory muscles of respiration

3. Flaring of the ala nasi

4. Supraclavicular and intercostal retractions

5. Noisy respiration

B. **Manifestations of inadequate ventilation**

1. Decreased breath sounds (unilateral or bilateral)

2. Absence of air exchange from the mouth or nose

3. Cyanosis

4. Minimal or absent chest wall motion

5. Airway obstruction

6. Restlessness, anxiety, and confusion

7. Hypoxia

8. Hypercarbia

C. **Manifestations of inadequate gas exchange**

1. Tachypnea

2. Cyanosis

3. Alveolar infiltrates on chest x-ray

4. Hypoxia

5. Increased dead space

D. **Therapeutic considerations**

1. Jaw thrust

2. Removal of foreign bodies from pharynx

3. Oral airway

4. Nasal airway

5. Translaryngeal intubation

6. Transtracheal intubation

7. Insertion of chest tube

8. CPAP

9. Respirator

3

EVALUATION CHECKLIST OF
THE MULTIPLE TRAUMA PATIENT

The following is a list of common injuries which should be evaluated in each multiple trauma patient and the findings which enhance confirmation of a specific diagnosis.

I. **Skull**

   A. **Scalp lacerations**

      1. Examine scalp under hair

   B. **Fracture**

      1. Seen through scalp laceration

      2. X-rays if decreased level of consciousness, ecchymosis, swelling, and/or cervical spine fracture

      3. Battle's sign, panda eyes

      4. Otorrhea

      5. Rhinorrhea

      6. Hemotympanum

II. **Face**

   A. **Fractures**

      1. Maxilla, mandible, and alveolus
         a. Dental malocclusion
         b. Intraoral ecchymosis
         c. Loose teeth
         d. Preauricular pain

      2. Orbit
         a. Deformity
         b. Swelling
         c. Diplopia
         d. Subconjunctival hemorrhage

    3. Zygoma
        a. Deformity
        b. Infraorbital hypesthesia
        c. Diplopia
        d. Subconjunctival hemorrhage

    4. Nose
        a. Deformity
        b. Swelling
        c. Epistaxis

B. **Facial lacerations**

C. **Facial nerve damage** (facial expression)

D. **Parotid duct** (consider with any cheek laceration)

III. **Brain**

A. **Level of consciousness**

    1. Oriented

    2. Agitated

    3. Follows commands

B. **Motor response to pain**

    1. Purposeful

    2. Semi-purposeful

    3. Spastic

    4. Decorticate

    5. Decerebrate

    6. Flaccid

C. **Brain stem**

    1. Pupils

    2. Calorics

    3. Corneals

    4. Doll's eye

IV. Neck

A. Larynx and cervical trachea

1. Hoarseness
2. Cervical subcutaneous emphysema
3. Hemoptysis
4. Cervical crepitus

B. Esophagus and pharynx

1. Dysphagia
2. Hematemesis
3. Contrast study
4. Subcutaneous emphysema

C. Spinal column

1. Neck pain
2. Decreased motion
3. Deformity
4. X-ray

D. Spinal cord

1. Decreased sensory and/or motor response of extremities
2. Decreased rectal tone
3. Priapism
4. Bradycardia

E. Carotid and jugular vessels

1. Cervical hematoma
2. Altered level of consciousness
3. Hemiparesis
4. Bruit

V. Chest

A. Hemothorax

1. Decreased breath sounds

2. Dullness to percussion

3. Shock

B. Pneumothorax

1. Decreased breath sounds

2. Tympany

3. Shock

C. Diaphragm

1. "Elevated" or obscured diaphragm on x-ray

D. Pulmonary contusion

1. Hypoxia

2. Hemoptysis

3. Pulmonary infiltrate on chest x-ray

E. Rib fractures

1. Pain on inspiration

2. Subcutaneous emphysema

3. Crepitus

4. Paradoxical motion

F. Sternal fracture

1. Pain on inspiration

2. Crepitus

3. Paradoxical motion

G. Clavicular fracture

1. Deformity

H. Cardiac tamponade

1. Shock

2. Increased CVP (neck vein distention)

3. Arrhythmias

I.   **Cardiac contusion**

1. Shock

2. Increased CVP (neck vein distention)

3. Arrhythmias

J.   **Tracheobronchial injury**

1. Subcutaneous emphysema

2. Hemoptysis

3. Large pleural air leak

4. Pneumomediastinum

K.   **Esophagus**

1. Hematemesis

2. Pneumomediastinum

3. Pleural effusion

4. Pneumothorax

L.   **Aorta and great vessels**

1. Wide mediastinum; obscured aortic knob

2. Decreased carotid, brachial, or femoral pulses

3. Altered level of consciousness

4. Hemiparesis

5. Hemothorax

6. Hoarseness

M. **Thoracic spinal column**

1. Back deformity

2. Upper back pain

N.   **Thoracic spinal cord**

1. Decreased chest wall/abdominal sensation

2. Paraplegia

VI. Abdomen

A. Spleen

1. Positive mini-lap (blood)

B. Liver

1. Positive mini-lap (blood, bile)

C. Pancreas

1. Increased amylase (serum)
2. "Delayed" abdominal tenderness and ileus

D. Stomach

1. Hematemesis
2. Positive mini-lap (blood)

E. Duodenum

1. Vomiting
2. Positive mini-lap (blood, bile, amylase)
3. Peritonitis
4. Obscured right psoas shadow

F. Small bowel

1. Positive mini-lap (blood, bile, amylase)
2. Peritonitis

G. Colon

1. Positive mini-lap (blood, vegetable fiber, bacteria)
2. Peritonitis

H. Rectum

1. Blood on rectal examination
2. Proctoscopy
3. Perineal tear
4. Association with pelvic fractures

I.   **Lumbar spine**

   1.   Low back pain or deformity

J.   **Lumbar spinal cord—cauda equina**

   1.   Decreased rectal tone

   2.   Paraplegia

   3.   Inability to void

K.   **Abdominal vessels**

   1.   Positive mini-lap (blood)

   2.   Shock

L.   **Retroperitoneal vessels (aorta, vena cava)**

   1.   Shock; hematoma found at exploration

   2.   Decreased femoral pulses

VII.   **Urinary Tract**

A.   **Kidney**

   1.   Flank hematoma

   2.   Flank ecchymosis

   3.   Hematuria

   4. L_{1-2} fracture

   5.   Posterior lower rib fractures

B.   **Ureter**

   1.   Penetrating abdominal injury (IVP)

C.   **Bladder**

   1.   Hematuria

   2.   Associated with pelvic fracture

D.   **Urethra**

   1.   Blood at meatus

   2.   Pelvic fracture

   3.   Displaced prostate

E. **Perineum**

    1. Laceration

F. **Genitalia**

    1. Swelling

    2. Ecchymosis

    3. Laceration

VIII. **Pelvis**

    A. Perineal ecchymosis

    B. Pubic symphysis diastasis

    C. Iliac wing instability

    D. Pelvic pain

    E. X-ray

    F. Hematuria

    G. Rule out rectal injury

    H. Shock

IX. **Extremity**

    A. **Fracture**

        1. Pain

        2. Deformity

        3. Crepitus

        4. Decreased motion

        5. Ecchymosis

        6. Tissue wound

    B. **Neural**

        1. Decreased sensory and/or motor function

C. **Vascular**

    1. Decreased pulse

    2. Hematoma

    3. Pallor/cyanosis

    4. Bruit

    5. Paresthesia

    6. Swelling

    7. Compartment tension

D. **Soft tissue**

    1. Defect

    2. Swelling

4

EMERGENCY RADIOGRAPHY

The radiology service is an integral part of the traumatology unit. The radiologist, a member of the trauma team, is best trained to interpret radiographs and is available on a 24-hr basis.

A radiologic technologist is assigned to the trauma unit around the clock. Processing facilities are available in the Triage area.

We primarily use portable radiographic equipment, which is adequate for most studies. The Admitting Area has access to the following modalities: whole body computerized axial tomography, a fully equipped angiographic suite with biplane cut film and C-arm mounted equipment, nuclear imaging, and ultrasonography.

In order to maximize patient management and care, all present and past radiographs of in-house patients are filed in the patient care area until the patient is transferred. Facilities for radiographic storage, interpretation, and consultation are available within the area.

I. The following is a brief discussion of radiographic procedures that are routinely performed in the evaluation of the post-trauma patient. As a rule, lateral cervical spine, chest, and pelvic x-rays are performed routinely on blunt trauma victims.

A. **Lateral cervical spine x-ray** A lateral projection of the C-spine is obtained on virtually all deceleration or crush accident victims. Over 90% of dislocations and fractures are best identified on the lateral projection. In our experience, 98% of significant cervical spine pathology is identified on a lateral film. If the patient has incurred multiple trauma, if the seventh cervical vertebra is not visualized, and if there is no evidence of spinal cord deficit on examination, a Philadelphia (hard) collar is applied and the remaining evaluation is completed; the lower cervical spine is cleared at a later time. Evaluation of the lateral cervical spine includes:

1. Alignment of the anterior and posterior borders of the cervical vertebrae

2. Alignment of the spinolaminal lines

3. Vertebral body, spinous process, laminae, pedicles, and odontoid for evidence of a fracture

4. Preodontoid space (should be ≤ 3 mm)

5. Prevertebral space (exclude swelling)

6. Normal lordotic curve

If the cervical spine film is abnormal and/or the patient complains of neck pain, neurosurgical/orthopedic consultation is obtained. A complete examination of the C-spine is indicated in a patient who complains of neck pain. This includes an AP, lateral, both oblique, flexion-extension, and odontoid views, and a swimmer's view in the alert patient. Occasionally, tomography in AP, lateral, or oblique projections is necessary.

B. **Chest x-ray** In deceleration or crush injuries, an upright chest radiograph is optimal. An **upright film** provides a nondistorted view of the superior mediastinum, which allows evaluation for the presence of a mediastinal hematoma. This view is optimal for visualizing a pneumohydrothorax and diaphragmatic contour changes. If the patient has a complaint of back pain, or if a pelvic fracture or spinal cord deficit is suspected, a supine chest x-ray should be obtained initially. If needed, a 5–10° oblique radiograph is obtained in order to identify the aortic component of the superior mediastinum on a supine film. (See p. 33.)

C. **Pelvic x-ray** Commonly, there may be no external manifestations associated with a pelvic fracture; therefore, an AP pelvic x-ray is considered routine in the deceleration or crush accident victim.

II. The following is a brief survey of the emergency radiographic techniques that may be clinically indicated in the post-accident victim.

A. **Excretory intravenous pyelography** (IVP) (see p. 177 for indications) Only gross information is sought from the emergency IVP in the trauma patient. Information is sought regarding presence or absence of one or both kidneys, renal parenchymal defect, or gross extravasation of contrast material. Frequently, these patients are hypovolemic, which results in renal arterial constriction and poor visualization on pyelography. It is suggested that 1½ to 2 times the standard contrast dose be administered. Following the exposure of a scout film, it is suggested that the patient be administered 76 or 60% iodine contrast as a single bolus of 100–150 cc, depending on the patient's size. A flat plate of the abdomen is then performed following the injection and one is performed at approximately 5 and 10 min following the contrast. If the patient must go immediately to the operating room, a single kidney, ureter, and bladder (KUB) film is exposed 5 min after the injection.

B. **Cystogram** (see p. 177 for indications) Following exposure of a scout film, 200–400 cc of 30–60% contrast material is dripped into the bladder via a Foley catheter. AP and lateral pelvic radiographs are obtained pre- and post-voiding. Oblique pelvic views may be indicated for further evaluation of the urinary bladder.

C. **Extremity arteriogram** (see p. 250 for indications) The following are suggested guidelines to be used in performing preoperative or intraoperative, hand-injected extremity arteriography. Gross anatomical alignment of fractures should be attempted before arteriography is performed. The suggested contrast material is 60% iodine solution. For a femoral arterial injection, 50 cc of contrast material should be rapidly injected. To evaluate the vasculature of the thigh, the x-ray should be exposed immediately before the completion of the injection. To visualize the vasculature of the lower leg, the x-ray should be exposed approximately 1–3 sec following injection, depending on the age of the patient. For axillary arterial injection, 30–40 cc of contrast material (60% iodine) should be rapidly injected. To evaluate the vessels of the upper arm, x-ray exposure should be performed at the termination of the injection. To evaluate the vascular structures of the lower arm, x-ray exposure should be performed 3–4 sec following the injection in the average patient.

D. **Carotid arteriogram**   A CAT scan is the gold standard by which intracranial pathology is evaluated. If a patient is too unstable to be transferred to the radiographic suite, a one-shot percutaneous carotid arteriogram is performed in order to evaluate vascular displacement from intracranial hemorrhage or edema. Radiographs of the skull are obtained in AP and lateral projections.

E. **Thoracic aortogram**   This study is indicated when there is presence of a mediastinal hematoma following deceleration trauma. Other indications are

   1. Transmediastinal penetration

   2. Cervical or supraclavicular hematoma

   3. Brachiocephalic pulse deficit

   It may be inadvisable to sit a patient up if a spine or pelvic fracture is suspected. If the superior mediastinum cannot be properly evaluated by a supine or upright chest x-ray, oblique views of the aorta may be obtained. If the superior mediastinum cannot be cleared with oblique 5–10° views, a thoracic aortogram is indicated (see p. 126).

F. **Pelvic angiography**   This study may be considered in massive pelvic bleeding and may be followed by embolic tamponade, if indicated (see p. 197).

G. **Esophagogram**   This study is usually indicated for penetrating neck or mediastinal wounds. Diatrizoate sodium (Gastrografin) is the contrast of choice (see p. 119).

H. **Skull x-rays**   The following is a list of relative and absolute indications for obtaining skull radiographs. Minimal projections are AP and lateral films. Tangential views to confirm a depressed skull fracture may be indicated.

   1. History of unconsciousness

   2. Skull penetration with foreign body

   3. Suspected depressed skull fracture

   4. Rhinorrhea

   5. Otorrhea

   6. Blood in the middle ear cavity

   7. Battle's sign

8. Raccoon's eyes

9. Coma or stupor

10. Focal neurologic signs

11. Cervical spine injury

I. **Extremity radiographs**   If there is physical evidence of fracture or dislocation, or subjective complaints, AP and lateral radiographs of the affected area should be obtained. The joint above and the joint below the suspected injury should be included on the same radiograph.

J. **Facial radiographs**   If there are signs or symptoms of facial injury, the appropriate radiographs should be obtained. These films usually consist of AP and lateral facial views, Waters' view, Towne's view, and/or mandibular series. Tomograms may be needed for complete evaluation.

K. **Thoracic spine**   Radiographic evaluation should be obtained if there is presence of upper back pain, paraplegia, upper back deformity, or missile trajectory in this region. AP and lateral films should be obtained.

L. **Lumbar spine**   Films should be obtained if there is low back pain, a lower extremity or pelvic neurologic deficit, low back deformity, or missile trajectory in the region. AP, lateral, and oblique radiographs are desirable.

5

TRANSFUSION

I. **Resuscitative Transfusion** In resuscitative transfusion, the major goal is to restore the intravascular compartment as rapidly as possible with components that match its losses.

In the multiple trauma patient where the main cause of hypovolemia is blood loss, colloid replacement and blood component therapy is the procedure of choice. In the multisystem trauma patient, this is part of the primary treatment which begins prior to or concomitant with diagnosis. The speed with which resuscitation is initiated is a major factor contributing to the patient's successful outcome.

The initial resuscitation priority of establishing adequate ventilation is carried out in conjunction with acquiring hemodynamic stability. At the same time, venous and arterial blood samples are drawn as indices of systems function: hemoglobin, hematocrit, fibrinogen, prothrombin time (PT), partial thromboplastin time (PTT), platelets, sodium, potassium, osmolality, blood urea nitrogen (BUN), glucose, creatinine, blood gas, and type and crossmatch.

A. The goals of active blood component therapy in the first 1–2 hr are:

1. **Restore intravascular volume** We assure adequate volume expansion by the infusion of plasma protein fraction (PPF).

2. **Maintain adequate oxygen-carrying capacity of the blood** We assure adequate circulating hemoglobin (at least 12 gm/dl) by infusing red blood cells (RBC).

3. **Maintain coagulability of the blood** We provide fresh frozen plasma, platelets, and/or cryoprecipitate, as dictated by guidelines described below.

B. Resuscitative transfusion is divided into five phases: vascular access, volume infusion, red blood cell infusion, maintenance of coagulability, and appropriate surgical intervention.

1. **Vascular access** The number, site, and size of lines are dictated by the patient's hemodynamic instability (see p. 9).

2. **Volume infusion** The first 1,500 cc of resuscitation fluid (PPF) is administered at a speed dictated by the patient's condition. In an institution where approximately 250 units of blood are used each week, availability of blood components is often impaired, despite valiant efforts by the Blood Bank. For this reason and because the physician is unable to await type and crossmatching, it is routine to commence resuscitation with a volume expander (PPF) rather than with whole blood.

3. **Red blood cell infusion** Following the first 1,000–1,500 cc of PPF, the average patient will be significantly hemodiluted; red blood cell infusion is indicated if further resuscitation is necessary. If massive hemorrhage and recalcitrant shock are evident, O Rh-positive red blood cells are infused until typed or crossmatched blood is available. Uncrossmatched blood is given if the initial hematocrit is less than 30, if a systolic blood pressure of < 100 fails to respond to resuscitation, or if rapid volume expansion is required, subsequent to an initial infusion of 1,500 cc of PPF. Initially, the O Rh-positive red blood cells may be uncrossmatched. O Rh-positive RBC are truly universal donors because they contain neither plasma antibodies nor cell antigens of a major ABO group, which may be associated with incompatibility. Immediately after type or crossmatch, type-specific red blood cells may be infused. The problem in administering O Rh-positive blood to an Rh-negative woman of childbearing age is the possibility of developing antibodies to the Rh antigen. The primary concern, however, is to save the patient's life by obtaining hemodynamic stability. If the patient's condition is stable, time might allow blood typing to identify the Rh-negative woman in order to provide her with Rh-negative red blood cells. If Rh-positive blood is given to an Rh-negative woman in her childbearing years, the Blood Bank should be notified within 48 hr for treatment with Rh immune globulin.

4. **Maintenance of coagulability** If more than 5 units of red blood cells are infused within a 24-hr period, serial PTT, PT, fibrinogen, and platelet counts are indicated in order to assess coagulability. Platelets, fresh frozen plasma, and/or cryoprecipitate may be infused as indicated by laboratory and clinical evaluation and/or may be prophylactically administered during massive transfusion (see p. 37).

5. **Surgical intervention** To avoid the metabolic complications frequently associated with massive transfusion requirements, "surgical bleeding" must be aggressively interrupted by pressure, suture ligation, removal of a massively bleeding organ, or must be controlled by embolic tamponade. Aggressive diagnostic evaluation will lead the surgeon to the source of hemorrhage and result in its control, with subsequent minimization of transfusion. If significant postoperative hemorrhage occurs, the patient should be returned to the operating room to control active bleeding.

Perspective
Resuscitation of the trauma patient with blood component therapy dictates the use of only those factors that are necessary. For example, hemorrhagic shock is rapidly reversed and controlled for some patients after they have received only resuscitative fluids without red cells; thus, the use of blood and its hazards are avoided. When needed, blood cells and coagulation factors are administered in components that provide optimum biologic activity in comparison with whole blood. This practice results in more red cells, platelets, and active clotting factors per volume infused. By avoiding the infusion of stored plasma, there are fewer protein

breakdown products, potassium, ammonia, citrate, plasma antibodies and antigens, and less potential thromboplastic activity. Furthermore, by using packed red blood cells from which the unprocessed plasma has been removed, transfusion reactions are less common. After using O Rh-positive red blood cells, rapid and safe return to type-specific blood is permitted at any time. Crystalloid solutions are used to maintain interstitial and intracellular compartment expansion.

C. **Preexisting disease and therapy** Patients with von Willebrand's disease and the hemophilias occasionally are encountered. These conditions are discovered not only by history but also by clinical evaluation and coagulation testing, which reveal unusual needs for corrective blood components. Cryoprecipitate is specific therapy for **von Willebrand's disease** and for **hemophilia A,** although for the former and for mild cases of the hemophilias, fresh frozen plasma (FFP) is often sufficient therapy even in the trauma patient. **Hemophilia B** is usually a milder bleeding disorder and its deficiency of factor IX often responds to FFP. However, the freeze-dried concentrate of factors II, VII, IX, and X, prothrombin complex concentrate (Konyne), may have to be used in spite of its high hepatitis risk. Hematology consultation should be obtained for patients with hemophilia or von Willebrand's disease.

Patients taking warfarin (**Coumadin**) for prevention of thrombosis have depressed hepatic synthesis of the vitamin K-dependent coagulation factors with a resultant prolongation of the PT. These factors are readily supplied by giving FFP (3–5 cc/kg of body weight). Vitamin K, even when given i.v., takes several hours to reverse the depressed production, but is given in addition to FFP.

II. **Massive Transfusion** Massive transfusion is defined as the infusion of 10 units of blood within a 24-hr period. Massive transfusion may be associated with coagulopathy, hypothermia, citrate intoxication, acidosis, or hyperammonemia.

A. **Coagulopathy** **Dilutional coagulopathy** is the most common cause of "nonsurgical bleeding" associated with massive transfusion. **Disseminated intravascular coagulopathy** is a less common, but not rare, cause of "nonsurgical bleeding" in the massively transfused post-trauma patient. Prothrombin time, partial thromboplastin time, fibrinogen, and platelet count should be monitored with at least every 10 units of packed red blood cells infused. Two units of group-specific fresh frozen plasma are usually administered with every 5–6 units of red blood cells, but the administration should be based on the results of coagulation parameters, clinical evaluation of bleeding, and evidence of an ongoing hemorrhagic process. In our experience, patients with craniofacial injury, major liver injuries, or severe pelvic fractures associated with massive blood loss frequently develop a coagulopathy. Coagulation factors should be monitored frequently. In the initial phase, fresh frozen plasma and packed cells should be administered in a ratio of 1:1 or 1:2. **Fresh frozen plasma** contains all of the soluble plasma clotting factors with biologic activities that are approximately equivalent to that found in fresh plasma. Fresh frozen plasma must be infused within 2 hr after thawing. If the fibrinogen level is less than 100 mg/dl and does not respond to fresh frozen plasma, **cryoprecipitate,** which contains concentrated fibrinogen, should be given. Four units of cryoprecipitate for each 10 kg of body weight will raise the fibrinogen level by approximately 150 mg/dl. Hypothermia, which may perpetuate the coagulopathy, should be aggressively controlled. In summary, the primary therapy for prolongation of the PTT, PT, and/or hypofibrinogenemia is administration of fresh frozen plasma and/or cryoprecipitate and aggressive and expeditious control of surgical bleeding.

The decision to infuse **platelet concentrates** is dictated by the platelet count in combination with the clinical situation. Thrombocytopenia may be secondary to dilutional effects and/or disseminated intravascular coagulopathy. After administering 10 units of red blood cells, a platelet count should be obtained. "Excessive bleeding" associated with a platelet count of less than 50,000/mm^3 usually indicates the need for platelet transfusion therapy. In nonbleeding patients, we accept a platelet count of 30,000/mm^3 before platelet infusion. The general guidelines are that a platelet count of greater than 30,000 is not associated with spontaneous hemorrhage due to platelet deficiency and that surgery can be performed satisfactorily when the platelet count is greater than or equal to 50,000–60,000/mm^3. A unit of platelet concentrate will usually increase the platelet count by 5,000–8,000/mm^3. The complete presentation of **disseminated intravascular coagulopathy** (DIC) manifests as: prolongation of the prothrombin time and partial thromboplastin time, hypofibrinogenemia, thrombocytopenia, and elevation of fibrin split products. Frequently, the trauma patient manifests with a less fulminant form of disseminated intravascular coagulopathy and may only present with aberrancy of any one or a multitude of these parameters. The primary treatment of DIC in the post-trauma patient is specific replacement by infusion of fresh frozen plasma and/or cryoprecipitate, platelet infusion, and expeditious control of surgical bleeding.

B. **Hypothermia** Hypothermia is commonly associated with massive transfusion. The degree of hypothermia is proportional to the rapidity and volume of stored blood infused. The body temperature may drop 3–10°C. Blood should be warmed through a long coil of tubing that has been inserted into the infusion line and immersed in a warm water bath. The patient's core temperature should be frequently monitored and therapy should be administered, as described on p. 375.

C. **Citrate intoxication** Citrate maintains anticoagulation of blood during its storage. With massive transfusion, there is some concern for the development of ionized hypocalcemia with citrate infusion, a clinically unusual situation. The manifestations of citrate intoxication are myocardial dysfunction (bradycardia), arrhythmias, and hypotension. Prophylactic calcium is not administered. However, should the patient develop manifestations of cardiac instability, 1 gm i.v. of calcium chloride should be considered.

D. Acidosis Whole blood is acidic and might add to the metabolic acidosis of hypo-perfusion in the shocked patient. We do not find acidosis to be associated with red blood cell transfusion; therefore, we do not advocate prophylactic administration of bicarbonate. The primary treatment of metabolic acidosis for the posttraumatic patient is intravascular volume expansion.

E. Hyperammonemia Ammonia is found in stored blood and may present a problem when infused in a patient with hepatic dysfunction. We do not find this to be a problem when red blood cells are used.

The metabolic complications associated with massive transfusion are best managed by rapid surgical control of blood loss, adequate restoration of intravascular volume, prevention of hypothermia, and appropriate infusion of fresh frozen plasma, cryoprecipitate, and platelets.

III. Autotransfusion

A. Rationale and general description A logical step for blood conservation is the collection and retransfusion of the patient's shed blood. An effective autotransfusion system can provide a blood source that is immediately available and, in addition, decrease the tremendous demand placed on the Blood Bank for blood products. This blood is obviously type-specific and crossmatch-compatible. The risk of infection such as hepatitis and syphilis is avoided, viable platelets and labile clotting factors are retained, and the metabolic alterations of stored blood are avoided. An exception is blood from the chest, which is depleted of fibrinogen. The blood collection may be

1. **Intraoperative** with the collection of blood in cardiac, vascular, thoracic, and abdominal procedures

2. **Postoperative** with the utilization of shed mediastinal or pleural blood, post-cardiac surgery or post-chest surgery

B. Intra- and postoperative autotransfusion

1. **Technique** The Sorenson autotransfusion system consists of a rigid outer canister, which is reusable, and a disposable sterile liner. The liner is made of a single 1,900-ml plastic bag containing two 170-μ filters to remove blood aggregates and gross particulate matter. Gravity causes blood to flow into the bag, which serves as a reservoir during collection. Controlled suction is applied in the canister and the partially collapsed liner. During early collection, the liner remains contracted, reducing the blood-air interface. The weight of the collected blood distends the bag. When a suitable volume of blood (400–1,500 ml) has been collected, the liner is removed and replaced. The bag is gently compressed to expel any air through the upper filter. **Removal of air from the bag is important because it eliminates the possibility of air embolism.**

Blood administration is accomplished through a second port of the bag. A 40-μ Pall filter can be used during infusion of the autotransfused blood. The suction pressure should not exceed -40 cm H_2O. An Emerson chest tube vacuum pump is set to maintain suction at -20 cm H_2O, although regulated wall suction would serve as well. The Sorenson autotransfusion system is assembled in the operating room and attached to mediastinal drains during closure of a sternal wound in cardiac/chest surgery. Blood collected from the pleural space or shed mediastinal blood is defibrinogenated; thus, it does not require anticoagulation. In adult patients, if a volume of shed blood in the postoperative period exceeds 250 ml during a 4-hr period, it can be autotransfused as necessary for intravascular volume replacement. Because of the theoretical risk of bacterial contamination, blood collected during a period exceeding 4 hr is not returned to the patient.

This system is simple and easy to follow and requires minimal training. Red cell survival is normal and platelets and labile clotting factors are retained; however, fibrinogen may be lost. Fibrinogen is typically absent from mediastinal or chest cavity blood. Intraperitoneal sources do have fibrinogen and thus require anticoagulation. Acid citrate dextrose (ACD) or citrate phosphate dextrose (CPD) is used as an anticoagulant in a ratio of 1:7, i.e., 100 ml of ACD or CPD to each 700 ml of collected blood. Where possible, the anticoagulant should run into the collection system and mix with the blood before reaching the bag. Objections to the use of shed abdominal and chest blood are derived from concern with the infusion of particulate debris, free hemoglobin, and the possible infusion of contaminated blood. However, the incidence of postresuscitative pulmonary insufficiency is not increased following resuscitation with shed abdominal or chest blood. Although significant volumes of free hemoglobin are infused as a result of red cell injury during collection or reinfusion, this does not increase the incidence of renal failure.

a. **Hemothorax** Patients with a hemothorax should be attached directly to the Sorenson system for blood collection and subsequent reinfusion. The routine chest drainage system should only be utilized once the decision has been made to discontinue autotransfusion.

   A maximum of 4 hr may elapse between collection and reinfusion. All air must be vented from the blood bag prior to administration to minimize the possibility of air embolism. If necessary, a pressure infusion cuff may be used after air is excluded from the bag. "Pushing blood" with a syringe causes hemolysis and raises the plasma free hemoglobin level.

b. **Hemoperitoneum** The danger of bacteremia following autotransfusion is minimized if shed abdominal blood is infused only in patients whose wounds are free from fecal contamination. Shed abdominal blood should be collected and held until examination of the abdominal cavity confirms the absence of colonic or ileal perforation. The presence of enteric contamination is usually an absolute contraindication for autotransfusion. However, if the situation demands immediate autotransfusion, the patient is treated with prophylactic antibiotics. Periodic blood cultures should be obtained in addition to culturing the contaminated blood.

2. **Complications** The complication rate related to transfusion of blood is reduced when comparing autotransfused with stored blood.

IV. **Transfusion Reactions** An adverse response to transfusion may occur as the result of an in vivo combination of antigen and antibody. Types of reactions include acute (10% death rate) hemolytic, usually secondary to ABO blood incompatibility; delayed hemolytic which occurs after 24 hr; allergic or urticarial (3% of all transfusions); and febrile in which leukoagglutinins are demonstrated in about 50% of the patients.

A. **Acute hemolytic reaction** This usually represents incompatible donor cells agglutinating with preexisting recipient antibodies, most often a clerical mistake which results in the administration of blood to the "wrong" recipient.

   1. **Manifestations** Clinical signs and symptoms usually begin after 50 ml or less of blood has been given. Jaundice may appear within a few minutes to a few days. The patient may develop flushing, chills, fever, tachypnea, tachycardia, and flank, back, or extremity pain. Bleeding from wounds may occur. The patient may develop hemoglobinuria or become oliguric (renal failure).

   2. **Treatment** Blood infusion should be terminated immediately. Repeat crossmatching and obtain a Coombs test. Decreased or absent serum haptoglobin implies hemolysis. A blood specimen should be obtained for the determination of free hemoglobin. Urine should be evaluated for free hemoglobin. If the patient requires additional blood, washed and crossmatched red blood cells should be administered. The urine should be alkalinized to reduce renal damage. Force diuresis should be employed to maintain a urinary output of 100 cc/hr. Shock and disseminated intravascular coagulopathy may develop rapidly. Heparinization may be life saving in DIC. If the patient has developed DIC, fresh frozen plasma, cryoprecipitate, and/or platelets are administered as dictated by coagulation parameters.

B. **Delayed hemolytic reaction**

   1. **Manifestations** Jaundice may develop from one to several days after transfusion. Chills and fever may accompany the icterus.

   2. **Treatment** Treatment is the same as for the acute state.

C. **Allergic reaction** This phenomenon occurs in about 3% of all transfusions.

   1. **Manifestations** Flushing, chills, fever, urticaria, and pruritus are clinical manifestations. Bronchospasm and laryngospasm rarely occur.

   2. **Treatment** Diphenhydramine (Benadryl) is usually adequate to treat the symptoms. The infusion should be terminated. Antipyretics may be beneficial. Blood should be cultured and plasma should be examined for bacteria. Prophylactic benadryl may be beneficial if additional blood is indicated.

D. **Febrile reaction**

1. **Manifestations**   This reaction is characterized by chills and fever that rarely exceeds 103°F.

2. **Treatment**   The infusion should be terminated and aspirin or acetaminophen (Tylenol) given. Benadryl may be of benefit if the fever persists. Blood should be cultured and plasma examined for bacteria. If additional blood is required, the patient should receive buffy coat-poor blood.

E. **Evaluation of transfusion reactions**

1. Stop the transfusion **immediately.**

2. Perform a careful clerical check to confirm the identity of the recipient and the accuracy of blood bank and clinical records.

3. A blood sample is drawn into a tube containing an anticoagulant and is centrifuged. The supernatant fluid is examined for visible evidence of hemoglobin.

4. A blood sample is drawn for repeat crossmatch, a Coombs test, and haptoglobin.

5. A urine sample is checked for hemoglobin.

6. Septicemia must be considered in the differential diagnosis; therefore, blood cultures are indicated for allergic and febrile reactions.

7. An incident report should be submitted to the Risk Manager and a copy to the Blood Bank Director.

6
ANESTHETIC CONSIDERATIONS

Trauma victims who have suffered multiple system damage present a unique challenge to the anesthesiologist. The patient who is undergoing anesthesia and has multiple system failure must be monitored as closely as in the Intensive Care or Critical Care Recovery Unit. In addition to the sophisticated monitoring required, there are several precautions that must be taken into consideration when anesthetizing a trauma victim.

I. Preanesthetic Phase

A. Assessment

1. Neurologic assessment must be completed and recorded on the anesthesia record before drugs are administered and/or intubation is performed.

2. Cervical spine x-ray is done before sitting a patient up or before intubation is attempted, if possible.

3. Chest x-ray in the upright position should be done to rule out mediastinal abnormalities, lung contusion, and pneumothorax.

4. Pelvic x-rays are obtained in all patients to rule out a fracture.

5. An admission arterial sample is obtained on room air for blood gas analysis.

6. In smoke inhalation patients, direct measurement of arterial oxygen saturation must be made, since arterial oxygen tension does not reflect saturation in these cases.

7. An assessment of vital signs provides information regarding cardiovascular instability, hypothermia, or respiratory distress.

B. Management

1. The patient is met at the Heliport by the Anesthesia Staff and Admitting Area Nurse for immediate airway stabilization and assessment.

2. If the patient arrives with an esophageal obturator airway (EOA) in place, leave it in place and intubate the trachea before removing the EOA.

3. Do not remove Military Anti-Shock Trousers (MAST) before lines are inserted, fluids are begun, and assessment is complete.

4. Place a Philadelphia collar on all patients until the cervical x-ray is read.

5. Insert adequate i.v. lines (see p. 9).

6. Thirty-five percent of our trauma victims have hypokalemia, ($K^+ \leq 3.5$ mEq/liter). Use digitalis and hyperventilation with care to prevent premature ventricular contractions (PVCs).

7. Coagulation studies should be ordered in virtually all patients.

8. Uncrossmatched O Rh-positive or O Rh-negative cells may be necessary (see p. 36).

9. Aspiration is common.

II. Anesthetic Phase

A. General principles

1. All procedures are done during one operation, if possible.

2. Orthopedic procedures have to be tailored to the patient's postoperative respiratory requirements, e.g., use Hoffman stabilization devices or Neufeld traction (see p. 245).

3. Operation is immediate if an urgent indication is present; evaluation of other systems proceeds simultaneously with surgery.

4. Do not reverse muscle relaxant at the end of the procedure.

5. Blunt trauma generally produces more profound physiologic impairment than penetrating trauma.

6. General anesthesia may be required to expedite the diagnostic work-up with or without subsequent surgery.

7. An intensive care environment must be provided for the patient in the operating room.

B. Drug contraindications

1. Opiates and thiopental (Pentothal) are used with caution in hypovolemic patients.

2. Ketamine (Ketalar) is contraindicated in patients with increased intracranial pressure.

3. Avoid succinylcholine (Anectine) in burns, eye injuries, spinal cord injuries, and massive soft tissue injury.

4. Halothane (Fluothane) and enflurane (Ethrane) should be avoided when increased intracranial pressure is detected. If they are used, it should be in low concentrations and **with hyperventilation.**

5. Avoid nitrous oxide if there is a pneumocephalus or a possibility of a pneumothorax, even if the chest x-ray is negative.

6. Avoid enflurane or methoxyflurane (Penthrane) in shock, oliguria, and renal trauma.

7. Use of pancuronium bromide (Pavulon) or curare is determined by hemodynamic needs and cardiac rhythm, not by the need for muscle relaxants.
   a. Pavulon creates arrhythmias and hypertension.
   b. Curare creates afterload reduction and hypotension.

C. **Airway problems**

1. In patients with facial trauma, cervical fractures, intraoral bleeding, or a fracture of the larynx, be prepared to provide either oxygenation by jet needle ventilation or a cricothyroidotomy if an airway is needed and cannot be performed by translaryngeal intubation. Muscle relaxants are contraindicated in patients who have these specific problems. If jet needle ventilation is used, a Y piece should be inserted in the line; occlusion of the side port allows insufflation while nonocclusion allows tracheal decompression in the case of upper airway obstruction. See p. 15.

2. All patients requiring general anesthesia should be intubated.

3. A small pneumothorax may develop into a tension pneumothorax after the anesthetic is begun; therefore, chest tubes should be inserted before draping in any patient with a pneumothorax.

4. Endobronchial tubes are useful for patients with a ruptured aorta, a ruptured bronchus, or severe ipsilateral hemoptysis.

D. **Hemodynamic**   Monitoring is discussed on p. 46.

1. Blood filters are not used.

2. Large bore catheters or feeding tubes are used for volume replacement.

E. **Pulmonary**   Minimum prophylactic positive end-expiratory pressure (PEEP), 3–5 cm H_2O, is always used with controlled ventilation in a patient with a lung contusion. After resuscitation, the contusion produces a more profound low $\dot{V}/\dot{Q}$ area (shunt) and causes a relative hypoxemia. PEEP helps to minimize this effect (see p. 316).

F. **Renal**

1. Do not use fluoride-releasing anesthetics (methoxyflurane and enflurane) if there is renal trauma, hypotension, or oliguria.

2. Pigment present in the urine may be myoglobin and/or hemoglobin.

3. Use fluids and/or diuretics to maintain urine output ≥ 0.5 cc/kg/hr; ≥ 1.5 cc/kg/hr, if there are pigments in the urine.

G. Hematologic

1. Dilutional coagulopathy commonly occurs after approximately 6 units of packed red cells.

2. Two units of fresh frozen plasma are given per 6 units of packed cells transfused (see p. 37).

3. Platelet transfusion is given for platelet counts $\leq 50,000/mm^3$ (see p. 37).

4. If hypotension occurs and hypocalcemic EKG changes are present after multiple transfusions, give 0.5–1.0 gm of $CaCl_2$ i.v. slowly (see p. 38).

H. Metabolic

1. Hypothermia is common. Correct arterial blood gas values for temperature changes. Warm the patient with heated humidifier in the ventilator circuit (see p. 375).

2. Alcohol and/or drugs such as phencyclidene (PCP), marijuana, and methamphetamine (speed) frequently are present in trauma patients; a toxicology screen may be helpful.

3. Metabolic acidosis is common and is usually corrected by volume infusion.

4. The metabolic acidosis that sometimes accompanies carbon monoxide intoxication is due to decreased oxygen utilization. The PvO_2 is frequently high in these patients, indicating a utilization deficit (see p. 508).

I. Neurologic

1. ICP monitors are used in closed head injuries when other trauma requires surgery so that changes may be detected during anesthesia.

2. Steroids, hyperventilation ($PaCO_2$ to 25 Torr), mannitol, sedation, and the head-up position are used to lower intracranial pressures.

3. Head injury has first priority for surgery in multiply injured patients; respiratory and cardiovascular stability must be concomitantly maintained.

4. Barbiturates are the anesthetic of choice in patients with closed head injuries.

J. Monitoring

1. The following instruments are ideal for monitoring:
   a. Calculator or computer
   b. Respirometer
   c. End tidal CO_2 monitor
   d. Dedicated stat lab, 24 hr/day, 7 days/week

2. Insert a PA line if
   a. Massive trauma is present.
   b. Massive volume replacement is needed.

c. History of coronary artery disease is obtained.

d. Myocardial contusion is present or suspected.

e. Pulmonary contusion requires PEEP > 10 cm H_2O to maintain PaO_2/FiO_2 ≥ 250.

f. Toxic substances are present in the blood, such as CO, propane, gasoline, sulfur, etc.

g. In general, the more systems involved (unstable) and the older the patient, the greater the need for a PA line.

3. Measure
   a. Pulmonary arterial pressures
   b. Systemic arterial pressures
   c. Wedge and central venous pressures
   d. SaO_2, PaO_2, $P\bar{v}O_2$, pH, $PaCO_2$, $P\bar{v}CO_2$, and $S\bar{v}O_2$
   e. Cardiac output, Hb, temperature, estimated weight and height, and body surface area

4. From the above values, calculate quickly and accurately with a computer or calculator:
   a. Systemic Vascular Resistance Index
   b. Pulmonary Vascular Resistance Index
   c. Double Product, Triple Product (myocardial oxygen consumption)
   d. Transmyocardial gradient (myocardial oxygen supply)
   e. $\dot{V}O_2$
   f. $CaO_2 - C\bar{v}O_2$
   g. $\dot{Q}s/\dot{Q}t$
   h. SV, SI, CI
   i. LVSWI, RVSWI
   j. Base excess
   (See p. 335.)

5. Electrolytes
   a. Serum K^+ and Na^+
   b. Urine K^+ and Na^+

6. Urine volume; serum and urine osmolality and creatinine

7. Coagulation studies
   a. Prothrombin time (PT)
   b. Partial thromboplastin time (PTT)
   c. Platelets

8. Hb/Hct

9. Blood glucose

10. Intracranial pressure, if indicated

Our ability to collect, record, and use the above-mentioned variables is facilitated by our Clincal Stat Lab, which is connected directly to our computer terminals, one of which is in the operating room. A programmable hand calculator also will work well.

III. **Postanesthetic Phase**   The patient is transferred to a nearby unit in which monitoring is done by a system identical to the one used in the operating room. Our computer has the ability to plot on an X-Y graph the relationship between any two of several variables. For example, a ventricular function curve of LVSWI on the Y axis and PCWP on the X axis is frequently used for hemodynamic tracking. The Critical Care Staff and Anesthesia Staff are one and the same group, which provides continuity of anesthesia/critical care from admission to discharge.

7

PEDIATRIC TRAUMA

Accidents are responsible for more than one-half of all deaths among boys and for nearly two-fifths of all deaths among girls of school age in the United States. There are an estimated 50,000 children permanently crippled by accidents every year and another 2 million who are incapacitated for several weeks or months.

The most common group of injuries in the childhood age group is blunt as opposed to penetrating injuries. Approximately 80% of life-threatening injuries in children occur as a result of blunt trauma. Since blunt injuries are frequently associated with head injuries, the evaluation of a patient with a depressed level of consciousness creates an additional problem in thoroughly evaluating the patient. As in the adult, blunt trauma in the child frequently is associated with minimal external evidence of injury, yet may be associated with life-threatening internal injuries. As a result of the difficulty in evaluating these patients, highly experienced professionals should be involved in the initial evaluation and resuscitation. Because of the devastating physical insult suffered by the child with blunt trauma, a team approach should be developed to rapidly assess and manage the child with multiple injuries. The Trauma Team should consist of a pediatric or general surgeon, an anesthesiologist, a pediatrician, and subspecialists such as an orthopedist, neurosurgeon, urologist, or plastic surgeon. The Trauma Team should be directed by the general or pediatric surgeon. A pediatrician is mandatory for the proper management of small children and infants to appropriately manage fluid, electrolyte, and drug administration. Even if the patient has no apparent general surgical injury, the general surgeon should oversee the initial assessment, resuscitation, and continuing general care. The surgeon should coordinate the recommendations from the pediatrician and surgical subspecialist according to the priorities dictated by the patient's needs.

A regional trauma center for children is desirable
—As an area for efficient evaluation of children with serious injuries
—As a center for resuscitation
—As an environment which is designed specifically to manage the injured child

Children brought into this unit have the advantage of centralized diagnostic facilities and specialty consultation in all the surgical and pediatric disciplines. A regional trauma center for children should include
—Appropriate means of transportation of the injured child to the facility, including ambulance and helicopter service
—A resuscitation area within the trauma unit for evaluation and life-saving treatment of a child with multiple injuries
—Core diagnostic facilities, including x-ray and blood and chemistry laboratories
—Experienced physicians and nursing staff available on a 24-hr basis within the unit and consultants in the various specialties available on immediate call

—Adjacent intensive care areas especially designed for children and their unique problems

—Available operating rooms for the treatment of serious injuries which require general anesthesia

I. **Special Considerations in the Child** The basic principles in the management of major injuries of the child are the same as those for the adult. There are many differences related to diagnosis and treatment that are unique to the child.

A. Because of the small size of the injured child, the margin for error is diminished relative to the adult. The loss of a small amount of blood in a young child assumes dramatic importance when considering the child's small blood volume. A closed fracture of the femur in a 10-year-old child may be associated with 300 or 400 cc of blood loss, which may represent 15–25% of circulating blood volume and contribute to hypovolemic shock.

B. Because of the increased surface area of the infant relative to weight, excessive heat may be lost into the environment. Following injury, the child is stripped of clothing in order that adequate assessment may be made. During this exposure, the child may become significantly hypothermic, especially if the room is cooled excessively with an air conditioner. The thermal regulatory mechanism of the child often is unable to meet the requirements of such a situation. The infusion of large quantities of cold blood will contribute to heat loss. A drop in core temperature may interfere with normal enzymatic function and other metabolic processes. Hypothermia is an additional metabolic insult superimposed upon the stress of trauma. The child should be placed in a warm environment and covered as soon as feasible, in order to combat hypothermia. Infused fluids should be warmed through a warming coil.

C. The management of fluid and electrolyte balance in the child is much more taxing than in the adult. Because of the small compartments of the child's body, the quantity of water and electrolytes must be precise in keeping up with maintenance and excessive losses. Frequently, a pediatrician will be invaluable in assisting in the management of the child's fluid and electrolyte balance. The pediatrician is also helpful in managing the nutrient requirements of the child.

D. The pediatrician is helpful in recommending specific drugs and their dosages for the young patient. Drug interactions and idiosyncrasies of drugs in the child must be well known.

E. A potential source of complications in the management of the injured child is the coexistence of a congenital anomaly. Cardiac defects may particularly complicate the child's course. Pulmonary, gastrointestinal, and urologic anomalies must be considered as possibilities when these systems become unstable.

F. From an anatomic and physiologic standpoint, the infant has a much lower respiratory reserve compared to the adult. Since the tracheobronchial tree is short and narrow, there is little room for error during intubation and manipulation of the trachea. Due to the small caliber of the trachea, there is difficulty in evacuating tracheobronchial secretions by tracheal suction.

G. Because of the frequent inability of young children to express pain and to localize symptoms, they are placed almost in the category of veterinary medicine. Even the older child may have difficulty in communicating with the physician, if frightened. Evaluation of the injured child demands patience upon the part of the examining physician and a desire to win the confidence of the child.

H. A paralytic ileus following blunt abdominal trauma is common. The frightened child frequently becomes aerophagic and develops an acute gastric dilatation. Because of the likelihood of acute gastric distention and the development of a paralytic ileus, gastrointestinal decompression should be performed early. If the gastrointestinal tract is not decompressed, abdominal distention will cause elevation of the diaphragm, which will minimize the vital capacity of the lungs. Gastric decompression will diminish the not infrequent complication of vomiting with associated aspiration.

II. Initial Evaluation The initial priority in managing the traumatized child is to assess and stabilize immediate life-threatening injuries. Respiratory instability, cardiovascular instability, and major central nervous system insult are the immediate threats to the child's life. The physician must assess the airway, chest, respirations, heart rate, blood pressure, and the peripheral circulation. The central nervous system is assessed by noting the patient's level of consciousness, response to verbal commands, response to pain, and the status of the brain stem. Once these systems are assessed and stabilized, a more thorough examination may be performed to precisely define the patient's injuries.

Resuscitation begins concomitant with the initial assessment. If there is airway obstruction, it should be alleviated and adequate ventilation should be maintained. If a hemothorax or pneumothorax is present, the pleural space should be decompressed. Venous lines should be inserted and volume infusion initiated.

III. Respiratory Assessment and Stabilization If the child is making no effort to breathe, artificial ventilation should be instituted immediately. If the child is trying to breathe but is moving little or no air, there may be airway obstruction. The mouth should be opened and the airway suctioned free of blood, mucus, vomitus, or foreign bodies. The chest should be auscultated to detect a diminution in breath sounds on either side. If there are diminished breath sounds and the patient is hypotensive, the pleural space should be decompressed rapidly. Generally, translaryngeal intubation provides optimal security for the patient with a tenuous airway. The stomach should be decompressed with a gastric tube to prevent vomiting and aspiration.

IV. **Cardiovascular Assessment and Stabilization**   The chapter on "Cardiovascular Assessment and Stabilization" (p. 7) in principle is germane to management of the child. Immediately upon admission, the pulse should be palpated for rate and intensity. The blood pressure should be rapidly obtained and the patient should be inspected for evidence of vasoconstriction. Venous access should be obtained by percutaneous or cutdown technique. Since the blood volume of the child is so small, hemorrhage must be completely and promptly controlled and volume deficits rapidly corrected to prevent cellular damage and cardiac arrest. Severe hypotension in a child is virtually always a result of hemorrhage. Cardiac contusion and tension pneumothorax must be excluded. Until blood is available, physiologic saline or lactated Ringer's solution may be used for volume expansion. Crystalloid (10 cc/pound) may be safely administered as an intravenous push to correct moderate to severe hypovolemia.

The response of the central venous pressure (CVP) is a valuable guide by which to monitor volume infusion. If the CVP is less than 4 cm of water, volume may be infused at a rapid rate of 5 cc/pound/hr. If the CVP is greater than 15 cm of water, cardiogenic shock or inaccurate placement of the central venous catheter must be excluded. If 20 cc of crystalloid/kg has been infused, blood must be administered to prevent marked hemodilution (see p. 36). Volume is infused until the CVP begins to rise and clinical manifestations of hypoperfusion are reversed. If there is adequate intravascular volume expansion and peripheral perfusion, the hourly urinary output should be approximately ½–1 cc/kg/hr.

Concomitant with respiratory and cardiovascular stabilization, the patient must be assessed to locate the source of shock. Generally, blood loss may be external or into the chest, intraperitoneal cavity, or retroperitoneal space, or associated with a femoral or pelvic fracture. Tension pneumothorax, cardiac tamponade, and cardiac contusion must be excluded in all cases.

Infused blood should be warmed in order to prevent hypothermia. Hypothermia may cause myocardial depression and cardiac arrhythmias. If the patient has received massive transfusion, calcium administration may be necessary to prevent acute hypocalcemia.

V. **Evaluation and Management of the Multiply Injured Child**   After cardiovascular and respiratory stabilization has been obtained, a more thorough examination is performed.

A. **Skull**   The child is evaluated for the presence of scalp lacerations; the skull is examined through the laceration to exclude a fracture. The skull is evaluated for the presence of ecchymosis, localized swelling, Battle's sign, otorrhea, rhinorrhea, and hemotympanum. X-rays are obtained if these signs are present.

B. **Face**   The face and intraoral cavity are examined for evidence of ecchymosis, swelling, deformity, and malocclusion, which is likely to represent a fracture. Facial hypesthesia and paresis are evaluated to exclude a peripheral nerve injury. Damage to the parotid duct should be considered with any cheek laceration.

C. **Brain** A more thorough neurologic examination is performed after initial stabilization. The child should be evaluated for the presence of orientation, agitation, or inability to follow commands. The child's motor response to pain should be noted to be purposeful, decorticate, decerebrate, or flaccid. The brain stem reflexes are evaluated to assess brain stem function. The clinician should seek evidence of lateralization of extremity movement or brain stem responses.

D. **Neck** Evidence of hoarseness, cervical subcutaneous emphysema, hemoptysis, or hematemesis may be evidence of damage to the larynx, trachea, esophagus, or pharynx. Neck pain, decreased cervical motion, or deformity may represent damage to the spinal column. Decreased sensory or motor response of the extremities, decreased rectal tone, priapism, or bradycardia may be manifestations of spinal cord injury. A cervical hematoma with altered level of consciousness or hemiparesis is suggestive of carotid arterial damage.

E. **Chest** Decreased breath sounds and dullness to percussion in association with hypotension is usually indicative of a hemothorax. The presence of unilateral decreased breath sounds and tympany to percussion is suggestive of a pneumothorax. Tachypnea, hypoxia, hemoptysis, and a pulmonary infiltrate on chest x-ray are diagnostic of pulmonary contusion. Rib fractures are clinically apparent by the presence of pain on inspiration, subcutaneous emphysema, crepitus, or paradoxical chest wall motion. A sternal fracture is identified by the presence of pain on inspiration, presternal crepitus, and sternal paradoxical motion with respiration. Cardiac tamponade is suggested when the patient is persistently hypotensive and the neck veins are distended in association with an increased CVP. Cardiac contusion is suggested by the presence of cardiac failure or arrhythmias. Tracheobronchial injury is likely when there is subcutaneous emphysema, hemoptysis, a large pleural air leak, pneumomediastinum, pleural effusion, or pneumothorax. A wide mediastinum, decreased extremity or carotid pulses, altered level of consciousness, hemiparesis, hemothorax, and hoarseness are commonly associated with injury to the aorta or great vessels. Injury to the thoracic spine may be manifest by the presence of upper back pain or deformity. A patient with injury to the thoracic spinal cord usually presents with decreased chest-abdominal wall sensation and paraplegia.

F. **Abdomen** Splenic, hepatic, and mesenteric injuries are diagnosed by a bloody peritoneal lavage. Hollow viscus injuries are usually identified when a laparotomy is performed for a bloody peritoneal lavage, which occurs secondary to injury of other organs, or for abdominal tenderness (peritonitis). Since the duodenum and pancreas are retroperitoneal, the child may present with delayed abdominal findings of ileus, tenderness, and hemodynamic or respiratory instability. The perineum and rectum should be evaluated in all children to exclude the possibility of a rectal or perineal injury.

G. **Urinary tract**   The presence of a flank hematoma, flank ecchymosis, hematuria, L_{1-2} fracture, or posterior lower rib fractures may be associated with a renal injury. The presence of hematuria may be associated with urinary tract injury at any level. If the child has a pelvic fracture, a urethral or bladder injury is likely. The presence of hematuria mandates a cystogram and intravenous pyelogram.

H. **Pelvis**   The child should be evaluated for the presence of perineal ecchymosis, pubic symphysis diastasis, iliac wing instability, and pelvic pain. A pelvic x-ray should be considered as part of the routine evaluation of the child, to exclude a pelvic fracture. A cystogram should be performed in children with a pelvic fracture.

I. **Extremity**   The extremity should be evaluated for the presence of pain, deformity, crepitus, decreased motion, or ecchymosis. If these manifestations are identified, it is likely that the patient has a fracture or dislocation. The extremities should be evaluated for impairment of sensory or motor function or decreased circulation. A thorough examination of the extremity will reveal the presence of a laceration. The clinical examination may be more diagnostic than an x-ray.

The principles governing the management of injuries in the child are essentially the same as those in the adult. The following laboratory parameters should be obtained in the multiply injured child: hematocrit, white blood cell count, amylase, electrolytes, calcium, magnesium, glucose, urinalysis, type and cross match, and arterial blood gases. To thoroughly evaluate the injured child, the following x-rays should be obtained: skull, spine, chest, abdomen, and pelvis. Extremity deformity or abnormality mandates an x-ray of that extremity. An intravenous pyelogram should be obtained if the patient has hematuria. A cystogram is indicated if the patient has hematuria or a pelvic fracture. A CAT scan is necessary if the sensorium is impaired. Tetanus immunization must be considered in all children with cutaneous defects secondary to trauma.

J. **Procedural comments**
   —Nasogastric intubation should be performed prior to evaluation of the child's abdomen. Gastric decompression will minimize abdominal distention and enhance the ability of the examiner to identify abdominal pathology.
   —If there is a question regarding the presence of abdominal pathology, a peritoneal lavage should be performed. The technique described for the adult is used in the older child or teenager. If the patient is an infant or child, a plastic catheter is inserted into the peritoneal cavity and 15 cc of saline/kg is instilled into the peritoneal cavity and aspirated. The presence of blood, bile, or intestinal content in the aspirate is an indication for surgical intervention. The pitfalls of this technique are the same as those described for the adult.
   —The presence of blood in the patient's chest requires a tube of at least a 20-French caliber in the infant and a 24- to 28-French caliber in the older child.

—Bleeding through a chest tube of greater than 2 cc/pound/hr without evidence of slowing is usually an indication for thoracotomy.

VI. **Monitoring**   Monitoring the child's physiologic systems is the same, in principle, as for the adult. The reader is referred to p. 487.

Section II
SHOCK

8

PRACTICAL MANAGEMENT OF SHOCK

Many types of major illness such as trauma, heart disease, sepsis, hemorrhage, and burns are associated with shock.

Shock is a complex pathophysiologic process initiated by altered hemodynamic function, which produces poor tissue perfusion. The lack of adequate tissue oxygenation and the accumulation of waste products impair normal cellular metabolism, ultimately leading to circulatory deterioration, organ failure, and death.

I. **Pathophysiology** Shock should be considered as a continuum of pathophysiologic alterations which become progressively more severe. Patients with shock pass through these successive phases at a rate determined by the severity of the initial insult.

A. **Mild to moderate shock** With a decrease in tissue perfusion, an early nonspecific clinical sign of shock is rapid, shallow breathing. The hyperventilation is generally associated with a normal arterial PO_2 and hypocarbia.

In response to hypoperfusion, baroreceptor reflexes elicit a powerful sympathoadrenal response, resulting in vasoconstriction and tachycardia. Vasoconstriction is initially beneficial in diverting blood from tissues such as skin and muscles to more vital organs. If hypoperfusion worsens, blood flow is further diverted from the gut, kidney, and liver. Arterial vasoconstriction combined with constriction of the large veins reduces vascular capacity, thereby increasing venous return.

When hypovolemia initially develops, compensatory mechanisms tend to return the blood volume back toward normal. Fluids tend to move rapidly from the interstitial space into the vascular space. In sepsis, capillary permeability may increase very early, which enhances the movement of fluid into the interstitial space. Consequently, septic patients often require much more fluid and become more edematous than patients with comparable hypotension from other causes.

Increased platelet aggregation is another mechanism that is often evoked in mild or early shock. Platelet aggregates or vasoactive substances released from platelets may occlude small vessels and impair microcirculatory perfusion. Platelet aggregates that embolize to the lungs may be a contributing factor to respiratory failure often seen following prolonged shock.

B. **Severe shock** If the depth of shock is more severe, or mild to moderate shock is protracted, disastrous physiologic changes occur. As shock continues, irrespective of the cause, there is swelling and rupture of the lysosomes with intracellular release of proteolytic enzymes and subsequent loss of cell wall integrity. These enzymes activate kinins and prostaglandins which cause local vasodilation and increase capillary permeability. The vasodilation may cause relative hypovolemia and contribute to maldistribution of organ perfusion. Increased capillary permeability leads to interstitial edema and organ dysfunction. Histamine is released from tissues in response to injury, which causes microcirculatory changes which compound perfusion abnormalities. Circulatory function may be further depressed by a circulating myocardial depressant factor released following splanchnic ischemia.

With tissue hypoxia, the cells must function under anaerobic conditions. Normally, glucose is converted to acetyl coenzyme A from pyruvate and enters the Krebs cycle to produce energy (38 mol of ATP for each mol of glucose). With hypoxia, pyruvate accumulates and is converted to lactic acid instead of acetyl coenzyme A. The transformation of glucose to lactic acid is a much less efficient mode of energy production (2 mol of ATP for each mol of glucose). In this process, accumulation of lactic acid is the main cause of metabolic acidosis seen with shock.

Due to the energy deficit of anaerobic metabolism, the sodium/potassium pump fails to maintain normal extracellular sodium and intracellular potassium levels. With pump failure, there is an intracellular accumulation of sodium and water which pulls fluid from the extracellular space, causing intracellular edema. This fluid shift plus the vasodilation caused by the accumulation of lactic acid and the release of vasodilatory substances, and leakage of the capillary endothelium causes significant hypovolemia in late or severe shock, regardless of its etiology.

Hypoperfusion results in pooling of blood in the capillaries. This stagnation, coupled with local chemical changes in the capillaries, causes red cell aggregation or "sludging" and intravascular clotting. Prolonged shock can cause consumption of clotting factors. This condition, known as disseminated intravascular coagulopathy, can be detected by serial clotting studies long before the full-blown clinical symptoms appear.

The progressive pathophysiology of shock eventually produces dysfunction of multiple systems, cell necrosis, and death. The brain, liver, kidney, heart, gastrointestinal tract, lungs, and immunologic system may deteriorate secondary to the cellular insults associated with shock. Physiologic alteration of these systems may be apparent early, e.g., as overt pulmonary or renal failure, or may present at a later time with sepsis and sequential systems failure.

II. **Therapeutic Concepts** Regardless of the etiology, the management of shock must be prompt, correct, and sustained. A preconceived plan of attack that can be implemented immediately upon a patient's arrival to the hospital is needed so that the progression of the shock process can be halted. Without a definitive plan, the outcome can be lethal. Even with a preconceived plan, procrastination in implementation can be detrimental to the patient's survival. Accurate monitoring together with early, appropriate treatment can, in many cases, result in complete reversal of the fundamental disorder before permanent organ damage occurs.

A tentative diagnosis of shock based on hemodynamic and clinical observations should be made as soon as possible and cardiopulmonary resuscitation started **immediately.**

At the time when medical treatment is initiated, a patient can be in any phase of the pathophysiologic continuum of shock. Hemodynamic stability can be achieved in many patients with severe or prolonged shock. With aggressive therapy, the process can be reversible, even when there is some degree of organ failure. However, with some severe cases, it may be impossible to generate an adequate blood pressure and perfusion level. This patient is in a state of "refractory" shock and usually dies within minutes to hours. There are other patients who, despite the restoration of hemodynamic stability, gradually deteriorate and expire days to weeks later, usually as the result of sequential multiple systems failure or sepsis. In this case, physiologic disruption has occurred beyond a critical level which has initiated an irreversible process. Since it cannot be determined when a patient passes from a state of reversible to irreversible shock, all patients with shock need maximal pulmonary and cardiovascular support.

The goal of the physician treating shock is to maintain vascular expansion, optimal cardiac filling, and adequate oxygenation to provide optimal microcirculatory blood flow. Packed red blood cells must be given early in the course of shock to provide optimal oxygen-carrying capacity. An adequate number of vascular lines must be inserted to infuse volume rapidly and reverse the hemodynamic instability associated with hypovolemic and septic shock. Early surgical intervention is necessary to promptly control hemorrhage and prevent early death or multiple systems deterioration. If the patient has evidence of left ventricular failure, inotropic-chronotropic support is indicated. The specific etiology of shock must be identified and reversed.

In addition to monitoring cardiovascular and pulmonary function, other biochemical parameters must be monitored frequently to detect insult to vital organ systems and to monitor the effectiveness of therapy. For example, liver enzymes, creatinine clearance, coagulation parameters, blood gases, etc., should be sequentially followed. If there is progressive deterioration in these systems, the clinician must assess cardiovascular performance as the origin of the systems dysfunction (see pp. 335 and 369).

A patient in shock can be given the best chance for survival when the causative factor is corrected and subsequent therapy is based on following trends in serial biochemical and physiologic measurements and evaluating the patient's response to therapy.

III. **Classification** The purpose of a shock classification is to facilitate rapid recognition of the underlying cause and to promote correct and specific therapy as quickly as possible. Shock may follow such diverse conditions as severe trauma, burns, major surgery, massive hemorrhage, dehydration, myocardial infarction, overwhelming infections, poisoning, and drug reactions. If shock is not rapidly controlled, a hemodynamic and cellular response develops that is similar in all cases, regardless of the initial etiology.

Commonly overlooked is the fact that more than one type of shock is frequently present in the same patient. There may be an element of left or right ventricular dysfunction associated with any type of shock. For example, an elderly patient with a history of coronary artery disease may incur hypovolemic shock following an accident; poor left ventricular performance is likely to compound the hemodynamic instability. In another instance, a patient with hemorrhagic shock may be successfully resuscitated, but develop septic shock from catheter contamination. This dual pathology multiplies the cellular insult.

To organize the clinical approach to diagnosis and treatment, shock can be divided into three main categories: hypovolemic, cardiogenic, and septic.

A. **Hypovolemic shock** Blood loss, plasma loss, or water loss is the result of a number of causes, including burns, hemorrhage, multiple trauma, and severe diarrhea. Hypovolemic shock occurs when the intravascular volume relative to vascular capacity is markedly decreased. It is generally associated with a blood volume deficit of at least 15–25%.

Hypovolemic patients usually have an increased heart rate, decreased cardiac filling pressure, increased diastolic pressure, low pulse pressure, low cardiac output, oliguria, increased peripheral vascular resistance, and pale, clammy skin. These clinical signs are the direct and indirect result of a blood volume deficit and intense sympathoadrenal discharge.

Vasoactive substances and lysosomal enzymes released following severe tissue injury can cause vasodilation and alter microcirculatory blood flow. These patients may be hypotensive in spite of a normal or increased cardiac output. Peripheral shunting occurs as microcirculatory perfusion falls.

B. **Cardiogenic shock** is the result of inadequate tissue perfusion secondary to failure of the heart as a pump. Although acute myocardial infarction and other heart disease are common causes in patients admitted to a specialized trauma unit, cardiogenic shock is usually the result of pulmonary embolism, cardiac tamponade, cardiac contusion, or ventricular, septal, or valvular rupture. Most patients with cardiogenic shock have low cardiac output, increased pulse rate, increased peripheral resistance, increased cardiac filling pressures, and pale, clammy skin.

C. **Septic shock** is the result of a widely disseminated infection affecting almost every physiologic system. The development of peritonitis from gut wounds, generalized infection from the spread of simple streptococcal or staphylococcal skin infection, and the spread of gas gangrene infection are examples of causes of septic shock that threaten patient survival.

Many of the responses to septic shock are due to vasoactive peptides or lysosomal enzymes released from damaged, ischemic, or infected tissues. These substances increase membrane permeability and decrease vascular resistance, thereby increasing vascular capacity. If there is a corresponding increase in blood volume, cardiac output tends to be high, causing hyperdynamic ("warm") septic shock. If the patient's blood volume does not increase, a relative hypovolemia exists and cardiac output will fall, resulting in a hypodynamic ("cold") type of septic shock.

D. **Other causes** of shock include anaphylatic, hypoglycemic, and neurogenic shock, and shock due to drug overdose. Shock in the patient with a head injury is almost never the result of central nervous damage. However, neurogenic shock can occur with spinal cord trauma secondary to a sympathectomy effect.

IV. Clinical Considerations

A. **Hypovolemic shock** develops as a result of decreased intravascular volume, secondary to external and/or concealed blood loss. Blood loss results in a decrease in the preload volume to produce a fall in the cardiac output. Initial vasoconstriction maintains the blood pressure; however, after a loss of approximately one-fourth to one-third of the intravascular volume, hypotension develops.

1. **Manifestations**
   a. Pallor
   b. Cool extremities
   c. Tachycardia
   d. Hypotension
   e. Diaphoresis
   f. Oliguria
   g. Decreased sensorium
   h. Decreased capillary refill
   i. Metabolic acidosis
   j. Hyperpnea

   | Note | Hypotension may not occur in the early stages of decreased tissue perfusion; however, aggressive therapy is indicated at this time before hypovolemia progresses.

2. **Hemodynamic parameters**
   a. Increased arterial-venous O_2 content
   b. Increased systemic vascular resistance
   c. Decreased to normal cardiac output
   d. Decreased wedge pressure
   e. Decreased central venous pressure
   f. Decreased oxygen consumption

   > **Perspective**
   > The initial hematocrit is not low unless there is massive hemorrhage. If the patient is seen early after trauma and the hemorrhage is not severe, the diminished red blood cell mass has not had time to equilibrate with the interstitial fluid which has moved into the vascular tree. Therefore, the initial hematocrit may be normal.

3. **Treatment**
   a. Oxygenation should be supported at all times.
   b. Intravenous fluids should be rapidly administered to restore intravascular volume.
      (1) An initial volume of 1,500 cc of intravenous fluid as plasmanate should be administered.

(2) Hemoglobin should be maintained at 12 gm %. If rapid fluid resuscitation is required after the initial 1,500 cc of plasmanate, red blood cells must be administered to maintain oxygen-carrying capacity (see p. 36).

(3) After the intravascular volume has been restored and hemorrhage is controlled, crystalloid is administered to replace interstitial and intracellular water.

> Note The end point of rapid volume infusion is a reversal of the manifestations previously described.

c. During shock, the following should be monitored: blood pressure, central venous pressure, urinary output, electrocardiogram, hematocrit and hemoglobin, arterial blood gases, coagulation profile, and electrolytes. The clinical manifestations of shock should be repeatedly evaluated to assess the adequacy of therapy.

d. External and internal hemorrhage must be controlled. Control may require early and aggressive operative intervention (see p. 10).

e. Immobilize fractures to reduce blood loss.

f. The patient should remain recumbent, preferably in the Trendelenburg position.

g. Avoid unnecessary movement, since rough handling and undue manipulation may precipitate profound hypotension.

h. Treat physiologic abnormalities that may intensify the diminution in tissue perfusion, such as electrolyte imbalance, hypoxia, hypothermia, and acidosis.

i. **Refractory shock** The following factors may perpetuate the "shock state":

(1) Inadequate volume replacement; continued bleeding
(2) Hypoxia and/or hypoventilation
(3) Tension pneumothorax
(4) Cardiac tamponade or contusion
(5) Hypokalemia or hypocalcemia
(6) Acidosis
(7) Hypothermia
(8) Central nervous system trauma (severe)
(9) Prolonged hypoxia which leads to myocardial insufficiency and possibly brain stem dysfunction (vasomotor regulation)
(10) Myocardial infarction

If the patient does not rapidly stabilize after initial volume infusion and operative control, a Swan-Ganz catheter should be inserted, if possible. If the central venous or wedge pressure rises during therapy for persistent shock, dopamine (Intropin) or dobutamine (Dobutrex) may be useful drugs. With refractory shock, the previously mentioned causes of persistent shock must be individually and aggressively excluded.

B. **Septic shock** may occur secondary to Gram-negative or Gram-positive aerobes or anaerobes. Common sources of bacteremia are the gastrointestinal tract, abdominal abscess, genitourinary tract, infected wounds, vascular lines, and pulmonary infection. Any septic focus has the potential of producing septic shock.

1. **Manifestations**
   a. Tachypnea (respiratory alkalosis)
   b. Pallor (constriction)
   c. Flushed (dilated) skin
   d. Oliguria
   e. Decreased mean arterial pressure
   f. Tachycardia
   g. Hyperthermia
   h. Decreased level of consciousness
   i. Diaphoretic or dry skin
   j. Metabolic acidosis (late finding)

2. **Hemodynamic parameters (usual)**
   a. Cardiac index increased (may be decreased)
   b. Arteriovenous (AV) O_2 content difference usually decreased (may be normal or increased)
   c. Systemic vascular resistance decreased (warm shock)
   d. Wedge pressure decreased (may be increased)

3. **Management** (see Table 1)
   a. Plasmanate and/or blood are administered, depending on the patient's hematocrit. A large bore i.v. (central line) should be inserted.
   b. Dopamine (Intropin) is useful if cardiac filling pressures are rising and perfusion is inadequate (oliguria).
   c. Broad-spectrum antibiotics should be administered (see p. 415).
   d. After fluid resuscitation has begun, methylprednisolone (Medrol) (30 mg/kg) should be administered i.v. over 20 min. This dose may be repeated once or twice in a 2- to 4-hour interval, if the patient has not stabilized.
   e. **The source of sepsis must be sought and eradicated if possible.** Blood cultures should be obtained immediately before beginning antibiotics (see p. 411).
   f. Sodium bicarbonate should be administered if the pH is less than 7.3.
   g. Respiratory support should be tailored to meet the needs of the patient (see p. 313).
   h. The following parameters should be monitored during the course of septic shock: vital signs, central venous pressure, urinary output, electrocardiogram, hematocrit and hemoglobin, arterial blood gases, electrolytes, coagulation profile, white blood cell count, creatinine clearance, urinary output, chest x-ray, serial blood cultures, and physical examination (see pp. 335 and 369).

Table 1. Hemodynamic stabilization in septic shock

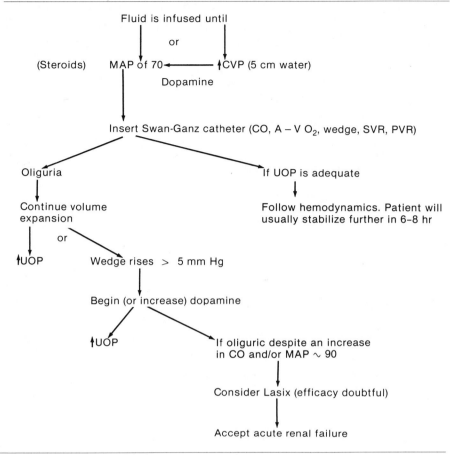

C. **Cardiogenic shock**   In cardiogenic shock, the tissue oxygen demands of the body are not met secondary to cardiac failure. The following are causes of or contributors to cardiogenic shock:
—Myocardial infarction
—Severe congestive heart failure
—Tamponade
—Contusion
—Hypoxia
—Sepsis
—Severe tachycardia or bradycardia
—Pulmonary embolus
—Valve or septal disruption
—Drug induction

1. **Manifestations**
    a. **Hypoperfusion**
        (1) Pallor
        (2) Tachycardia

(3) Diaphoresis

(4) Oliguria

(5) Decreased sensorium

(6) Cool extremities

(7) Hypotension

(8) Decreased capillary refill

(9) Tachypnea

(10) Metabolic acidosis

b. **Increased hydrostatic pressure (congestion)**

(1) Dyspnea

(2) Gallop

(3) Rales

(4) Distended neck veins

(5) Hepatomegaly

(6) Sacral and peripheral edema

2. **Hemodynamic parameters**

a. Decreased cardiac output

b. Decreased oxygen consumption

c. Increased systemic vascular resistance

d. Increased wedge pressure

e. Increased central venous pressure

f. Increased $A - V\,O_2$ content

3. **Diagnosis**

a. Radioisotope angiocardiography and/or echocardiogram (decreased ejection fraction)

b. Thallium-201 or technetium pyrophosphate scan (infarction)

c. CPK isoenzymes (infarction)

d. Ventilation/perfusion scan (pulmonary embolus)

e. EKG

f. Chest x-ray

g. Cineangiography

4. **Management** Specific therapy depends upon the hemodynamic parameter that is primarily affected. Therefore, the clinician must evaluate the preload (wedge), afterload (systemic vascular resistance), heart rate, and contractility (cardiac output versus wedge; ejection fraction). To assess these factors, a Swan-Ganz catheter is inserted.

a. Fluids should be administered until the wedge pressure rises, to make certain that the intravascular volume is optimal. Should the patient be on levels of positive end-expiratory pressure (PEEP) that are above physiologic levels, PEEP should be reduced, if at all possible, to improve venous return. Diuretics may be beneficial if the wedge is markedly elevated and the patient has significant manifestations of congestion. The intravenous administration of nitroglycerin may be helpful if the patient has ischemic changes on EKG and the wedge is markedly elevated (see p. 343).

b. Dobutamine (Dobutrex) is useful in improving myocardial contractility (see p. 342).

c. Sodium nitroprusside (Nipride) or nitroglycerin may be helpful if the patient is markedly hypertensive or the cardiac output fails to respond to fluid administration and/or dobutamine. Nipride and nitroglycerin may precipitously lower the wedge pressure, which may further impair cardiac output; these drugs should not be used if the wedge is ≤ 15 mm Hg. The primary goal in afterload reduction is to decrease the resistance to left ventricular ejection, thus improving aortic flow and systemic circulation (see p. 342).

d. Intra-aortic balloon pump assistance is indicated when drug therapy has failed. The principal use of the aortic balloon pump is to improve coronary flow and to decrease the afterload on the left ventricle.

e. Support oxygenation based on the patient's needs (see p. 313).

f. Relieve cardiac tamponade, if present.

g. Digoxin may be indicated for supraventricular tachycardia or congestive heart failure, if hypoperfusion is minimal.

h. A pacemaker may be required for profound bradycardia.

i. Propranolol (Inderal), lidocaine (Xylocaine), and/or cardioversion may be necessary to treat ventricular tachycardia.

j. The hemoglobin should be maintained at approximately 12–13 gm % to maintain arterial O_2 content.

k. Heparinization, vena caval interruption, or pulmonary arterial embolectomy may be indicated for pulmonary embolization.

l. The following parameters should be monitored:
   (1) Left ventricular stroke work index
   (2) $A - V\ O_2$ content
   (3) Oxygen consumption
   (4) Systemic vascular resistance
   (5) Pulmonary vascular resistance
   (6) Wedge pressure
   (7) Central venous pressure
   (8) EKG
   (9) Myocardial oxygen consumption (heart rate × systolic blood pressure)
   (10) Myocardial oxygen supply (transmyocardial gradient)
   (11) Systolic, mean, and diastolic systemic pressures
   (12) Systolic, mean, and diastolic pulmonary pressures

When a therapeutic maneuver is initiated, each of these parameters must be evaluated to determine whether the therapeutic intervention improved oxygen consumption and myocardial oxygen consumption or altered myocardial oxygen availability.

Section III
SYSTEMS INJURY

INTRODUCTION

There is no system of the body that is immune to external trauma. Trauma may damage systems that cause an immediate threat to life, such as the cardiovascular, pulmonary, or central nervous systems, or it may affect systems that are usually not life-threatening, but that may cause morbidity, such as soft tissue or bony injuries. In general, the more systems that are insulted the greater the morbidity and mortality. Also, the severity of the injury to a given organ will determine the patient's outcome.

The primary goal of the physician is to stabilize the pulmonary, cardiovascular, and central nervous systems. Immediate operative intervention may be necessary in order to gain stabilization. Once these systems are stable, less life-threatening injuries are assessed and managed. It is essential that all injuries be identified at the time of admission. Major injuries are usually easily identified; however, more subtle injuries may not be detected initially. These relatively minor injuries, however, may lead to later morbidity, e.g., a perineal laceration may be missed on admission and not become evident until the patient develops sepsis 5–7 days later. On the other hand, if an obvious peripheral injury, such as an open femoral fracture, receives the primary attention, life may be lost from an unsuspected, undiagnosed thoracic aortic tear.

It is important that one physician, a surgeon, supervise the multidiscipline care of the trauma patient. The surgeon is best qualified to coordinate management of the patient since he has experience in providing physiologic support and understands the principles associated with physical injury to all organ systems. The general surgeon is the individual most capable of integrating the input from the various medical and surgical disciplines, placing each injury into appropriate perspective, and dictating a plan of management that is in the overall best interest of the patient. Even if the patient has no general surgical problem, the general surgeon should be in charge until the patient is stable, injuries are clearly delineated, and the patient is assuming a course of recovery.

The postoperative management of the severely injured patient is just as important as the initial care. The frequently complex postoperative course is best managed by the surgical and critical care physician. There is little consolation in expeditiously controlling massive liver hemorrhage if the patient dies from a pulmonary contusion which was poorly managed in the postoperative period. The multiply injured patient requires expert surgical care and meticulous physiologic support to survive the multiple insults that follow major trauma.

9

HEAD AND NECK INJURIES

The head and neck contain many vital structures essential to life. Injuries that may immediately threaten the patient's life are trauma to the brain, the airway, and vascular structures. There are numerous other structures that may not threaten the patient's life immediately, but may cause significant morbidity if damaged. Injuries to the skeleton and soft tissues of the head may cause impairment of the airway, mastication, or swallowing. Injuries to the eyes and ears are seldom a challenge to the patient's life, but may severely mitigate the individual's functional capacity. The primary significance of a scalp or skull injury is that there may be underlying injury to the brain or a meningeal tear which may result in meningitis. As with any other injury, life-threatening injuries must be addressed first to prevent immediate death. Many injuries to the head and neck will require surgical subspecialist input. The injuries should be assessed in a prompt and thorough manner and repaired as soon as possible after the injury. Many injuries that are not life-threatening may have to be relegated to later management if there are other life-threatening injuries present that preclude prolonged operative management of these lesions. Multiple specialist input should be channeled through the general surgeon (Team Leader in charge), who can then develop a management plan that is in the overall best interest of the patient.

I. **Scalp**

A. **Contusions and lacerations** The scalp is the hair-bearing, vascular, and tenacious soft tissue covering of the calvarium. The scalp is subject to contusion and laceration. To make the diagnosis of a scalp injury is important to properly manage the soft tissue defect, but most importantly, a scalp injury may be an indication that there is underlying damage to intracranial structures. Small lacerations, contusions, and hematomas may not be detected unless they are actively sought, since they may be hidden under the hair. Larger lacerations are usually made apparent by the presence of blood in the hair. Since the scalp is quite vascular, it is a common source of major hemorrhage and shock. The clinician frequently fails to appreciate the amount of blood that has been lost at the scene and in the ambulance, which compounds the blood loss that is seen at the time of admission. The excellent vascularity of the scalp is a major reason why the scalp tends to heal rapidly and is associated with a low incidence of infection.

The principles applied to soft tissue injuries are germane to the management of scalp lacerations (see p. 260). Initially, compression is applied to the scalp defect to control hemorrhage. The hair around the wound should be shaved to allow technical access to the wound edges. The wound should be copiously irrigated and the skin washed with soap. The patient may require infiltration of the wound with

Xylocaine to allow adequate, pain-free cleansing. Devitalized wound margins should be debrided. The surface of the skull should be palpated and inspected to detect the presence of a skull fracture. If there is no fracture present, the wound is closed in one layer with nylon or stainless steel sutures. If the galea is disrupted and the wound is relatively clean, separate closure of the galea and skin may offer better cosmesis and minimize scarring. An absorbable suture is used to close the galea if it is repaired separately from the skin. As in all soft tissue wounds, tetanus immunization should be considered.

B.   **Avulsion**   Traumatic loss of the scalp represents a potentially serious and even fatal injury. Early closure of the wound under optimum conditions is the goal in the management of these patients. Improper management of these injuries will lead to death from prolonged infection or intracranial complications. The concepts of open wound management apply, as discussed on p. 261. A few additional points should assure proper management of this unique injury.

The mechanism of injury is almost always industrial, with the patient's hair being caught in belts or gears of power-driven machinery. The amputated scalp is most frequently destroyed or damaged to the point that its replantation by microvascular technique is not possible. Even in situations in which the detached scalp is not mangled and in which it has been properly managed during its transportation from the accident scene to the hospital (management of amputated distal elements is discussed on p. 274), the results of attempted revascularization of the scalp are usually unsuccessful. The reason for this is that the avulsive nature of the injury stretches the vessels beyond their normal capacity prior to their tearing. This creates a long segment of intimal and medial damage, which is unrecognized and results in subsequent thrombosis and failure of the revascularization. Under ideal circumstances, scalp replantation and revascularization should be considered; when this is successful, it represents the most suitable method for wound closure.

In the more usual circumstances, however, in which revascularization is not a consideration, treatment depends upon one of two situations: the periosteum or pericranium remains intact over the skull; or the periosteum is destroyed or removed.

Treatment when the periosteum is intact   The early conversion of the open wound to a closed wound by split thickness skin grafting remains the method of choice in treating this type of scalp avulsion. The ability of the intact periosteum to support a split thickness skin graft is well established. The use of thick, rather than thin, split thickness skin grafts provides a more stable cover, but requires careful suturing and anchoring techniques to ensure a full take of the graft. Attempts to utilize the scalp as a skin graft have generally met with failure, even when the scalp has been completely defatted.

Treatment when the periosteum is destroyed or absent   The blood supply to the outer table of the calvarium is derived exclusively from the overlying periosteum. If the periosteum is destroyed, the underlying bone must be immediately covered or desiccation and sequestration will soon follow. Moderate-size defects and even some large defects can be closed by local scalp flap techniques. The blood vessels in the scalp extend to the vertex and freely anastomose with one another so that long and relatively narrow flaps can be raised without delay. The mobility of the scalp allows its transfer to cover fairly large defects. The donor site is closed with a split thickness skin graft, since pericranium is left behind when the scalp flap is raised. To gain further reach of the flap, the nonstretchable galea can be serially incised; thus, additional length to the flap can be gained.

In extensive losses of the scalp, tissue must be brought in from a distance. Classically, this has been done with an abdominal jump flap using the arm as a carrier to transfer a flap of abdominal wall skin and subcutaneous tissue to the calvarium. This is a multistage technique and requires several weeks of immobilization for success. Recently, microvascular free flaps utilizing a groin flap have been used as a single stage technique for closing these defects. The use of a free omental flap with split thickness skin graft coverage of the omentum has been used successfully.

An alternative to flap coverage is removal of the outer table of the skull and exposure of the diploe beneath; this area is then allowed to granulate and subsequently is covered with a split thickness skin graft. The technique of boring holes through the outer table and allowing the granulation tissue to grow up through these holes and spread over the outer table is a very time-consuming and often frustrating and unsuccessful procedure, and is to be avoided, if possible.

II. **Skull** Skull fractures may be open or closed and may be linear or depressed. The primary concern with any skull fracture is that it is likely to be associated with intracranial pathology. Skull fractures may involve the calvarium or the base of the skull and may be identified radiographically or by clinical examination. A skull fracture of the vault may be seen or palpated through a scalp or facial wound. A fracture of the cranial vault should be suspected if there is a history of alteration in level of consciousness, a focal neurologic sign, a scalp laceration or hematoma, or a cervical spine injury. A basilar skull fracture may be suspected in the presence of a Battle's sign, "panda eyes," cerebral spinal fluid rhinorrhea or otorrhea, or hemotympanum.

Linear, nondisplaced calvarial fractures indicate that significant energy has been delivered to the skull; thus, intracranial pathology is likely. **Depressed skull fractures** are commonly associated with meningeal and brain lacerations and require elevation and repair of the dura if the depression is significant. **Open fractures** may be linear or depressed. Management of the soft tissue wound is discussed on p. 261. Since the patient with a **basilar skull fracture** usually has a meningeal tear, he or she must be observed for evidence of meningitis and cessation of an ongoing cerebrospinal fluid leak (see p. 227).

III. **Eye**

A. **Lid injuries** All lid injuries should be carefully inspected to determine if the eyeball is also involved. If only the lid is involved, a sterile dressing can be used to protect the area and repair can be delayed until a convenient time, depending on other injuries present. (See p. 86.)

1. **Lid margins** Vertical lacerations through the lid margins require meticulous repair to avoid postoperative complications such as lid notches or corneal ex-

posure. Repair can be delayed up to 36 hr, until a surgeon with experience in ophthalmic plastic surgery is present, the patient's condition is satisfactory, and the proper instruments, suture material, and anesthesia are available.

2. **Lacrimal area**   An experienced consultant should determine if the lacrimal system is disrupted. Repair can be delayed up to 36 hr, if necessary, to be sure that continuity of the lacrimal system can be maintained with appropriate stents, silicone tubes, etc. Any lid laceration involving the inner canthal area may also involve the lacrimal system.

3. **Horizontal lacerations**   Horizontal lid lacerations along the skin line can be closed with interrupted fine sutures, whenever convenient, up to 36 hr after the injury. Fat in the wound indicates that the laceration involves the deeper structures in the orbit, possibly the levator palpebra, and requires ophthalmologic consultation. Fat in the wound should also arouse suspicion regarding possible perforation of the bony orbit, with penetration into the intracranial space.

4. **Lid hematoma**   See p. 86.

B. **Conjunctival lacerations**   Conjunctival lacerations usually do not require surgical repair. If the laceration is very severe and extensive, there is a good chance that the eyeball is also injured, and ophthalmologic evaluation is necessary.

C. **Subconjunctival hemorrhage**   Subconjunctival hemorrhage does not require treatment. It clears spontaneously, without residual damage. Visual acuity determination and/or ophthalmoscopic examination of the fundus should be done to rule out ocular injury.

D. **Ocular injuries**

1. **Penetrating**
   a. **Lacerations**   In all instances, full thickness lacerations of the globe require **repair by an ophthalmic surgeon as soon as possible.** A perforating laceration can be recognized by the dark uveal tissue that appears in the wound in scleral lacerations, or by prolapse of the iris in corneal lacerations. Protect the eye with a metal protective shield, until repair can be done. If a metal shield is not available, tape an eye pad over the eyelid. Do not put any ointment in the eye. Use anesthetic drops, if necessary, to examine the eye; antibiotic drops then may be used if immediately available.
   b. **Missile injuries**   Penetrating missiles may either lodge in the globe or pass through the anterior and posterior part of the eye and on into the orbit. Such double perforations have a poor prognosis. Protect the eye with a metal shield. X-ray or CAT scan localization of the foreign body will be necessary before definitive treatment is possible and should be done within 12 hr. An ophthalmologist should examine the patient as soon as possible to determine if immediate repair of the globe is necessary.

2. **Nonpenetrating**

   a. **Blunt injury**   Blunt injuries often result in a nonreactive and dilated pupil. This may be temporary or permanent and may cause confusion if head trauma is also significant.

      Causes of **unilateral dilation of the pupil** in an alert patient include direct trauma to the iris and damage to the third cranial nerve. If the patient is comatose, compression of the third cranial nerve from an intracranial mass lesion is an additional consideration.

      A **hyphema,** blood in the anterior chamber, may also be caused by a blunt injury. Immediate treatment is limited to protection of the eye with a shield and/or eye pad. All hyphemas require ophthalmologic consultation to rule out other ocular injury and to prevent serious sequelae from the hyphema.

   b. **Missiles**   High speed missiles may pass adjacent to the globe and cause severe contusion injury. If there is no perforation of the globe, and if the missile is localized outside the globe but in the orbit, as determined by x-ray or CAT scan examination, there is no reason to remove the missile surgically. The prognosis for good vision after severe contusion is poor.

E. **Orbital fractures** (see p. 91)

   1. Fractures of the **orbital rim or zygoma** do not cause functional changes to the eye. If there is no direct ocular damage, such fractures should be treated by appropriate consultants.

   2. Fractures of the **floor or medial wall** of the orbit require ophthalmologic evaluation. Entrapment of an extraocular muscle may result in permanent diplopia. Optimal time for repair is 5–7 days after the injury, allowing adequate time for x-ray tomography and careful clinical evaluation. **Not all** orbital floor fractures should be repaired. Surgical intervention carries the risk of serious complications, including loss of vision.

   3. Fractures of the **roof of the orbit or the optic nerve canal** should be evaluated jointly by a neurosurgeon and ophthalmologist. Although not usually indicated, there are rare occasions when surgical decompression of the optic nerve by a neurosurgeon might preserve vision.

F. **Head injuries**

   1. **Corneal exposure**   This is one of the most common ocular complications of head trauma and may be the result of seventh nerve palsy or coma. Regardless of the cause, prevention of corneal damage is preferable to treating corneal ulcers after they occur.

      The corneal epithelium is the primary protective structure of the cornea. If the epithelium is intact, simple measures are adequate to maintain ocular integrity. Sterile fluorescein strips (**do not use fluorescein drops,** which are easily contaminated and may introduce virulent bacteria into corneal abrasions) can be used to determine if the epithelium is intact. Moisten the strips with the patient's tears, anesthetic solution, or sterile saline, and place just inside the lower lid long enough to introduce fluorescein into the space. Close the lids for 5–10 sec, then wash the excess fluorescein from the eye with sterile saline or antibiotic drops. Any defects in the epithelium will stain green; normal epithelium will not stain. If there is a defect in the epithelium, proper protection of the cornea will result in healing. Careful and frequent evaluation is necessary to prevent corneal ulcers and subsequent corneal scars.

a. **Tape lids** The lids provide protection for the cornea, and one of the simplest procedures is to tape the upper lid shut. Use plastic tape, ½ inch wide; apply to the upper lid, pulling it closed; press the tape onto the lower lid. This effectively keeps the lid closed. Simply putting a pad over the eye **does not** always close the lid and may actually cause an abrasion by rubbing directly on the cornea.

b. **Lid sutures or glue** Temporary and effective closure of the lids can be achieved by a double-armed 4-0 nylon suture. Each needle is first passed through a rubber or silicone peg about 2 × 4 mm, then passed through the skin of the upper lid about 5 mm from the lid margin, coming out at the margin of the upper lid. The peg prevents the suture from eroding through the skin of the lid. The needles are removed, and the long ends of the suture are pulled to close the lid and taped to the skin of the cheek. The lid can be opened as needed to put drops or ointment in the eye or to inspect the cornea. The suture will last about 2 or 3 weeks.

Another temporary method is to use tissue glue to glue the upper lashes to the skin on the lower lid. The skin should be dry before the lids are closed. This procedure will keep the lids closed for about 2 weeks.

c. **Semipermanent lid adhesions** If the corneal exposure appears to be more permanent, or if there is also involvement of the fifth cranial nerve causing corneal anesthesia, lid adhesions are indicated. This is a procedure by which the lid margins are cut and joined so that the upper lid is fused to the lower lid. The adhesions can be done on the lateral side only, or on both the lateral and medial side to give more complete protection. Although the lid may appear to be completely closed when using both medial and lateral adhesions, there is an opening in the middle that permits good vision. The only disadvantage is cosmetic. The lids can be separated surgically at a later date if the original condition requiring the lid adhesions clears. Lid adhesions can be done at the bedside and are a very effective way to provide protection to the cornea.

d. If continual vision by the patient is required, a good protective mechanism is **plastic wrap**, taped around the eye, to provide an airtight seal. An alternative device is a pair of swim goggles with a watertight seal around the eye. Air cannot dry out the cornea, and drops and ointment can still be used.

e. **Ophthalmic ointment** and/or **eye drops** may be used temporarily for protection in patients with corneal exposure. If a corneal erosion does not show evidence of healing in 48 hr, or if it appears to be increasing in size, switch at once to a more effective method. Prevention of corneal complications is much easier than treating a corneal ulcer.

2. **Ocular muscle paralysis**   If diplopia (double vision) occurs because of cranial nerve palsy, patch each eye alternately, on a daily basis. Spontaneous recovery usually occurs within 6 months. Periodic ophthalmologic evaluations should be arranged to determine progress.

3. **Carotid cavernous fistula**   A fistula from the carotid artery to the cavernous sinus may occur because of trauma. The first symptom is a hissing sound heard by the patient. A bruit can usually be heard by placing the bell of the stethoscope over the closed eyelids. The eye is usually proptotic and may be pulsating, and the conjunctival vessels are engorged. No emergency treatment for the eye is required. Neurosurgical and ophthalmologic consultation should be obtained.

G. **Intraocular infection**   Patients with intravenous lines over an extended time period may develop **candidiasis,** with the first evidence of infection evident in the eye. Vitreous haze, with diffuse whitish lesions on the retinal surface, may be the first indication of candidiasis. Regular ophthalmoscopic examination will reveal early changes.

See **IV** for additional information relating to maxillofacial trauma.

Perspective

The ophthalmologist should be consulted immediately for the following conditions:

—When an actual or suspected globe injury has occurred
—When eye examination in suspected eye injury is not possible

Less urgent conditions which require ophthalmologic consultation are:

—Corneal abrasions
—Orbital floor or roof fractures
—Any pupillary abnormality, not explained by neural trauma
—Any ocular muscle paralysis
—Any suspected carotid-cavernous fistula

Any faciomaxillary injury, whether it involves the eyes or not, requires prompt consultation from the Maxillofacial Injury Service.

IV. **Maxilla, Mandible, and Face**   The patient with multiple system injuries requires a simultaneous coordinated effort of multiple specialty teams, while the patient with apparently isolated maxillofacial injuries requires examination and continuous monitoring of all organ systems during the resuscitation and treatment of the facial injury. A coordinated team effort saves lives and achieves maximal functional rehabilitation. Continuous comprehensive monitoring of all organ systems allows safe observation of ancillary injuries throughout the immediate operative management of maxillofacial trauma.

The treatment of maxillofacial trauma is conceptualized into three categories: emergent, early, and delayed. **Emergent assessment and stabilization** are directed toward immediate life-threatening events:
—Airway obstruction
—Major hemorrhage
—Aspiration
—Evaluation of the cervical spine
—Evaluation for intracranial injury

Early management of maxillofacial injuries involves clinical and radiographic assessment and definitive treatment. The maxillofacial injury is managed soon after admission, if possible, in order to ensure an optimal result. If the patient's general condition is not good, then certain facets of maxillofacial trauma may be treated later. For example, a patient with a lung contusion and a high shunt is better served by frequent postural changes and chest percussion rather than being maintained in the supine position for several hours for interosseous wiring of facial fractures. Early treatment is indicated for:
—Application of arch bars for mandibular and/or maxillary fractures
—Reduction of nasoethmoid fractures and drainage of the frontal sinus
—Reduction of orbital fractures which cause proptosis and corneal exposure
—Debridement and closure of soft tissue wounds

Other injuries may be treated at a later time.

Delayed treatment is generally performed within 10–14 days, prior to fibrous union. Delayed treatment, 7–14 days after injury, may be optimal for certain situations:
—Periorbital fractures associated with severe globe injuries
—Excessive swelling
—Poor result after an initial closed procedure
—Application of a head frame
—The need for complex x-rays, which are not safe to obtain in the first few hours after injury, since it would require transportation of a critically ill patient from the receiving area
—Splints which must be constructed prior to adequate stabilization
—Soft tissue reconstruction
—A patient who is "unstable" on admission

Note Oral placement of gastric tubes is preferred to minimize nasal or sinus obstruction and to prevent inadvertent intracranial placement through a fractured cribriform plate. Nasal tubes increase the incidence of sinusitis and are thought to increase the incidence of meningitis if there is a cerebrospinal fluid (CSF) rhinorrhea.

A. **Emergency treatment of maxillofacial trauma**

1. **Airway obstruction** Airway obstruction is expected in those patients with facial fractures that compromise the airway, that result in significant swelling

in the pharynx, floor of the mouth or neck, or result in fractured denture segments. Respiratory obstruction may result in rapid demise; only a short period of time exists between the onset of significant symptoms of respiratory obstruction (stridor, hoarseness, retraction, drooling, inability to swallow) and total inability to breathe. Thus, an alert clinician anticipates respiratory problems and performs prophylactic intubation or tracheostomy. Tracheostomy should be strongly considered in patients with facial injuries who have

a. Pan-facial fractures (maxillary, mandibular, and nasal)
b. Multiply fractured mandible (where the floor of the mouth and neck are swollen and the tongue falls back to occlude the pharynx)
c. Rigid fixation of the mandible to the cranial vault with a headframe or suspension wires (easy reintubation is prevented)
d. Massive soft tissue swelling
e. Significant burns of the head and neck area
f. Intermaxillary fixation in comatose patients or those with chest pathology (see p. 95).

2. **Life-threatening hemorrhage**

a. **Facial lacerations** Bleeding from facial lacerations can result in significant hemorrhage. It is usually controlled with **digital pressure** or **circumferential pressure bandage**. Because of the presence of facial nerve branches adjacent to major facial arteries, blind clamping is avoided.

b. **Closed maxillofacial injuries** Major hemorrhage is usually the result of laceration of arteries or veins in the walls of fractured pneumatic cavities of the face. The following mechanisms are used to control hemorrhage:

   (1) **Anterior-posterior nasal packing** (most important). Efficient anterior-posterior nasal packing can be achieved with two 30-cc balloon Foley catheters. One is inserted through each nostril, inflated in the pharynx, and pulled to occlude the posterior choana on each side (posterior obturator). Several packs of terramycin-soaked petroleum jelly gauze are then inserted into each nasal cavity, care being taken to pack the recesses carefully. This provides an anterior-posterior compression which can be fixed more rigidly by tying or clipping the catheters under tension at the columella. Necrosis of the columella must be avoided by intermittently relaxing this pressure. Usually a period of several hours of pressure is sufficient to stop the bleeding. The pressure must then be relaxed and the packing removed after 24–48 hr. (See Figure 1.)

   (2) **External compression dressing** (Barton's and circumferential bandage) is usually not necessary. Bleeding into the soft tissues of the face usually stops when tissue pressure equals arterial pressure. An external compression dressing assists in achieving this objective and can be used temporarily. Extensive **localized hematoma** within facial soft tissue should be aspirated to speed healing and prevent tissue necrosis.

   (3) **Selective arterial ligation** (internal maxillary, ethmoidal, or bilateral external carotid ligation) is a last resort. Selective arterial ligation is

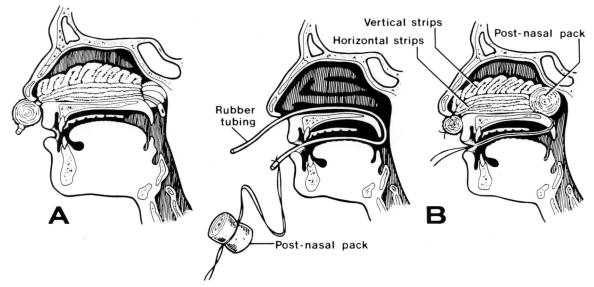

Figure 1. Anterior-posterior nasal packing.

reserved for those patients who continue to hemorrhage, despite the above measures. Massive uncontrolled hemorrhage secondary to closed maxillofacial trauma occasionally occurs; one must be prepared to administer multiple transfusions and to monitor hourly the state of coagulation for abnormalities and thoroughly correct any depleted factors. Coagulation abnormalities are frequently observed in patients with combined cerebral and maxillofacial injuries.

3. **Aspiration** Pulmonary aspiration of oral secretions, gastric contents, or blood frequently accompanies maxillofacial trauma, especially if there is concomitant cerebral injury. Noisy respirations, a low arterial oxygen content, and a decrease in lung compliance are seen. Tracheal suction reveals the contaminant. A chest x-ray usually shows an infiltrate (see p. 323).

4. An x-ray must be obtained in patients with maxillofacial trauma to exclude a **cervical fracture.**

5. Patients with maxillofacial trauma are at risk for an **intracranial injury.** If the patient has any alteration of consciousness, a CAT scan should be obtained. If a "minor" lesion is present, and the patient is going to be under general anesthesia for a prolonged time, consider inserting an intracranial pressure monitor.

B. **Early treatment of maxillofacial trauma** Definitive maxillofacial treatment is usually rendered during the initial treatment of other injuries. Management consists of

1. **Clinical examination** Appropriate clinical examination is performed when emergency resuscitation is complete. The diagnosis of most facial injuries is best accomplished by thorough clinical examination. X-rays should serve, in most cases, to **confirm** the clinical observations. Facial injuries must be suspected in anyone who has contusions, bruises, or discoloration visible in the

craniofacial region; pain or localized tenderness; lacerations (clues to underlying facial injuries); numbness; paralysis; malocclusion; visual disturbance; or facial asymmetry or deformity.

Assume there is a fracture under <u>any</u> laceration or bruise. Thorough examination of the face should be accomplished in an orderly fashion progressing from either superior to inferior or inferior to superior and consists of

a. Evaluation for symmetry and deformity

b. Palpation of all bony surfaces (nose, orbital rims, zygomatic arch, malar prominence, border of mandible) to detect crepitation, bony irregularity, or tenderness

c. Evaluation of facial nerve function

d. Evaluation of facial sensation noting the presence of supraorbital, corneal, infraorbital, or mental nerve anesthesia or hypesthesia.

e. Search for occult lacerations (the ear canal, nose, mouth, pharynx)

f. Evaluation of occlusion. Note the excursion of the jaw, relationship of the teeth, arch form, intercuspation of the teeth, fractured or missing teeth, and gaps or level of discrepancy in maxillary or mandibular dentition (Figure 2).

g. Evaluation of globe turgor, extraocular motion, and the presence of hyphema or visual abnormalities such as field defect, diplopia, and decreased vision.

2. **Simple x-rays** The multiply injured patient should not be taken from the receiving area for extensive radiographic evaluation of facial injuries. Simple bedside x-rays, combined with a thorough clinical examination, provide almost all the information necessary for emergency operative treatment. A concerned radiologic technician can take appropriate facial films in the treatment area (albeit reversed from their usual projection) with surprising quality. A systematic interpretation of these films is necessary.

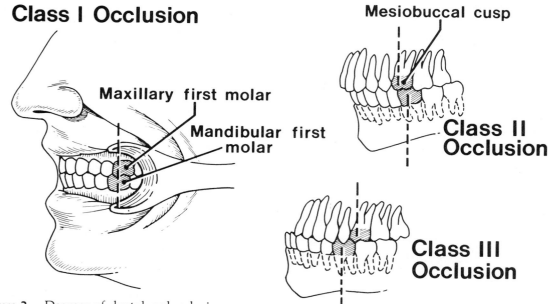

Figure 2. Degrees of dental malocclusion.

Types of emergency radiographs include

a. **Waters' view** (reversed)—frontal, supraorbital, orbital, and zygomatico-maxillary and nasal areas
b. **Towne's view** (reversed)—condylar and subcondylar region of the mandible and floor of the orbit
c. **Lateral and AP skull**—sinuses, and frontobasilar and nasoethmoid areas
d. **AP and lateral oblique mandible films**—body, symphysis, condylar, and coronoid mandibular areas.

An emergency CAT scan, arteriogram, or myelogram are the only radiographic examinations that require transporting the patient from the receiving area for the emergency diagnosis of craniofacial injuries in the multiply injured patient.

3. **Maxillary and mandibular impressions** Maxillary and mandibular impressions are obtained for construction of models when jaw fractures cannot be managed by intermaxillary fixation or interosseous wiring, i.e., in edentulous or partially edentulous patients. The models are used to study occlusion between fracture fragments and to construct splints to maintain fractures in reduction. The impressions are best taken at the time of the initial anesthesia. Wallet photographs assist in the comparison of the post-injury and pre-injury condition.

4. **Grossly displaced fractures are manually reduced.**

5. **Intermaxillary fixation is applied.** Early immobilization of fractures of the jaw with the use of arch bars and intermaxillary fixation is desirable. One can apply the intermaxillary wires or elastics during the operation or after several days in those patients who are prone to vomiting or respiratory obstruction. Arch bars can be applied under local anesthesia as a separate procedure or when abdominal, chest, or lower extremity injuries are being definitively dealt with in the operating room (see p. 95).

6. **Wounds are appropriately debrided and closed.**
   a. **Inspect the wound** for
      (1) Foreign bodies
      (2) Depth
      (3) Assessment of deep structures likely to be injured
   b. **Timing of soft tissue closure** Wounds of the face should be closed as soon as possible, but closure may be performed up to 24 hr following injury. Closure of soft tissue lacerations should be accomplished **after** fracture reduction to prevent manipulating the wound closure. Arch bars should be applied **before** closing lacerations.
   c. **Debridement** Conservative debridement of devitalized or crushed tissue is performed. Debridement of devitalized tissue should be quite conservative in the region of the vermillion, oral commissures, eyelids, and distal nose, because the apparently devitalized tissue often survives and deformities created by excision can seldom be appropriately reconstructed. More aggressive debridement, however, in the forehead or cheek areas

84   Systems Injury

can convert a ragged area of scarring into a more desirable clean linear laceration.

d. **Pressure irrigation** of wounds (through a 30-cc syringe and No. 22 needle) helps dislodge dirt, foreign material, and bacteria.

e. **"Tattoo" or "road dirt"** Foreign material **must** be removed **at the time of the initial examination.** It **cannot** be satisfactorily removed following healing and presents a permanent tattoo. Scrubbing with a brush (dermabrasion) removes the imbedded material.

f. **Closure** Approximation of wounds is usually accomplished with a layered closure.

(1) Subcutaneous sutures

(2) Inverted dermal stitch (usually 4-0 vicryl or 4-0 dexon)

(3) Interrupted skin sutures (6-0 nylon).

Cutaneous facial sutures are usually removed on the 3rd to 5th postoperative day (sometimes alternate sutures). In patients on steroids, a delay in wound healing can be anticipated and suture removal should be delayed.

g. **Prophylactic antibiotics** Antibiotics are generally not administered for uncomplicated facial lacerations. Prophylactic penicillin, which must be given preoperatively, is administered only to **multiple trauma** patients with fractures that open into the mouth. For patients with **isolated facial trauma,** such as an open intraoral fracture, a fracture involving the teeth, a sinus fracture, or a laceration communicating with the intraoral environment, prophylactic antibiotics are given.

h. **Meticulous alignment of facial tissues** with a layered repair assures the most satisfactory appearance and minimizes the need for secondary procedures. Late revisions are seldom as satisfactory as proper initial treatment.

i. **Postoperative wound hygiene**

(1) **Cutaneous wounds** All suture lines are cleansed several times a day with a 50:50 peroxide-saline mixture on cotton swabs. Bacitracin (for facial suture lines) or ophthalmic (pH corrected for ocular use) ointment (for periorbital suture lines) is applied after cleansing to prevent drying and crust formation, which increases infection and inflammation and contributes to increased scarring.

(2) **Intraoral wounds** Intraoral hygiene is performed with repeated (q4h) irrigations of either half-strength 3% peroxide-saline or a mixture of 10% povidone-iodine (Betadine), 40% peroxide, and 50% saline when an intraoral infection is being treated with irrigations.

j. **Late scarring from wounds** It takes approximately 1–2 yr for a scar to mature. A red, raised scar that is quite prominent and often displays soft tissue contracture is seen initially. A frank discussion with the patient regarding the time course of scar maturation helps the patient to understand the healing process. Early scar revisions are not indicated unless there is gross malalignment of tissues or contracture of a type that will cause ectropion and corneal exposure. Many scars whose initial appearance is startling will improve sufficiently so that revisional surgery which seemed necessary in the early phase of scar maturation is not required.

7. **Special wounds**
    a. **Eyelid and periorbital soft tissue wounds and hematoma**   The presence of an eyelid or periorbital hematoma, laceration, or contusion should prompt a thorough examination of the globe for possible penetration, hyphema, retinal injury, or accompanying orbital fracture. A small, apparently superficial laceration can be the only visible evidence of a penetrating wound into the globe or an intraocular foreign body. The early detection of such injuries is of great concern. Examination of the globe in these cases should be handled only by the ophthalmologist if the globe is difficult to see because of lid edema. Rough manipulation may cause extrusion of ocular contents. Superficial soft tissue lacerations of eyelids (involving skin and orbicularis) are easily closed in layers. Full thickness, soft tissue losses exceeding one-fourth of the length of the eyelids are generally managed with **advancement flaps** for reconstruction of the lower lid and with **transposition flaps** from the lower to upper for losses of the upper lid.

    Eyelid marginal lacerations, or those through the tarsal plate, are best handled as a two-layer repair with a conjunctivotarsal repair (inverted absorbable sutures) and an orbicularis skin repair. Three sutures at the lid margin facilitate alignment of the cilia, gray line, and global lid margin. Alignment of the global surface of the lid margin is most important in preventing corneal irritation. Suspect lacrimal gland involvement if a deep laceration of the superior, outer upper lid is present, or lacrimal canalicular involvement if a laceration is near the medial canthus. Suspect deep structure involvement (intraocular muscles) if orbital fat is present in the wound. Injury of the cornea secondary to exposure must be prevented (see p. 77).

    b. **Lacrimal system**   Lacrimal injury must be suspected in any laceration near the medial canthus or in any fracture that involves the bones adjacent to the lacrimal canal. Lacrimal system injuries are caused by
    (1) Lacerations (with direct transection of the lacrimal system within the canthal ligaments or soft tissue)
    (2) Fractures of the medial maxilla and nasoethmoid region which obstruct the lacrimal system by bone displacement or fracture healing

    Lacrimal integrity is assessed with a No. 22 angiocath by injecting fluorescein through a lacrimal punctum (after gentle dilatation), by using finger pressure to obstruct the opposing punctum. The presence of fluorescein either in the wound or in the nose would indicate lacrimal system transection or patency of the lacrimal system, respectively. The lower lacrimal canaliculus should **always** be repaired, since the upper canaliculus alone is often inadequate for satisfactory tear drainage. Repair of a canaliculus should be performed with a microrepair over fine silicone tubes.

    c. **Windshield lacerations**   Multiple small avulsive flap lacerations are usually seen and are managed by
    (1) Meticulous cleansing of road dirt and embedded foreign bodies (by scrubbing or abrasion)

(2) A choice of

    (a) Dermabrasion of the small, multiply avulsed flaps

    (b) Excision of small flaps and linear closure

    (c) Partial debridement of avulsed flaps and closure

d. Facial nerve injury Lacerations of the face can transect branches of the facial nerve, while contusions can cause temporary paralysis. Facial nerve injuries must be suspected when lacerations are present over facial nerve branches and can be confirmed by comparing motor activity on both sides of the face. Major branches of the facial nerve are:

(1) Temporal (located on a line between the tragus and 1 cm superior to the eyebrow)

(2) Orbital-zygomatic (located on a line between the tragus and the lateral canthus)

(3) Buccal (tragus to floor of nostril)

(4) Marginal mandibular (runs along the mandibular border)

(5) Cervical (does not require repair)

Lacerations of the facial nerve should be repaired at the time of the transsection under magnification with fine sutures. The distal segment will not respond to stimulation after 48 hr, making localization more difficult if a delayed repair is elected. Repair of branches need not be performed in the distal one-fourth of the buccal and mandibular branches. The electromyograph (EMG) will assist in the identification of a transection versus a lesion in continuity (contusion), where delayed management is necessary. Temporal bone fractures are a common cause of traumatic injury of the facial nerve, and consideration should be given to the use of steroids or decompression.

e. Lacerations of parotid gland or duct

(1) **Gland** Deep lacerations of the posterior cheek can involve the parotid gland, facial nerve, or parotid duct. Drainage from lacerations of the gland without major duct injury will cease spontaneously if the wound is drained and the skin is closed. We have not observed permanent fistula from glandular (without major ductal) lacerations, although some clear drainage with high amylase may persist from the wound for several weeks. Subcutaneous collections of fluid need not be aspirated or drained in the absence of fever or skin changes which signify impending fistulization.

(2) **Duct** Stensen's duct extends from the anterior margins of the gland (1 inch anterior to the tragus on a line between the tragus and floor of the nose) to the buccal surface opposite the second maxillary bicuspid. Ductal lacerations are nearly always accompanied by buccal branch facial paralysis. Ductal injuries can be managed by

    (a) Repair with fine sutures over an angiocath or silicone tube within the duct "splinting" the repair

    (b) Creation of a "fistula" into the mouth or relocating the proximal duct stump into the oral cavity

    (c) Ligation of the duct (expect considerable temporary swelling)

> Note | A nasogastric tube is inserted for postoperative nutritional support.

    f. Ear injuries

        (1) Lacerations The ear is very vascular; therefore, the result is usually favorable following repair of lacerations. The cartilage edge is trimmed and the soft tissue is debrided. The soft tissue is approximated without placing sutures in the cartilage. A light compression bandage is placed around the ear.

        (2) Avulsion A plastic surgery consult should be obtained for ear avulsions. The ear may be replanted or the cartilage may be buried into subcutaneous tissue and used for reconstruction of the ear at a later time.

        (3) Hematoma A hematoma of the ear should be drained in order to prevent a "cauliflower ear." A light compression bandage is applied after drainage.

C. Definitive x-ray examination is provided by

    1. Facial series consisting of

      a. Waters' view

      b. Caldwell's view

      c. Lateral skull

      d. Submentovertex skull

      e. Towne's view

    2. AP and lateral tomograms Polytomography is utilized in the evaluation of fractures involving the frontal sinus, the thin bones of the orbit, the mandibular condyles, and the frontobasilar and nasoethmoid regions.

    3. Computerized axial tomography (CAT) is helpful in the evaluation of frontobasilar, cranio-orbital, orbital, and nasoethmoid injuries.

    4. Xeroradiography can disclose foreign bodies, soft tissue densities, or fractures within the thin bones of the facial skeleton.

    5. Mandible films Specific films are ordered for the mandible or for involved teeth.

      a. PA mandible (symphysis, angle, ramus)

      b. Lateral oblique mandible (body, angle, ramus, condyle)

      c. Panorex examination (full lower maxilla and the complete mandible)

      d. Occlusal, palatal, or apical views of teeth involved in a fracture

D. Definitive fracture management by region

    1. Nasal fractures

      a. Diagnosis—bruising, swelling, deviation (lateral impact), or retrusion and flattening (frontal impact) of the nasal pyramid, deviation of the septum, difficulty breathing, nasal or periorbital hematomas, small lacerations

      b. Radiographic evaluation—nasal series, Waters' view, and sinus films

c. **Treatment**—closed reduction of the septum and nasal pyramid; anticipate late corrective rhinoplasty

  (1) A laterally displaced nasal fracture requires completing the fracture and restabilizing the nasal pyramid in the midline. The septum is straightened with an Asch forceps and supported by light packing.

  (2) Frontal impact injuries exist in several degrees of severity, depending on the comminution of the nasal-supporting processes of the maxilla, septum, and the medial orbital walls (see **Nasoethmoid fractures,** below).

2. **Zygomatico-maxillary complex injuries** The body of the zygoma has five attachments to adjacent structures: the arch, frontal bone, medial maxilla, maxillary alveolus, and anterolateral orbit.

  a. **Diagnosis**
    (1) Periorbital and subconjunctival hematoma
    (2) Depression of the lateral canthus
    (3) Depression of the malar prominence
    (4) Orbital rim step and/or tenderness
    (5) Unilateral epistaxis (secondary to hemorrhage through the maxillary antrum)
    (6) Difficulty chewing (impingement of the zygomatic arch on the coronoid)
    (7) Intraoral hematoma in the upper buccal sulcus
    (8) Impairment of extraocular muscle function
    (9) Infraorbital nerve hypesthesia

  b. **Radiographic evaluation** Caldwell's view (fronto-zygomatic junction); Waters' view (lateral wall of the maxillary antrum, inferior orbital rim, and orbital floor); submentovertex view (posterior displacement of the body of the zygoma; zygomatic arch)

  c. **Treatment** Indications for reduction are
    (1) Deformity
    (2) Enophthalmos
    (3) Diplopia
    (4) Dystopia (vertical malposition of the globe)
    (5) Loss of malar prominence
    (6) Anesthesia of the infraorbital nerve
    (7) Significant displacement

    Closed or semi-closed reduction is used infrequently, since many fractures show recurrent displacement. Displaced fractures are treated with open reduction and wiring along the orbital rim and fronto-zygomatic areas. Support for the body of the zygoma (if unstable) is obtained by packing the maxillary antrum or K-wire fixation (third point of stabilization). Zygomatic arch fractures usually exhibit a classic W-shaped depression and are usually stable after semi-closed reduction.

3. **Nasoethmoid fractures** result from a direct blow to the glabellar and upper nasal area.

a. **Diagnosis**
   (1) Depression or comminution of the nasal dorsum
   (2) Pain
   (3) Bilateral eyelid hematoma
   (4) Laceration
   (5) Deformity
   (6) Crepitation
   (7) CSF rhinorrhea
   (8) Traumatic telecanthus (increase in the distance between the medial canthal ligaments)
   (9) High index of suspicion
   (10) Epistaxis
   (11) Lateral movement of the canthus when lateral traction is applied to the eyelid

   Nasoethmoid fractures are usually accompanied by a comminuted nasal fracture and often coexist with a frontal sinus or frontobasilar injury.

b. **Radiographic evaluation**
   (1) Waters' view, Caldwell's view, lateral skull x-rays
   (2) Tomograms
   (3) CAT scan

c. **Treatment**   Immediate or early (within 96 hr) anatomic reconstruction for significant displacement or mobility. A fracture that involves the frontal sinus is associated with a high incidence of sinusitis due to inadequate drainage created by fracture deformity. If the posterior wall of the frontal sinus or cribriform plate is fractured, the patient is at risk for meningitis. Displaced frontal sinus fractures are ideally promptly reduced and drainage is provided. If the patient's general condition is unstable, the sinus should be drained to prevent sinusitis and the fractures reduced at a later time. This can be done under local anesthesia.

4. **Frontobasilar fractures** consist of a frontal skull fracture and fractures of the anterior cranial base and exist with combinations of supraorbital fractures, nasoethmoid fractures, and frontal sinus fractures.
   a. **Diagnosis**
      (1) Periorbital hematoma or swelling
      (2) Frontal contusion or laceration
      (3) CSF rhinorrhea
      (4) Associated nasoethmoid, supraorbital, or orbital fractures
      (5) High index of suspicion
      (6) Epistaxis
   b. **Radiographic evaluation** (most important to confirm the diagnosis)
      (1) Waters' view, Caldwell's view, lateral skull x-rays
      (2) Tomograms
      (3) CAT scan
   c. **Treatment**   Those injuries with a comminuted nonreconstructible posterior frontal sinus wall or nasofrontal duct benefit from cranialization or nasalization of the frontal sinus. Consideration for direct (intradural)

repair of any dural leak is not an immediate concern, and is rarely required. If the brain needs to be resected, the frontal sinus should be decompressed or exenterated, especially if a large dural patch is present. The purpose of frontal sinus decompression is to prevent sinusitis, which may infect the meninges.

5. **Frontal sinus fractures**
   a. **Diagnosis**
      (1) Epistaxis
      (2) Contusion, bruise, or laceration of the forehead
      (3) Depression in the glabellar area
      (4) Suspect when a frontal, supraorbital, orbital, or nasal fracture is present
      (5) CSF leak
   b. **Radiographic evaluation**
      (1) Waters' view, Caldwell's view, lateral skull x-rays
      (2) Tomograms are a must in order to exclude damage to the nasofrontal duct and posterior wall of the sinus.
   c. **Treatment**
      (1) Anterior wall or simple posterior wall fractures. Reposition fragments and drain the sinus.
      (2) Posterior wall or ducts. If satisfactory reconstruction is not possible, exenteration, cranialization, or nasalization is indicated. Cranialization consists of removal of mucosal lining, leaving the anterior bony wall intact, and obliterating the opening to the nose (nasofrontal duct). Nasalization consists of widely removing the floor of the frontal sinus and the nasofrontal duct and mucosa.

6. **Supraorbital fractures**
   a. **Diagnosis**
      (1) Bruise
      (2) Laceration
      (3) Deformity
      (4) Orbital rim step or irregularity
      (5) Supraorbital hypesthesia
      (6) Downward and outward protrusion of the globe
   b. **Radiographic evaluation** Waters' view, Caldwell's view, lateral skull (orbital roof irregularity) x-rays
   c. **Treatment** Direct interosseous wiring following fracture reduction

   Note Make certain that the orbital roof is intact.

7. **Orbital fractures** An orbital fracture or a globe injury should be suspected whenever there is an injury to the ocular or periorbital area. The basic visual screening examination consists of visual acuity, confrontation fields, extra-ocular motion, and examination of anterior and posterior chambers.

a. **Orbital floor fracture**
   (1) **Diagnosis**
       (a) Periorbital and subconjunctival hematoma or swelling
       (b) Anesthesia of the infraorbital nerve
       (c) Diplopia during vertical gaze (entrapment of inferior rectus and inferior oblique muscles)
       (d) Enophthalmos
       (e) Dystopia (vertical malposition of the globe)
       (f) Orbital emphysema
   (2) **Radiographic evaluation**
       (a) Waters' view, Towne's view, Caldwell's view
       (b) Tomograms
       (c) CAT scan
   (3) **Surgical treatment** Indications for surgery are vigorously debated, but, in general, consideration for exploration should be given when any of the following exists:
       (a) Enophthalmos
       (b) Entrapment, with positive forced ductions, which is not resolving
       (c) Vertical malposition of the globe (dystopia)
       (d) Anesthesia, which is not resolving
       (e) Massive loss of orbital floor on radiographs
       Treatment consists of removal of incarcerated tissue from the maxillary antrum with replacement or reconstruction of the orbital floor.
b. **Medial orbital wall fracture**
   (1) **Diagnosis**
       (a) Enophthalmos
       (b) Diplopia when looking laterally (restriction of medial rectus muscle)
       (c) Orbital emphysema
   (2) **Radiographic evaluation**
       (a) Waters' view and Caldwell's view
       (b) AP and lateral tomograms
       (c) CAT scan
   (3) **Treatment**
       (a) **Surgical treatment** Indications for surgery are entrapment with positive forced ductions and enopthalmos. Surgery includes removal of incarcerated tissues from the ethmoid sinuses and repair or reconstruction of the medial orbital wall.
       (b) **Nonsurgical treatment** involves the use of antibiotics and restricted nasal breathing and nose blowing for patients with orbital emphysema to decrease contamination of orbital tissues with nasal organisms.
c. **Infraorbital rim fracture**
   (1) **Diagnosis**
       (a) Palpable step deformity of rim
       (b) Signs of floor fracture

(2) **Radiographic evaluation**
    (a) Waters' view, Towne's view, Caldwell's view
    (b) Tomograms
    (c) CAT scan
(3) **Treatment** Repair if there is significant displacement. Exclude a possible associated maxillary or zygomatic fracture.

8. **Sinus fractures**
  a. **Diagnosis**
    (1) Swelling
    (2) Paranasal fractures
    (3) Epistaxis
  b. **Radiographic evaluation** is performed by a sinus series.
  c. **Treatment** Sinus fractures have the potential for obstruction and infection. A Caldwell-Luc approach for sinus packing is the treatment of choice in those maxillary sinus fractures needing reconstruction; a simple nasal antrostomy provides drainage. The mere presence of an air fluid level in a fractured sinus does not necessarily mean that drainage is indicated. However, decongestants are indicated.

> **Note** **Fever in the presence of any facial injury** should prompt a **sinus evaluation** and appropriate aspiration. Adequate surgical drainage is indicated if infection is confirmed.

9. **Le Fort's (maxillary) fractures** Maxillary fractures are grouped according to the Le Fort classification (Figure 3).
    —**Le Fort I (horizontal)** fracture separates the maxillary alveolus from the upper facial skeleton.
    —**Le Fort II (pyramidal)** fracture separates a central, pyramidal-shaped nasomaxillary segment from the zygomatic and orbital portions of the facial skeleton.

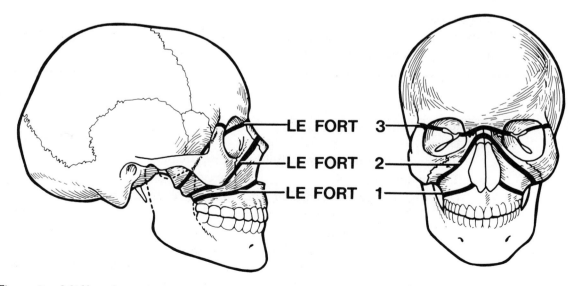

Figure 3. Midface fractures.

—**Le Fort III** (**craniofacial dysjunction**) fracture separates the facial bones from the cranial skeleton through the orbits (the upper portion of the zygomaticofrontal junction, the orbital floors, and the nasoethmoid areas). Le Fort III fractures usually exist as comminuted lesser Le Fort fragments, namely Le Fort I, II, and zygomatic fractures. Single fragment Le Fort III fractures are uncommon.

a. **Diagnosis**
   (1) Mobile maxillary alveolus
   (2) Zygomatic, orbital, nasal, or nasoethmoid fractures are commonly associated.
   (3) Malocclusion
   (4) Elongated and depressed midface
   (5) Profuse nasopharyngeal bleeding
   (6) Facial swelling
   (7) CSF leak in Le Fort II and III fractures
   (8) Approximately 10–15% of Le Fort fractures are accompanied by a palatoalveolar fracture (split palate).
b. **Radiographic evaluation**
   (1) Waters' view, Caldwell's view, lateral skull x-rays
   (2) Tomograms or CAT scan for orbital and upper facial involvement
c. **Treatment**   Placing the patient in intermaxillary fixation in occlusion for 6–8 weeks reduces the maxilla so that it is in proper relationship to the mandible. Midface elongation can be shortened by the use of suspension wires (wires from the maxillary or mandibular arch bar to a point on the facial skeleton that is above the highest level of fracture). Open reduction of upper facial fractures (zygoma, orbit, and nasoethmoid) is performed reducing these fractures to intact frontal bone structures. (See individual fractures.)

Perspective
Suspect a CSF leak, a frontal sinus, nasoethmoid, or frontobasilar injury, or a lacrimal system involvement in Le Fort II or III fractures.

---

10. **Complex facial fractures**
   a. **Diagnosis**   Complex facial injuries (pan-facial fractures) are diagnosed by integrating the above individual components.
   b. **Treatment** (Figure 4)
      (1) Reconstruct the mandible and relate it to the cranial base.
      (2) Relate the maxilla to the mandible through proper occlusion (splints are used to stabilize the dental arches or substitute for important missing teeth in partially or fully edentulous patients).
      (3) Reduce upper facial fractures individually, as described, and stabilize them to an intact portion of the frontal cranium.

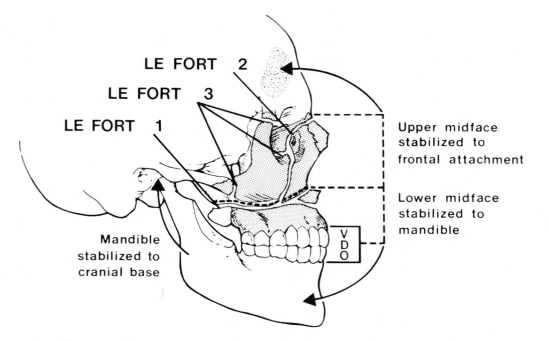

Figure 4. Reconstruction of midface fractures.

External fixation devices (usually a headframe or Joe Hall Morris biphasic mandibular fixation device) are used occasionally to stabilize the mandible in proper relation to the cranial base, to stabilize a comminuted mandible fracture, or to correct retrusion of facial bones. Internal wiring is preferable to external fixation devices in most cases.

11. **Intermaxillary fixation and occlusion**   The treatment of maxillary or mandibular fractures usually involves ligating arch bars to the maxillary and mandibular dentition, placing the patient in occlusion (teeth in proper relationship and in maximal intercuspation), and holding this relationship by the use of elastics (rubber bands) or wires between the maxillary and mandibular arch bars. (See **Definitive airway management,** below.)

Mandibular fractures are generally kept in intermaxillary fixation for 4–6 weeks, until immobility (union) has been achieved. Maxillary fractures are kept in intermaxillary fixation for 6–8 weeks.

Appropriate dental hygiene must be continued despite the presence of arch bars and elastics and is facilitated by proper cleaning of the teeth at the time of placing the arch bars. Care of the patient in intermaxillary fixation involves intermittent observation of the occlusion and intermittent adjustment of the wires or elastics for cleaning or exercise, if indicated, and replacement of worn elastics. Intermaxillary fixation is accomplished with wire if elastic fixation does not achieve stability. In the partially or fully edentulous patient, acrylic splints are constructed to serve the function of partial or full dentures. The splints allow the jaws to be placed in occlusion, without fracture segment tipping, collapsing, or overriding.

12. **Definitive airway management**   The patient with maxillofacial injury often has an inadequate or tenuous airway. If a patient with maxillofacial injury also

has head or chest pathology, respiratory function may not be secure unless precautionary steps are taken. The head-injured patient who is briskly purposeful on admission is likely to be alert enough to protect the airway and spontaneously mobilize secretions in about 5–7 days after injury. If the admission motor examination reveals a semipurposeful or rigid (decorticate/decerebrate) extremity posture to pain, then the patient is likely to need airway protection and access for removal of tracheobronchial secretions for greater than a week. If the airway is maintained with a translaryngeal tube and there is major intraoral or facial edema, accidental extubation may result in a severe hypoxic insult due to a difficult reintubation. Jaw fractures (maxilla or mandible) should be initially treated with at least the application of arch bars. If the fractures are unstable, usually comminuted, then intermaxillary fixation is also required initially.

With the above considerations, the following is a suggested set of guidelines for the definitive management of the airway in the patient with maxillofacial trauma:

a. An **oral-translaryngeal tube** should be used with any patient who has:
   (1) Head injury (briskly purposeful) or chest injury **and**
   (2) Minimal intraoral/facial swelling **and**
   (3) In whom intermaxillary fixation may be performed after extubation, i.e., not unstable.

b. **Tracheostomy** is performed on
   (1) Any patient who must have intermaxillary fixation, i.e., unstable jaw fracture, and has a head or chest injury
   (2) Any patient with major intraoral/facial swelling who has a head or chest injury
   (3) Any patient with a combination of a nasal, maxillary, and mandibular fracture
   (4) Any patient with a head injury who responds to pain with semipurposeful or rigid extremity posture and who has a mandibular or maxillary fracture.

c. A **nasal-translaryngeal tube** is used when there is
   (1) Major or minor intraoral/facial swelling **and**
   (2) Patent nose **and**
   (3) No posterior pharyngeal swelling **and**
   (4) No head or chest injury
   The above criteria usually describe an isolated mandibular fracture.

13. **Mandibular fractures**   The mandibular fracture is a very common facial fracture in the multiply injured patient. It is often compounded into the mouth, but is less commonly compounded through the skin. Fractures may occur in the condylar-subcondylar area, the region of the angle, or in the body and symphysis. More than one half of all mandibular fractures are multiple; therefore, the presence of a mandibular fracture should prompt a thorough search for a second fracture.

a. **Diagnosis**
   (1) Pain
   (2) Occlusal abnormality ("teeth don't feel like they are coming together correctly")
   (3) Numbness in the distribution of the mental nerve
   (4) Swelling, bruising, lacerations (extraoral or intraoral)
   (5) Bleeding from a tooth socket
   (6) Fractured or missing teeth
   (7) Trismus (pain on moving the jaw)
   (8) Open bite (inability to close the jaws) anteriorly, laterally, or bilaterally
   (9) Abnormality or irregularity in arch form or intercuspation of teeth
   (10) Irregularity along the mandibular border or a "gap" in dentition
   (11) Bleeding from ear (can indicate a laceration of the anterior wall of the ear canal from a condylar fracture or dislocation as well as a basilar skull fracture)
   (12) An alveolar fracture is a separation of the dental alveolus from the lower mandible.

b. **Radiographic evaluation**
   (1) PA of the mandible (symphysis, ramus, angle)
   (2) Lateral oblique of the mandible (body, angle, condyle, condylar neck, coronoid)
   (3) Panorex (mandible and lower maxilla)
   (4) Occlusal and apical films (symphysis, palate, and views of roots of teeth)

c. **Treatment**
   (1) Application of arch bars, splints, or dentures as appropriate to the state of the dentition
   (2) Intermaxillary fixation
   (3) Closed reduction is appropriate for most condylar, coronoid, and ramus fractures and those stable fractures in the angle, body, and symphysis (dentulous) portion of the mandible
   (4) Open reduction and internal wire fixation is necessary for displaced fractures and unstable fractures in the angle, symphysis, and body of the mandible. Intraoral splints may be used to facilitate the treatment of some unstable fractures.
   (5) Provision for nutrition with a blenderized diet or by a nasogastric (NG) tube is necessary.

14. **Gunshot or shotgun wounds** The following general principles of treatment are a necessity for maximal rehabilitation in these severe injuries.
   a. Immediate stabilization of bone fragments by region; stability often requires external fixation
   b. Soft tissue closure or skin to mucosa closure if tissue is missing after conservative debridement
   c. Delayed reconstruction of soft tissue or bony defects

E. **Maxillofacial Trauma Service**   The Oral Surgery Service and the Plastic Surgery Service function jointly to create the Maxillofacial Injury Center at MIEMSS. Joint rounds take place twice weekly. A conference on maxillofacial trauma is held once each month. The two services alternate daily first-call responsibility; a member of the other service is on second call.

Exceptions to the alternating responsibility system are listed below:

1. All soft tissue injuries in the head and neck area are treated by the Plastic Surgery Service at the discretion of the attending traumatologist.
2. All isolated mandibular fractures which are open to the skin are treated by the Plastic Surgery Service.
3. All isolated mandibular fractures not open to the skin are treated by the Oral Surgery Service.
4. All fronto-naso-ethmoidal fractures are treated by the Plastic Surgery Service with consultation of the Neurological Surgery Service.
5. All isolated alveolar fractures are treated by the Oral Surgery Service.
6. An ophthalmology consult is required for all orbital fractures with the potential for visual problems.

Perspective

The face is of obvious importance in communication, nutrition, perception, and interpersonal relationships. People unfortunately are judged by some of their associates according to the attractiveness of their facial structures. Although there are few facial emergencies, the literature has underemphasized the advantages of prompt definitive reconstruction of facial injuries and its contribution to superior aesthetic results. It is not unusual for the victim of multiple trauma to be principally concerned about facial deformity once life-threatening injuries have resolved. Early definitive care of maxillofacial injuries will repay the trauma surgeon with superior results and grateful patients. At MIEMSS, the Maxillofacial Team provides coordinated care beginning at admission. Additionally, time spent with the family and the patient explaining the injury, the steps necessary in the treatment, and the expected time course of healing will pay rich dividends in the ultimate adjustment that the patient makes to the injury. At MIEMSS, an educational pamphlet is available for patients and families which describes the injuries, treatment, nutrition, and time course of rehabilitation for the patient with major maxillofacial injuries.

V. **Neck**

A. **Penetrating neck trauma**   The neck compactly contains many vital vascular, visceral, and neural structures, which may be injured secondary to penetrating trauma. A penetrating neck wound is likely to be associated with damage to a vital structure. If a vital structure has been damaged, usually there are clinical manifestations of such injury. On the other hand, manifestations may be minimal or absent; therefore, a high index of suspicion should be maintained. Structures that may be involved are:

    —**Neural**
        Spinal cord
        Phrenic nerve
        Brachial plexus
        Recurrent laryngeal nerve
        Cranial nerves
        Stellate ganglion
    —**Vascular**
        Carotid artery
        Jugular vein
    —**Visceral**
        Thoracic duct
        Esophagus and pharynx
        Thyroid gland
        Larynx and trachea
    —**Associated Intrathoracic**

1. **Manifestations** The following is a list of the clinical manifestations that may occur secondary to injury of vital neck structures.

    a. **Spinal cord**
        (1) Quadriplegia
        (2) Brown-Séquard deficit (ipsilateral hemiparesis)

    b. **Larynx and trachea**
        (1) Hemoptysis
        (2) Stridor
        (3) Cervical subcutaneous emphysema
        (4) Sucking neck wound
        (5) Hoarseness
        (6) Dyspnea

    c. **Phrenic nerve** injury is indicated by an elevated diaphragm on the chest x-ray.

    d. **Brachial plexus**
        (1) Sensory/motor deficit in an arm
        (2) Horner's syndrome

    e. **Carotid artery**
        (1) Decreased level of consciousness
        (2) Contralateral hemiparesis
        (3) Hematoma
            (a) Frequently expanding
            (b) May cause dyspnea secondary to compression of the trachea
        (4) External hemorrhage
        (5) Hypotension
        (6) Thrill
        (7) Bruit
        (8) Pulse deficit

f. **Jugular vein**
   (1) Hematoma
   (2) External hemorrhage
   (3) Hypotension
g. **Recurrent laryngeal nerve** injury may be indicated by hoarseness.
h. **Cranial nerves**
   (1) Glossopharyngeal—dysphagia
   (2) Vagus—hoarseness
   (3) Spinal accessory—inability to shrug a shoulder and to laterally rotate the chin to the opposite shoulder
   (4) Hypoglossal—paresis of the tongue
i. **Thoracic duct** injury is usually asymptomatic and found at exploration.
j. **Esophagus and pharynx**
   (1) Dysphagia
   (2) Bloody saliva
   (3) Sucking neck wound
   (4) Bloody nasogastric aspirate
k. **Thyroid gland** injury may present as a hematoma.
l. **Stellate ganglion** injury is suggested by a dilated pupil.
m. **Associated intrathoracic injuries**
   (1) Esophagus
   (2) Tracheobronchial tree
   (3) Lung
   (4) Heart
   (5) Great vessels
      (See p. 128.)

2. **Diagnosis**
   a. **Neck x-ray**
      (1) Emphysema
      (2) Displacement of trachea
      (3) Fractures
      (4) Foreign body (e.g., bullet)
   b. **Chest x-ray**
      (1) Hemothorax
      (2) Pneumothorax
      (3) Widened mediastinum
      (4) Foreign body
      (5) Mediastinal emphysema
      (6) Apical pleural hematoma
   c. **Esophagogram**   The esophagogram may be helpful in ascertaining the presence of a disruption of the cervical esophagus. However, a negative study does not exclude an esophageal injury.
   d. **Endoscopy**
      (1) Laryngoscopy
      (2) Bronchoscopy

(3) Pharyngoscopy

(4) Esophagoscopy

$\boxed{\text{Note}}$ A negative evaluation does not totally exclude significant injury to the larynx, trachea, bronchus, pharynx, or esophagus.

e. **Arteriography** The neck is divided into three zones:

(1) **Zone 1** That portion of the neck inferior to a transverse line which passes through the cricoid ring

(2) **Zone 2** That portion of the neck lying between Zones 1 and 3

(3) **Zone 3** That portion of the neck superior to a transverse line which passes through the angle of the mandible

Arteriography is suggested for lesions that involve Zone 1 or Zone 3. Arteriography may reveal information regarding the adequacy of collateral circulation should the carotid artery need to be ligated in Zone 3; this would be important in deciding whether intracranial-extracranial bypass may be indicated. The arteriogram would also define the presence or absence of antegrade circulation and the presence of an arterial laceration. Arteriographic information would be helpful if there is extension of an injury from Zone 1 into the chest in order that the lesion may be identified preoperatively and the surgeon be prepared for the specific pathology to be encountered at surgery. It should be emphasized that the patient should not be taken to the arteriographic suite unless stable.

3. **Treatment** There is controversy regarding mandatory versus selective neck exploration for wounds that penetrate the neck. We adopt the policy of selective intervention so that a patient who has one of the above-mentioned manifestations is explored, while stable and asymptomatic patients are observed.

a. **Initial management**

(1) Intravenous lines are inserted. If there is difficulty in resuscitating the patient, most of the volume should be infused in lines below the diaphragm.

(2) If the patient is asymptomatic, an initial complete evaluation for the above-mentioned injuries is performed.

(3) If the patient is symptomatic

(a) Secure cardiovascular and respiratory stability.

(b) Rapidly assess the patient for gross evidence of cervical injuries while securing cardiovascular and respiratory stability.

(c) After respiratory and cardiovascular stability are obtained, a more complete survey for cervical trauma is performed.

(d) If a hematoma is rapidly expanding, immediate exploration is necessary.

(e) Difficulty in resuscitating a patient with a penetrating neck wound may be secondary to intrathoracic injury (massive hemothorax and/or tension pneumothorax); early thoracotomy is indicated if there is major intrathoracic hemorrhage.

b. Operative management

   (1) Skin preparation should include the entire neck, chest, and groin for procurement of a saphenous vein, if a vascular injury is likely.

   (2) A low transverse incision is selected for low cervical injury or injuries to midline structures when vascular injury is unlikely.

   (3) The neck incision should parallel vessels that are suspected to be damaged.

   (4) The surgeon should be prepared to perform a thoracotomy or median sternotomy to obtain proximal vascular control, if necessary.

c. Specific management

   (1) Spinal cord See p. 228.

   (2) Larynx and trachea

      (a) A tracheostomy should be performed for patients with a fractured larynx; exploration by laryngeal fissure should be performed under the guidance of the ear, nose, and throat (ENT) surgeon.

      (b) A small tracheal wound, if convenient, may be used as the site for a tracheostomy tube; cervical tracheal wounds are closed and protected by a tracheostomy tube inferior to the tracheal injury.

   (3) Cranial nerve Phrenic, vagus, recurrent laryngeal, glossopharyngeal, spinal accessory, hypoglossal
   (See p. 258.)

   (4) Brachial plexus See p. 254.

   (5) Carotid artery injury The primary issue regarding carotid arterial injuries centers around the choice of ligation versus repair. The primary consideration in deciding whether to ligate or repair a carotid arterial injury depends upon the presence or absence of a major neurologic deficit. If a patient has a **major neurologic deficit** (coma and/or hemiparalysis), the flow through the carotid vessel should not be reconstituted and is thus managed with ligation. If a patient has no neurologic deficit or only a minor deficit, revascularization should be performed. If there is **no antegrade flow and the patient has a minor neurologic deficit or is asymptomatic**, repair should be performed if proximal and distal vascular control is easily obtained. However, if there is difficulty in obtaining distal vascular control, the vessel should be ligated since excessive manipulation of that portion of the vessel may result in clot embolization to the brain and a neurologic deficit. If the patient has **antegrade carotid flow and there is no neurologic deficit**, repair should be performed, if possible. If back bleeding is not vigorous, a carotid shunt should be used, if the stump pressure is less than 50 mm Hg. In general, a young healthy patient will tolerate cross-clamping of the carotid, if there is adequate intravascular volume expansion. If a patient without neurologic deficit has antegrade carotid circulation, yet the vessel cannot be repaired, the vessel is ligated. Young patients with normal intravascular volume expansion will usually tolerate ligation of the carotid artery. An elderly patient without neurologic deficit who has the carotid artery ligated may require extracranial-intracranial bypass should a neurologic deficit appear following ligation.

(6) **Jugular vein**
  (a) The jugular vein should be repaired, if there is no difficulty in doing so.
  (b) If there is difficulty in repairing a jugular venous injury, ligation should be performed (continuity of at least one jugular vein should be maintained, if possible).
  (c) If there is a jugular venous injury, the patient's head should be kept lower than the heart to diminish the likelihood of air embolization.

(7) **Thoracic duct** If a thoracic duct injury is identified, the duct should be ligated above and below the injury.

(8) **Esophagus and pharynx**
  (a) Small wounds should be repaired by suture technique, preferably with two layers; debride the edges.
  (b) The esophageal wound should be drained by a stab incision. Do not place the drain on the suture line.
  (c) If the repair is questionable, it may be buttressed with sternocleidomastoid muscle.
  (d) A large or tenuous wound may be converted to a cervical esophagostomy or pharyngostomy.

(9) **Thyroid gland** Hemostasis is usually gained with suture ligatures or by lobectomy.

B. **Blunt neck injury** The manifestations and management of the patient with blunt neck trauma are, in general, the same as that described under "Penetrating Neck Trauma." The following injuries are the most commonly seen following blunt cervical trauma:

1. Laryngeal fracture
2. Fracture of the cervical trachea
3. Laryngotracheal separation (The patient may need emergency intubation by tracheostomy, or translaryngeal intubation over a flexible bronchoscope.)
4. Carotid arterial intimal injury or transection
5. Cervical spine injury

(See pp. 98 and 228.)

10
THORACIC INJURIES

Thoracic injuries may occur secondary to blunt or penetrating trauma. Penetrating injuries of the chest occur secondary to knife wounds, gunshot wounds, or other sharp objects. Blunt trauma to the chest is usually secondary to a compression (crush) or deceleration event. Events that are frequently responsible for causing blunt chest trauma are vehicular, industrial or farm accidents, falls, and altercations. Trauma that is inflicted upon the chest can result in damage to the chest wall, lungs, trachea, major bronchi, esophagus, thoracic duct, heart, diaphragm, mediastinal vessels, and spinal cord. Any combination of these injuries may occur.

There may not be external evidence of chest wall injury, yet intrathoracic injury can be extensive and life-threatening. The resulting disturbance in cardiac and pulmonary function can be fatal if not promptly diagnosed and corrected. Significant intrathoracic injuries are usually obvious. Even though there may be no obvious signs of chest injury, intrathoracic injuries must be excluded in all cases of blunt or penetrating trauma. Respiratory and circulatory stability are achieved by following these basic principles:

—Maintain a clear airway by removing retained blood, secretions, and vomitus.
—Provide sufficient minute ventilation volume for adequate oxygenation and removal of carbon dioxide.
—The lungs must be fully expanded and the pericardial space decompressed, if necessary.
—Blood loss must be assessed and appropriate volume infused.
—Continued blood loss may require surgical intervention to obtain circulatory stability.

The following findings should be noted during the initial evaluation:
—Blood pressure and heart rate
—Evidence of respiratory distress
—Asymmetrical breath sounds
—Distended or collapsed neck veins
—Chest wall or cervical wounds
—Pain secondary to palpation of the chest wall
—Chest wall splinting
—Paradoxical chest wall motion
—Subcutaneous emphysema
—Cervical hematoma
—A decreased carotid or brachial pulse

A chest x-ray, arterial blood gas, central venous pressure, and EKG are diagnostic tools that should be obtained on all trauma patients.

I. **Chest Wall** Chest wall injuries are generally manifested by pain, ecchymosis, abrasions, rib or sternal fractures, costochondral separations, or chest wall lacerations.

The major concern with trauma to the chest wall is related to the possibility that there may exist an intrathoracic injury or associated extrathoracic injury.

A. **"Sucking" chest wounds (open pneumothorax)**   A small wound involving the chest wall may act as a one-way valve, which results in an accumulation of air in the pleural space and compression of the lung, i.e., a tension pneumothorax. A large wound may prevent the development of negative pleural pressure and result in hypoventilation.

   1. **Manifestations**
     a. "Sucking" chest wound
     b. Decreased breath sounds
     c. Hyperinflation of the chest wall, if under tension

   2. **Treatment**
     a. **Immediately** insert a chest tube for all sucking wounds.
     b. Apply a moist, sterile airtight dressing over the defect.
     c. Exclude associated injuries.
     d. Debride and close wounds.
     e. If there is an intrathoracic injury, explore and repair, if necessary.
     f. Marlex mesh and/or muscle flaps may be necessary to close a large defect.

B. **Clavicular fractures**   The major concern with clavicular fractures is to exclude the possibility of a brachial plexus, subclavian vascular, or intrathoracic injury.

C. **Rib fractures**   Intrathoracic and extrathoracic injuries must be excluded in all cases in which rib fractures are identified. Chest wall splinting secondary to pain must be adequately controlled; otherwise, atelectasis will develop. Atelectasis may cause pneumonia or hypoxia secondary to increased shunting. Chest wall instability may result in regional hypoventilation.

   1. **Simple rib fractures**
     a. **Manifestations**
       (1) Chest wall pain with inspiration
       (2) Crepitus by palpation
       (3) Chest wall splinting by inspection

        | Note | A delayed pneumothorax may occur within the first 24 hr.

     b. **Diagnosis** by chest x-ray:
       (1) Fractures are usually visualized unless the cartilaginous portion of the rib is involved.
       (2) Fractures may be missed radiographically when there is minimal displacement.
       (3) Nonvisualized fractures usually become apparent radiographically in 7–14 days when displacement occurs.

c. **Treatment** If major intrathoracic injury has been excluded, the principal focus on treatment is the control of pain.
   (1) Parenteral morphine sulfate, meperidine (Demerol), or oral codeine can be administered. **Analgesics** should be titrated to induce pain relief without interfering with the cough reflex or causing stupor, either of which will enhance the development of atelectasis.
   (2) An **intercostal nerve block** may be necessary in order to control chest wall pain. The **technique** involves extending one rib above and one rib below the most superior and inferior fracture. Since ribs are most frequently fractured posterolaterally, injection is usually 4–5 inches lateral to the posterior midline. Bupivacaine (Marcaine), 0.25–0.5%, is used to anesthetize the intercostal nerves. Up to 225 mg of Marcaine with epinephrine or 175 mg without epinephrine may be used at a time. This dose may be repeated every 3 hr. A 22-gauge needle is used to strike the lower aspect of the rib. The needle is withdrawn slightly and directed immediately below the rib. If aspiration reveals no blood, 5–8 cc of Marcaine is injected. A chest x-ray should be obtained following the nerve block to exclude a pneumothorax.
   (3) Two or more rib fractures in an elderly patient is an indication for hospitalization. The patient should be observed for the development of atelectasis and/or a delayed pneumothorax.

2. **Multiple rib fractures**
   a. The same consideration for simple fractures applies to multiple rib fractures. However, chest wall pain is usually more severe.
   b. **Treatment**
      (1) Depending upon the constitution of the patient, chest wall pain may be controlled with oral or parenteral analgesics.
      (2) Intercostal nerve blocks are usually needed to control chest wall pain.
      (3) Epidural thoracic blocks may be useful. However, they are rarely used at MIEMSS because of a concern for septic complications.
      (4) Intramedullary stabilization of rib fractures is utilized if there is another indication for thoracotomy.
      (5) Intercostal nerve blocks may cause a pneumothorax in obese patients and/or patients with greater than five fractured ribs. These patients are also difficult to titrate with analgesics. They frequently require intermittent mandatory ventilation–positive end-expiratory pressure (IMV-PEEP) support until the chest wall pain is better tolerated.
      (6) See section on pulmonary insufficiency (p. 313).

3. **First rib fractures** imply that a major force has been applied to the chest. In this situation, the patient is at risk of having an associated intrathoracic injury, such as injury to the aorta or great vessels, brachial plexus, tracheobronchial tree, heart, or lungs.

4. **Flail chest** The major concern with flail chest is adequate control of chest wall pain and exclusion of associated intrathoracic injuries. The flail may involve the anterolateral, sternal, or posterior chest. The latter requires no treatment other than pain control since it is protected by the strong back muscles and scapula. Pulmonary contusion is frequently associated with flail chest.

   a. **Manifestations**
      (1) Findings are the same as those described for simple rib fractures (see p. 106).
      (2) Paradoxical chest wall motion
      (3) Tachypnea as a result of hypoxia

   b. **Treatment**
      (1) The control of chest wall pain is the same as described on p. 107 for multiple rib fractures.
      (2) Because of the frequent association of pulmonary contusion, the patient with flail chest is likely to require IMV-PEEP to normalize an increased pulmonary shunt (see p. 316), especially when multiple injuries are present.
      (3) An older patient (older than 55 years) will frequently require ventilatory support for 2–3 weeks, until chest wall stability is obtained.
      (4) See section on pulmonary insufficiency (p. 313).

Perspective

We tend to be aggressive with ventilator support and fluid restriction in patients who have flail chest and pulmonary contusion. Ventilator support is withdrawn as dictated by pulmonary parenchymal and chest wall function (see p. 321).

D. **Sternal fractures** are frequently associated with intrathoracic injury, especially cardiac contusion. The lesion results in severe pain causing chest wall splinting and may cause a flail chest.

   1. **Manifestations**
      a. Presternal ecchymosis or abrasions
      b. Crepitus by palpation
      c. Inspiratory pain
      d. Tenderness to palpation
      e. Paradoxical chest wall motion
      f. Chest wall splinting

   2. **Diagnosis** A lateral x-ray of the sternum will reveal a fracture if there is displacement.

   3. **Treatment**
      a. Analgesics are instituted as described on p. 107.

b. Infiltration of the sternal hematoma with a local anesthetic may decrease splinting.

c. IMV-PEEP, if necessary.

d. Sternal wiring is beneficial if there is gross displacement and instability; this should be delayed until associated injuries are managed and the patient is stable.

e. Associated injuries are appropriately managed.

E. Extrapleural hematomas The majority of extrapleural hematomas are usually associated with multiple rib fractures and usually represent hemorrhage from intercostal vessels. Apical or mediastinal extrapleural hematomas may represent injury to the great vessels.

1. Diagnosis The chest x-ray reveals a significant extrapleural density.

2. Treatment
a. Hematomas are generally managed in a conservative manner.
b. Drainage is indicated if
   (1) Superimposed infection is suspected
   (2) Lung compression causes significant impairment of pulmonary function

F. Shotgun blast A shotgun blast to the chest wall may create a major defect. The first priority of surgical management is to exclude major intrathoracic or intra-abdominal injuries. The wound must be adequately debrided to remove nonviable tissue. The shotgun wad should be removed. A lattice of pericostal sutures (nylon) or Marlex mesh should be used to bridge the defect. The lattice is then covered with omentum or adjacent muscle flaps.

II. Pneumothorax Those thoracic injuries that allow an accumulation of atmospheric air into the pleural space result in a rise in intrathoracic pressure and a reduction in vital capacity, depending on the amount of pulmonary collapse produced. Pneumothorax usually occurs following
—Chest wall laceration
—Gunshot wounds
—Fractured ribs
—Alveolar disruption
—Bronchial disruption
—Esophageal injury

These injuries may occur secondary to blunt or penetrating trauma. Essentially, any pneumothorax has the potential to develop into a tension pneumothorax.

A. Manifestations

1. The patient may or may not have obvious findings of chest wall injury.

2. Decreased breath sounds

3. Pleuritic pain

4. Tachypnea

5. Hyperresonance

6. Subcutaneous emphysema may or may not be present.

B. Diagnosis Chest x-ray shows that there is usually an apparent peripheral lucent rim as a result of visceral and parietal pleural separation. If there is equivocation, inspiratory-expiratory views should be obtained to resolve the question. A relatively small pneumothorax may be missed on a supine chest x-ray. Therefore, the x-ray should be obtained in the upright position when possible. Increased lucency superimposed over the diaphragm in a supine x-ray suggests the presence of a pneumothorax.

C. Treatment

1. A chest tube is indicated for any pneumothorax following trauma.

2. A chest tube is inserted at the time of admission if the breath sounds are decreased and the patient is hypotensive or in respiratory distress; otherwise, a chest x-ray is obtained first (see p. 113).

3. All patients with a pneumothorax should be followed with serial chest x-rays.

4. If a large air leak is noted following the insertion of a chest tube, a tracheal or bronchial tear must be excluded by bronchoscopy.

5. An air leak that is associated with alveolar disruption will almost always stop with time.

6. If the airway pressures are elevated secondary to decreased pulmonary compliance, alveolar leak is poorly controlled. Once ventilation is terminated and the patient is spontaneously breathing, the leak will usually stop. An air leak may be secondary to a leak in the chest tube system or may arise because the last hole in the chest tube is outside the pleural space. The following is a list of causes of inability to expand the lung:
   a. Improper position of the chest tube
   b. Nonfunctional chest tube
   c. Inadequate number of tubes
   d. Inadequate chest tube suction
   e. Retained bronchial secretions
   f. Bronchial tear or lung laceration

7. If the lung cannot be expanded with appropriate suction and tube position, bronchoscopy is performed to exclude endobronchial secretions or a bronchial tear.

8. The chest tubes should be frequently evaluated for function and the presence of air leaks. There should be fluctuation of fluid within the tubing, if

the tube is functional. See p. 471 for technique of insertion, care, and removal.

D. Complications

1. **Empyema**   See p. 419.

2. **Bronchopleural fistula**   See p. 138.

III. **Hemothorax** may occur secondary to blunt or penetrating trauma. Blood in the pleural space may result in
—Blood loss which results in decreased cardiac output
—Mediastinal shift which results in impairment of venous return
—Lung compression which results in decreased ventilation and hypoxia

The hemothorax may emanate from pulmonary vessels or systemic vessels such as intercostal vessels and other branches of the aorta. As in other cases of thoracic trauma, extrathoracic trauma must be excluded.

A. **Manifestations**

1. Asymptomatic if the hemothorax is small

2. Shock

3. Respiratory distress

4. Decreased breath sounds

5. Dullness to percussion

6. Mediastinal shift

B. **Diagnosis**   The chest x-ray findings depend upon the quantity of blood in the pleural space. An upright chest x-ray is a more adequate reflector of the quantity of blood in the pleural space than a supine film.

1. A small hemothorax will result in blunting of the costophrenic angles.

2. A moderate-sized hemothorax will produce partial opacification of the hemithorax and a lateral meniscus.

3. A large hemothorax will produce opacification of the hemithorax.

4. It is more difficult to identify a hemothorax on a supine film, but increased density is usually noted in the affected hemithorax.

5. The hemothorax may be "loculated" to produce a subpulmonic hemothorax.

6. If there is any question regarding the presence of a hemothorax, a lateral decubitus chest x-ray is obtained and should resolve the question.

C. Treatment The therapeutic goal is to completely evacuate the blood in the pleural space to normalize pulmonary function and to prevent the subsequent formation of a fibrothorax or empyema.

1. **Small hemothorax**
   a. If there is no pneumothorax and the patient is stable, the patient may be observed.
   b. If the patient is unstable or requires mechanical ventilation, a chest tube should be inserted.
   c. The patient should be followed with serial chest x-rays, monitoring of the vital signs, serial hematocrits, and serial coagulation studies.

2. **Moderate to large hemothorax**
   a. A chest tube should be inserted and suction (-25 cm) should be applied (see p. 471).
   b. A 32- to 36-French chest tube should be used to prevent tube occlusion. Stripping of the tube should be performed hourly to prevent tube occlusion with clots.
   c. The chest tube drainage should be followed to monitor the blood loss. Approximately 85% of pleural space bleeding will stop with conservative therapy. If the drainage decreases, the following should be considered:
      (1) Bleeding has terminated.
      (2) The tube is occluded.
      (3) The tube is not communicating with the source of the bleeding.
      (4) The clot has organized.

      Serial chest x-rays should be obtained to evaluate the patient for an undrained hemothorax. The patient should be followed with serial vital signs, coagulation parameters, hematocrits, urinary output, and arterial blood gases.
   d. Continued drainage is likely if a central pulmonary vessel, systemic arterial vessel, or large peripheral lung laceration is involved.
   e. The following are indications for thoracotomy
      (1) Greater than 200 cc of blood loss/hr for 3–4 hr
      (2) A trend of bleeding which is increasing over a 3- to 5-hr period
      (3) Greater than 300–500 cc of blood loss/hr for 2 hr
      (4) A large clotted hemothorax

      | Note | Surgical intervention should be more aggressive in the elderly patient, who is less able to survive blood loss. See p. 129 for a discussion of types of thoracotomy incisions. A single evacuation of greater than 800–1,500 cc of blood from the pleural space does not require surgery, but requires careful observation.

3. **Autotransfusion** should be used during thoracotomy or with closed thoracostomy (see p. 39).

4. **Decortication** Small to moderate quantities of clot remaining in the pleural space will usually resolve in 4–10 weeks with expectant management. If the patient has a large quantity of clot in the pleural space, a thoracotomy should be performed to prevent the formation of an empyema or fibrothorax. A thoracotomy is indicated for any undrained hemothorax in which pulmonary function is significantly compromised. A thoracotomy is indicated if there are multiple areas of empyema formation following a hemothorax (see p. 419).

IV. **Hemopneumothorax**

    A. Hemothorax and pneumothorax are commonly seen together in the trauma patient.

    B. **Treatment** Management of hemopneumothorax is the same as that described for isolated hemothorax and pneumothorax, except that two chest tubes are used: one tube (high) anterior for air, the second posterior (low) for fluid.

    Note See p. 471.

V. **Tension Pneumothorax** A tension pneumothorax is a pneumothorax associated with a progressive accumulation of air trapped in the pleural space. The following physiologic insults occur:
- —The pleural space is converted from a negative to an increasingly high positive pressure system impairing venous return.
- —Mediastinal shift compresses the inferior vena cava as it passes through its diaphragmatic hiatus.
- —Contralateral lung compression along with pulmonary collapse on the affected side results in severe hypoventilation.

These physiologic alterations can result in hypoperfusion, hypoxia, and sudden death.

    A. **Manifestations**

        1. Decreased breath sounds

        2. Hyperresonance to percussion

        3. Hyperinflation of the affected side associated with minimal chest wall excursion

        4. Tachypnea

        5. Agitation

        6. Hypotension

        7. Tachycardia

8. Hypoxia

9. Shift of trachea and apical heart beat to the unaffected side

B. **Diagnosis**   The chest x-ray usually reveals

1. Mediastinal shift

2. Flattening of the ipsilateral hemidiaphragm

3. Absence of lung markings

4. Increased widening of the intercostal spaces relative to the opposite side

5. Tracheal and cardiac border shift away from the affected lung

C. **Treatment**

1. The pleural space should be decompressed immediately. Initially, a 14- to 16-gauge needle is inserted into the fifth intercostal space, midaxillary line. Needle decompression converts the tension pneumothorax to a simple pneumothorax. This maneuver allows time to obtain the chest tube tray and for proper surgical technique. The chest tube is then inserted and connected to sealed underwater suction.

   | Note | The needle is inserted only 1 cm past the rib; otherwise, the lung may be punctured. This can be minimized by clamping the needle at the skin level.

2. If the breath sounds are decreased and the patient is stable, an x-ray is obtained prior to the insertion of a chest tube to exclude other causes of decreased breath sounds, such as a lung cyst or a ruptured diaphragm, neither of which requires a chest tube. Should the "stable" patient become acutely unstable, immediate thoracic decompression is indicated.

3. Following chest tube insertion, the lung should rapidly expand; the air leak will be minimal unless there is
   a. Ruptured bronchus
   b. Lacerated lung
   c. Esophageal perforation

VI. **Pulmonary Parenchyma**   Major pulmonary parenchymal injury usually occurs secondary to blunt trauma, but may be associated with penetrating injury. The pathology is usually a **pulmonary contusion**, but pulmonary hematomas or lacerations occasionally occur. Contusion of the lung results in the formation of interstitial edema and alveolar hemorrhage. **Pulmonary hematoma and lacerations** may be thought of as a more severe degree of hemorrhage, edema formation, and parenchymal disruption. The pulmonary contusion commonly produces enough pulmonary insult to cause a significant rise in the pulmonary shunt and hypoxia as a sequel.

A. **Manifestations**

    1. Respiratory distress is usually apparent.

    2. Chest wall abrasions and ecchymosis may or may not be present.

    3. Rib fractures are common, but not universal.

    4. Bloody secretions are seen on cough or when the trachea is suctioned.

B. **Diagnosis**

    1. The PaO_2/FiO_2 ratio is frequently less than 300 if the shunt is significantly elevated (see p. 316).

    2. Chest x-ray
        a. Nonsegmental pulmonary infiltrate
        b. Rib fractures $(+/-)$
        c. Hemothorax and pneumothorax are commonly seen.

> **Note** A chest x-ray infiltrate is almost always seen on the admission film if the contusion is clinically significant. However, there may be a 6- to 8-hr delay in appearance of the infiltrate.

    3. If the patient is intubated, the compliance may be calculated and is almost universally decreased.

> **Perspective**
> The chest x-ray findings frequently underestimate the degree of pulmonary parenchymal insult. The most important reflector of pulmonary parenchymal insult is the PaO_2/FiO_2 ratio and the compliance.

C. **Treatment** is titrated to the specific needs of the patient.

    1. Chest wall pain must be adequately controlled (see p. 107).

    2. Chest wall instability may be an important factor in the elderly patient, who frequently will require ventilation with IMV-PEEP (see p. 319).

    3. A hemothorax or pneumothorax is treated as described on pp. 109 and 111.

    4. The patient will usually require intubation and ventilation with IMV-PEEP if
        a. There is obvious respiratory distress
        b. The PaO_2/FiO_2 ratio is less than 200
        c. There is associated shock

    5. Extubation is dictated by the patient's pulmonary function (see p. 321).

6. Adjunctive therapy
   a. Steroids may be beneficial.
   b. **Cautious fluid administration** is necessary, since the injudicious administration of fluids will exacerbate the shunt effect caused by the pulmonary contusion.
   c. Tracheobronchial toiletry
   d. Chest physiotherapy and postural drainage (see p. 318).

7. The chest x-ray infiltrate usually begins to clear approximately 48–72 hr following injury. If the infiltrate does not begin to clear, this usually represents a superimposed pneumonia or a pulmonary hematoma. The sputum Gram stain should be followed daily to detect superimposed infection.

8. **A lung laceration** is generally managed by a procedure similar to that described for pulmonary contusion (see above). If blood loss is significant, the patient may require a thoracotomy. If air leak is significant, bronchoscopy should be performed to exclude a bronchial tear. The patient may require a thoracotomy if unable to expand the lung. If operative intervention is necessary, suture of the lung laceration may be all that is necessary; however, leaking bronchioles should be individually ligated with fine silk. If the lung is grossly destroyed, resection may be required.

9. A patient with a **pulmonary hematoma** is usually managed by a procedure similar to that described for pulmonary contusion. A lobectomy may be required if there is a superimposed abscess or if the pulmonary shunt progressively rises secondary to pulmonary consolidation from "internal hemorrhage" and/or transbronchial aspiration. The pulmonary shunt and lung compliance should be closely followed in these patients.

10. Significant pulmonary parenchymal disruption, usually a lung laceration, may result in a **bronchopulmonary venous fistula**. If the patient develops acute cardiovascular and/or pulmonary deterioration, systemic air embolization may have occurred. In this situation, an immediate thoracotomy is indicated to control the bronchial leak. See p. 513.

VII. Traumatic Lung Cyst

A. A traumatic lung cyst may occur after blunt or penetrating trauma. The parenchymal defect may be radiographically apparent immediately following injury. Often, the cyst is not visualized until parenchymal blood has been absorbed. The cyst may be the source of hemoptysis or sepsis, i.e., pneumonia or lung abscess.

B. **Treatment**

1. Tracheobronchial toiletry

2. Chest physiotherapy and postural drainage

3. Antibiotics if pneumonia develops

4. Rarely, excision of the cyst is indicated if sepsis cannot be controlled with medical therapy.

VIII. **Trachea and Bronchus** Tracheobronchial injuries may result from blunt or penetrating trauma. Tears may be complete or incomplete. Penetrating trauma may involve any region of the tracheobronchial tree. Lesions that result from blunt trauma occur primarily within 2.5 cm of the carina. Separation of the tracheobronchial tree may occur, but continuity may be maintained if the peribronchial or peritracheal tissue is not disrupted.

A. **Manifestations** The physical findings seen in the patient with tracheobronchial disruption suggest but do not confirm the diagnosis.

1. Subcutaneous emphysema

2. Cough

3. Respiratory distress

4. Hemoptysis usually secondary to a disrupted bronchial artery

5. Pneumothorax
   a. Frequently of a tension variety
   b. A major air leak is usually found after chest tube insertion if there has been disruption of the peribronchial tissue.
   c. The lung may not expand.

6. Mediastinal emphysema (Hamman's crunch)

7. Intercostal retractions

8. If the peribronchial tissue was not disrupted, a pneumothorax may be absent or minimal. Approximately 7–21 days following injury, granulation tissue will enter the bronchial segment and result in stenosis. The bronchial stenosis may result in lobar collapse, which may be associated with fibrosis and/or suppuration.

B. **Diagnosis**

1. **Chest x-ray** Radiographic findings may be specific or should increase the index of suspicion that a tracheobronchial tear may be present.
   a. Pneumothorax
      (1) Tension pneumothorax
      (2) Inability to expand the lung with chest tubes in place
   b. Progressive subcutaneous emphysema
   c. Deep cervical emphysema (an anatomical extension of the mediastinum)
   d. Mediastinal emphysema

    e. First or second rib fractures

    f. Peribronchial air

    g. "Dropped lung"—if the bronchus has been completely torn, the collapsed lung will drop toward the diaphragm.

  2. **Bronchoscopy** almost always identifies the extent and location of the tracheal or bronchial tear.

C. **Treatment**

  1. The first priority is to secure the airway and ventilate the patient.

    a. A chest tube is inserted if a pneumothorax is present. A major air leak is an indication for bronchoscopy.

    b. If there is difficulty in ventilating the patient, the normal bronchus should be selectively intubated by passing a translaryngeal tube over a flexible bronchoscope.

    c. If there is a cervical tracheal laceration, emergency security of the airway may be obtained by tracheostomy or by passing a translaryngeal tube over a flexible bronchoscope.

    d. If the thoracic trachea is lacerated and the patient cannot be ventilated, a translaryngeal tube is inserted over a flexible bronchoscope into a bronchus distal to the tracheal tear.

  2. Small tears (less than one-third of the circumference) may be managed conservatively if the lung can be reexpanded and the patient easily ventilated. If the patient requires ventilatory assistance, surgical repair may be necessary to ventilate the patient and prevent contamination of the pleural space and mediastinum. If the patient is spontaneously breathing, a tracheostomy is performed to prevent the generation of high airway pressures.

  3. Complete tracheobronchial disruption or partial tears involving greater than one-third of the circumference of the lumen require surgical intervention. Tracheal or right bronchial tears are approached by a right thoracotomy. Left bronchial tears are approached by a left thoracotomy.

  4. Tracheobronchial tears that are diagnosed late, when granulation tissue is proliferating into the lumen, should be debrided and sutured, since the failure to remove exuberant granulation tissue usually results in stenosis.

  5. Patients with tracheobronchial tears should periodically be bronchoscoped and the bronchi dilated, if necessary, to prevent stenosis.

D. **Complications** Sequelae of bronchial strictures are

  1. Atelectasis and fibrosis

  2. Bronchopulmonary suppuration

  3. Bronchiectasis

IX. **Esophagus** Esophageal injuries are uncommon and may occur secondary to blunt or penetrating trauma. However, blunt trauma is a rare cause of esophageal perforation.

A. **Manifestations** The physical findings seen in the patient with esophageal perforation are nondiagnostic, but should be highly suggestive of the lesion.

1. Dysphagia

2. Upper abdominal pain

3. Subcutaneous emphysema

4. Mediastinal emphysema

5. Pneumothorax

6. Hydropneumothorax

7. Hematemesis

8. Bloody nasogastric drainage

9. Transmediastinal penetration

B. **Diagnosis**

1. The chest x-ray may reveal findings associated with esophageal injury that are nonspecific:
   a. Pneumothorax
   b. Hydropneumothorax
   c. Subcutaneous emphysema
   d. Mediastinal emphysema

2. If a chest tube is inserted and a hydrothorax is evacuated, methylene blue should be instilled into the esophagus. If methylene blue drains out of the chest tube, the diagnosis of esophageal disruption is confirmed.

3. If the patient has physical or radiographic findings suggestive of an esophageal lesion, an esophagogram should be performed. Gastrografin (diatrizoate sodium) creates less tissue inflammation compared to barium if there is extravasation from the esophagus. On the other hand, Gastrografin is quite noxious if it is aspirated into the tracheobronchial tree. If the patient is unconscious or has pulmonary complications following trauma, barium should be used since Gastrografin aspiration may greatly exacerbate the pulmonary pathology. Since esophagography is associated with a significant false negative rate, a negative study with Gastrografin may be followed with barium, which gives better mucosal detail.

4. Esophagoscopy is indicated if the esophagogram is negative.

   Note In a significant percentage of cases, injury may be present despite negative endoscopic and radiographic findings.

5. An esophageal injury may be identified at the time of emergency thoracotomy if there has been inadequate time to evaluate the patient preoperatively. If there is a question regarding esophageal integrity at the time of thoracotomy, methylene blue or air may be instilled into the esophagus under pressure. If there is extravasation of methylene blue or air, the diagnosis is confirmed.

C. **Treatment**

1. Successful management of an esophageal injury is most likely when early surgical intervention takes place.

2. Small wounds can usually be repaired with primary closure. The wound should be debrided prior to closure. Transpleural drainage is obtained with chest tubes. The suture line may be covered with a pedicled intercostal muscle bundle or pleural flap, if possible. A distal esophageal lesion may be buttressed with the fundus of the stomach.

3. Large wounds or wounds more than 24 hr old are frequently not amenable to primary closure alone. If there is a question regarding the security of the wound by primary closure, the following should be performed:
   a. Suture of the wound
   b. Transpleural drainage
   c. Cervical esophagostomy
   d. Ligation of the esophagogastric junction and a gastrostomy
   e. Insertion of a needle catheter jejunostomy for nutrition
   f. Administration of broad-spectrum antibiotics to minimize mediastinitis

4. Distal esophageal wounds are approached through a left thoracotomy, while midthoracic wounds are approached through a right thoracotomy.

X. **Heart**

A. **Penetrating cardiac injuries** Assume that any penetrating injury of the chest involves the heart, until proved otherwise. Stab wounds of the heart are more likely to seal and result in tamponade without major hemorrhage. On the other hand, gunshot wounds are frequently associated with major hemorrhage into the chest. If the gunshot wound creates a small defect in the pericardium, tamponade and minimal hemorrhage may result. Atrial penetrations of any size are least likely to seal.

1. **Manifestations**
   a. **Tamponade** (usually secondary to small wounds such as stab wounds)
      (1) Hypoperfusion (decreased blood pressure)
      (2) Distended neck veins (increased central venous pressure (CVP))
      (3) Muffled heart tones (infrequently seen)

(4) Wound involving any portion of the chest or upper abdomen

(5) Paradoxical pulse—a decrease of the systolic blood pressure greater than 10 mm Hg during spontaneous inspiration

(6) The patient may be asymptomatic in a significant percentage of cases.

b. **Hemorrhage** (usually associated with large wounds such as a gunshot wound)

(1) Hypoperfusion (decreased blood pressure)

(2) Hemothorax

(3) Wound involving the thorax or upper abdomen

(4) Neck veins are usually not distended, since the patient is usually hypovolemic (CVP is usually decreased).

> Note | Patients with cardiac wounds may initially respond to volume infusion. Hypotensive patients who fail to respond to volume infusion following penetrating chest trauma usually have inadequate volume infusion secondary to ongoing hemorrhage or tamponade.

2. **Diagnosis**

a. **Tamponade**

(1) If the patient is hypotensive, has an elevated central venous pressure or distended neck veins, and pericardial aspiration of blood results in a rise in the blood pressure and a fall in the central venous pressure, the diagnosis of tamponade is confirmed.

(2) This is not a radiographic diagnosis.

(3) If tamponade is suspected and pericardiocentesis is negative, a subxiphoid incision is performed to exclude the diagnosis.

b. **Pericardiocentesis**

(1) **Paraxiphoid approach** An 18-gauge spinal needle is attached with an alligator clip to the V-lead of a grounded EKG machine. The needle is passed to the left of the xiphoid process and directed posteriorly, medially, and cephalad toward the right midclavicular line. Continuous aspiration is performed. If the heart is struck, the needle will transmit pulsations and the EKG will reveal acute changes. If 5–10 cc of blood is removed from the pericardial space and the hemodynamics improve, the diagnosis of tamponade is confirmed.

(2) **Subxiphoid approach** A negative pericardiocentesis does not exclude cardiac tamponade. In a significant percentage of cases, the tap is negative because of either an inability to maintain the needle point in the pericardial space or clots filling the pericardial space. A subxiphoid incision is performed and the xiphoid process is removed. The dissection is taken down to the pericardium and the pericardium is opened. If blood is removed from the pericardial space, a thoracotomy is performed.

c. **Hemorrhage** Chest x-ray may reveal a hemothorax or widened mediastinum.

3. **Treatment**
   a. Rapid and massive volume infusion should be initiated to obtain hemodynamic stability.
   b. Diagnostic evaluations should be performed in the operating room.
   c. Pericardiocentesis and/or subxiphoid approach to the pericardium should be performed if the diagnosis of tamponade is likely and the patient is relatively stable.
   d. If the patient arrests or is becoming bradycardic and/or hypotensive (systolic pressure less than 90), the pericardial tap should be circumvented and a thoracotomy performed. Thoracotomy is performed to massage the heart, compress the aorta, open the pericardium and control bleeding, and volume is simultaneously infused.
   e. The thoracotomy incision of choice is a left fourth or fifth space inframammary incision. The pericardium is opened anterior and parallel to the phrenic nerve. The wound is usually controlled with digital pressure. Occasionally, a Foley catheter must be inserted into the defect and the balloon inflated to tamponade the defect. A pursestring suture is then passed around the catheter. If the defect is controlled with digital pressure, horizontal 2-0 mattress sutures with pledgets are used to close the defect. The pericardium is loosely approximated and the mediastinum is drained with a chest tube.

   | Note | Transected **coronary vessels** are ligated. If a proximal, large coronary vessel is partially lacerated, it is repaired with suture technique. If the patient develops significant ischemia, the injury is managed with a coronary artery bypass graft. **Valvular and septal lesions** are treated conservatively if there is no evidence of heart failure. These lesions are repaired electively if cardiac insufficiency cannot be controlled by medical therapy.

4. **Complications**
   a. Pericardial effusion may develop postoperatively and cause tamponade.
   b. Postpericardiotomy syndrome
   c. Cardiac failure if there is
      (1) Valvular damage
      (2) Septal damage
      (3) Coronary insufficiency
      (4) Myocardial necrosis secondary to blast effect or an excessive number of sutures causing strangulation
      (5) Cardiac herniation

B. **Blunt cardiac injuries** Blunt trauma may cause myocardial contusion or disruption of a cardiac chamber and result in tamponade. Tamponade secondary to blunt trauma is uncommon. However, it occurs with enough frequency that it should be considered in the hypotensive patient who fails to respond to volume infusion, especially if the central venous pressure is elevated or the neck veins are distended. Cardiac contusion, if clinically significant, may cause arrhythmias, ventricular failure, conduction blocks, or myocardial ischemia. Septal defects or valvular damage occur rarely in the patient who presents to the hospital alive.

   1. **Cardiac tamponade and contusion**
      a. **Manifestations**
         (1) **Cardiac tamponade** See p. 120.
         (2) **Cardiac contusion**
            (a) Chest wall pain, abrasions, or ecchymosis may be present.
            (b) Arrhythmias
            (c) Cardiac failure (hypoperfusion and/or congestion)
            (d) Pericardial friction rub
            (e) Asymptomatic
            (f) Angina
            (g) Conduction blocks (EKG)
            (h) Myocardial ischemia (EKG)
      b. **Diagnosis**
         (1) **Cardiac tamponade**
            (a) If the patient is suspected of having cardiac tamponade, a subxiphoid incision is performed and the pericardium opened to secure the diagnosis.
            (b) If the patient is deteriorating, a left anterolateral thoracotomy should be performed.
            (c) If the patient is undergoing a laparotomy and deterioration suggests the possibility of a cardiac tamponade, the diaphragmatic pericardium is opened to exclude the diagnosis of tamponade.
         (2) **Cardiac contusion**
            (a) The EKG is usually nonspecific. Nonspecific changes are

usually ST-T segment abnormalities. The EKG may reveal evidence of ischemia, conduction blocks, or arrhythmias.

    (b) CPK-MB may be elevated.

    (c) The technetium pyrophosphate scan has not been helpful in identifying cardiac contusion in our patients.

    (d) Angina-like pain is not relieved by HNO_3.

c. Treatment The management of cardiac contusion is similar to that for a myocardial infarction. See p. 122 for management of tamponade.

    (1) All patients, following blunt chest trauma, should have cardiac monitoring.

    (2) Serial EKG should be obtained for 3–4 days if contusion is suspected.

    (3) Serial CPK isoenzymes should be obtained during the first 36 hr if cardiac contusion is suspected.

    (4) Arrhythmias are treated appropriately.

    (5) Cardiac failure is treated (see p. 342).

    (6) If cardiac contusion is likely, a cardiology consult is obtained.

    (7) Stress should be minimized to decrease the myocardial oxygen demand. For example, treat significantly elevated hypertension.

    (8) Maintain myocardial oxygenation

        (a) Hemoglobin 12–13 gm %

        (b) Appropriate pulmonary support

        (c) Maintain intravascular volume expansion

        (d) Judicious use of PEEP

    (9) If the patient requires operative intervention, a Swan-Ganz catheter is advisable to follow and maintain appropriate hemodynamics.

    (10) Always obtain an EKG 3–4 weeks postcontusion to rule out infarction.

2. Septal defects

  a. Manifestations

    (1) Cardiac failure

    (2) Murmur

    (3) Arrhythmia

    (4) Conduction disturbances

  b. Diagnosis

    (1) Chest x-ray may reveal pulmonary engorgement, if the patient has a left-to-right shunt.

    (2) A Swan-Ganz catheter may be used to sample blood from the right side of the heart. A step-up in the PO_2 in the right ventricle or pulmonary artery relative to the central veins is indicative of a left-to-right shunt.

    (3) Cardiac angiography (isotopic angiocardiography will also reveal a significant septal defect).

c.　**Treatment**
　　　　　(1)　Arrhythmias and cardiac failure are treated medically.
　　　　　(2)　If cardiac failure cannot be managed medically, the defect is repaired.
　　　　　(3)　Conduction blocks may require the insertion of a pacemaker.

　　　　　Note | Patients may be stable initially but develop cardiac failure days or weeks following injury.

　3.　**Valvular damage**　The aortic valve is the most commonly injured valve following blunt trauma (often secondary to ascending aortic tear).
　　　a.　**Manifestations**
　　　　　(1)　Murmur
　　　　　(2)　Heart failure
　　　b.　**Diagnosis**
　　　　　(1)　Echocardiogram
　　　　　(2)　Cardiac catheterization
　　　c.　**Treatment**　If the patient cannot be managed medically, valve replacement is indicated.

XI.　Aorta and Great Vessels

A.　**Blunt injuries of the aorta**　The incidence of rupture of the aorta in persons thrown from a vehicle is more than twice that in persons who are not ejected. Aortic injury occurs secondary to chest compression or deceleration accidents such as automobile or motorcycle accidents, car-pedestrian collisions, falls from great heights, airplane accidents, and burial by landslide.

　　The thoracic aorta may be injured at any location. There is a 15–20% incidence of multiple ruptures. Eighty-five percent of patients with this injury will die at the scene. Of the survivors, the vast majority of injuries are located at the aortic isthmus (immediately distal to the origin of the left subclavian artery). Of these, 20% will die within 6 hr and 72% will die within 1 week. The implications of these statistics are that early and aggressive diagnosis and intervention are mandatory.

Note | The surgeon should not become concerned with obvious, peripheral injuries, because the previously "sub-clinical" aortic injury may rapidly rupture and take the patient's life.

　1.　**Manifestations**　A high index of suspicion for aortic rupture must be maintained in all high-risk accident patients. There may be no external evidence of chest trauma. Clinical findings are often minimal or absent. Extrathoracic and other intrathoracic lesions are relatively common.
　　　a.　Retrosternal or interscapular pain
　　　b.　Dysphagia from esophageal compression

c. Hoarseness

d. Dyspnea

e. Upper extremity hypertension (acute coarctation)

f. Harsh systolic murmur over the precordium or interscapular area

g. Superior vena cava syndrome (infrequent)

h. Cervical-supraclavicular hematoma

i. Left hemothorax (late sign)

2. **Diagnosis**

a. **Chest x-ray**   The following findings are suggestive of a superior mediastinal hematoma:

   (1) **Ill-defined aortic knob**

   (2) **Superior mediastinal widening***

   (3) Depression of the left main stem bronchus

   (4) Tracheal deviation to the right

   (5) Obliteration of the aortopulmonary window

   (6) Deviation of the nasogastric tube to the right

   (7) Left apical "capping"

   Traumatic rupture of the aorta occasionally occurs in a patient with a normal chest x-ray.

   (See p. 32.)

b. **Aortography**   Plain radiographic findings usually suggest a mediastinal hematoma. In a large percentage of these patients, a ruptured thoracic aorta will be found. Aortography is the only mechanism to diagnose rupture of the aorta; therefore, any widened mediastinum or ill-defined aortic knob seen on x-ray is a ruptured aorta, until proven otherwise. **Indications** for aortography are

   (1) An ill-defined aortic knob

   (2) Widening of the mediastinum on an upright chest x-ray

   (3) A physical finding that is suggestive of a mediastinal hematoma

   (4) Inability to clear the superior mediastinum on a supine film in a patient who cannot be sat upright—for example, a patient with a thoracic or lumbar spine fracture.

Perspective
Aortography should precede thoracotomy, unless there is a rapid deterioration of the patient. Aortography is necessary to confirm the diagnosis and to determine the site or sites of rupture. A ductus diverticulum may be misinterpreted as an aneurysm.

---

3. **Treatment**   Sixty-five percent of all ruptured aortas also require a celiotomy. In multiply injured patients, thoracotomy should precede other procedures unless there is a rapidly progressing cranial-cerebral injury or

---

*Since a supine chest x-ray frequently distorts the superior mediastinum, making this structure look wider, an **upright AP chest x-ray** is recommended.

massive intra-abdominal bleeding. **Traumatic rupture of the aorta deserves the highest priority of treatment.** If there is massive hemoperitoneum, the abdomen should be opened, the source of hemorrhage packed, and the aorta rapidly repaired. If repair must be delayed, keep the systolic blood pressure less than or equal to 120 mm Hg with antihypertensive agents.

    a. A right radial arterial line should be inserted to monitor proximal aortic pressures.

    b. The aortogram catheter should be left in the abdominal aorta to monitor adequacy of aortic shunt blood flow.

    c. The aorta is approached through a left thoracotomy.

    d. Proximal and distal control of the aorta is gained by the use of umbilical tapes.

    e. A shunt is used to bypass the aortic injury to perfuse the distal thoracic aorta.

    f. The injury is repaired with a prosthesis or, rarely, by primary apposition.

> | Note | If the operator is well experienced, a shunt need not be used, but **speed is of the essence.** A shunt is the procedure of choice. Cardiopulmonary bypass requires systemic heparinization and is not recommended in the trauma patient.

4. Complications

    a. Atelectasis

    b. Pneumonia

    c. Hypertension, transitory or permanent

    d. Paraplegia

    e. Renal failure

    f. Mortality varies between 15 and 20%

B. Blunt injuries of the great vessels   Injury to the aortic arch vessels may occur secondary to blunt trauma, but it is uncommon. This type of injury is usually due to deceleration accidents. The subclavian artery may be damaged secondary to impingement from a first rib or clavicular fracture. An innominate or carotid artery injury generally presents as a tear at or near its origin from the aorta.

1. Manifestations

    a. Bruit

    b. Decreased or absent carotid pulse (innominate or carotid artery)

    c. Decreased or absent brachial pulse (subclavian or innominate artery)

    d. Cervical hematoma

    e. Supraclavicular hematoma

    f. Neurologic deficit (lateralization and/or coma)

    g. Extremity ischemia

    h. Precordial murmur

    i. External evidence of thoracic trauma may not be present.

2. **Diagnosis**
   a. Chest x-ray (upright) may reveal the following nonspecific manifestations of injury to the great vessels of the aorta:
      (1) Ill-defined aortic knob (left subclavian artery injury)
      (2) Mediastinal widening
      (3) Apical pleural "capping"
      (4) "Mass" to the right of the superior mediastinum
      (5) First rib fracture
   b. An aortogram is essential to define the site of injury.

3. **Treatment** Immediate surgery is indicated to prevent rupture and exsanguination.
   a. A median sternotomy is the incision of choice to approach the innominate artery or the proximal right subclavian or common carotid arteries. Extension of the incision into the neck may be necessary.
   b. A left anterolateral fourth intercostal space incision may be necessary to gain proximal control of the left subclavian artery. Resection of the medial clavicle may also be necessary to gain exposure to a subclavian injury.
   c. An aortocarotid shunt may be indicated for lesions of the innominate artery or the proximal common carotid artery (see p. 102).
   d. The vessel may be repaired with an end-to-end anastomosis or with a saphenous vein interposition.

C. **Penetrating injuries of the aorta and great vessels** The aorta, its proximal tributaries, and pulmonary hilar vessels may be injured secondary to penetrating trauma. Penetrating injuries of these structures usually result in a massive hemothorax. The patient usually has a gunshot wound or stab wound to the neck or chest. Patients with these injuries frequently expire prior to reaching the hospital.

1. **Manifestations**
   a. **Massive hemothorax and hypotension are the most common manifestations upon presentation.**
   b. Tamponade may occur if an intrapericardial portion of the vessel has been injured.
   c. The carotid or brachial pulse may be weak or absent.
   d. Bruit
   e. Cervical or supraclavicular hematoma
   f. Bleeding from the entrance wound
   g. Upper extremity ischemia
   h. Coma and/or hemiparesis
   i. Respiratory distress secondary to tracheal compression
   j. Stab or bullet wound of the neck or chest

   | Note | Transmediastinal penetration is associated with a lesion of the aorta or great vessels, until proved otherwise.

2. **Diagnosis**
   a. The chest x-ray is nonspecific for injury to the great vessels.
      (1) Hemothorax
      (2) Widening of the mediastinum
   b. An emergency thoracotomy may be necessary, at which time the diagnosis is made.
   c. If the patient is stable, an aortogram is indicated if there is
      (1) Mediastinal hematoma
      (2) Upper extremity ischemia
      (3) Neurologic deficit
      (4) Cervical or supraclavicular hematoma

3. **Treatment**
   a. Intubate and ventilate the patient; early control of the airway is essential, since a progressive hematoma may prevent subsequent intubation.
   b. Vascular access should be obtained and appropriate volume infusion begun.
   c. Insert a chest tube for a hemothorax.
   d. Exclude tamponade.
   e. Blood from the pleural space should be autotransfused.
   f. Emergency thoracotomy
      (1) If bleeding from the chest is massive and the patient is unstable, an inframammary anterolateral thoracotomy must be performed as an emergency.
      (2) Bleeding points should initially be controlled with pressure.
      (3) If the patient is bleeding from the hilum of the lung, the pericardium is opened and a clamp applied to hilar vessels to control hemorrhage.
      (4) If needed, the incision may be extended to gain proximal and distal control.
         (a) Vertically split the sternum.
         (b) Resect the medial clavicle.
         (c) Extend the incision to the neck.
         (d) Horizontal sternal transection into the opposite chest.
   g. Elective thoracotomy
      (1) Median sternotomy is the incision of choice for
         (a) Ascending aorta
         (b) Aortic arch
         (c) Innominate artery
         (d) Proximal common carotid artery
         (e) Hilar pulmonary vessels or the proximal right subclavian artery
      (2) The proximal left subclavian artery is approached through the anterolateral fourth intercostal space.
      (3) The descending thoracic aorta should be approached through the posterolateral fifth intercostal space.

h. After appropriate debridement, the vessel is repaired by end-to-end anastomosis or saphenous vein interposition. Occasionally, a large aortic defect must be replaced with a graft despite the concern for the use of "foreign bodies" in contaminated cases.

i. The need for a shunt during the repair of a carotid or innominate artery is discussed on p. 102.

XII. Diaphragm Diaphragmatic injuries may occur secondary to penetrating or blunt trauma. Penetrating injuries usually cause relatively minimal injury to the diaphragm. However, the significance is that there may be damage to vital structures within the thorax or abdomen (see p. 131). The majority of diaphragmatic injuries secondary to blunt trauma occur on the left side. Cardiovascular and/or pulmonary symptoms are commonly seen early after injury because of the effect of visceral herniation or damage to pulmonary or vascular structures. Patients are frequently asymptomatic. Bowel obstruction or strangulation with perforation may appear after a variable time if the lesion is not identified and repaired following injury.

A. Manifestations

1. Respiratory distress

2. Shock from associated injuries

3. "Asymptomatic"

4. Abdominal or thoracic wall abrasions or ecchymosis may or may not be present.

5. Hyperresonance to percussion and bowel sounds located in the left lower chest.

B. Diagnosis

1. The chest x-ray may reveal an obscured or "elevated" diaphragm.

2. Peritoneal lavage will usually produce a hydrothorax or result in efflux of the lavage through a previously placed chest tube. If there is question that the fluid is emanating from the peritoneal lavage, add methylene blue to the lavage and note its exit from the chest.

3. Bile may exit a previously placed right-sided chest tube.

4. A nasogastric tube may "enter the left chest."

5. Visceral herniation may be apparent on the chest x-ray.

6. Visceral herniation into the thorax may be confirmed by an upper gastro-intestinal (UGI) or barium enema study.

7. The chest x-ray may reveal a mediastinal shift.

C. **Treatment** A ruptured diaphragm is usually accompanied by a significant intraperitoneal injury.

1. Left-sided diaphragmatic hernias should be repaired by a transperitoneal approach to evaluate and repair possible abdominal injuries.

2. Right-sided diaphragmatic injuries
   a. If the peritoneal lavage is negative, the hernia is repaired through a right thoracotomy.
   b. If the peritoneal lavage is positive, the diaphragmatic injury is repaired by a transperitoneal approach with a supplementary thoracotomy, if needed.

3. Wounds are closed in two layers with "0" nonabsorbable suture following debridement of frayed wound edges.

4. Fluid and air should be completely evacuated from the pleural space before the diaphragm is completely closed. A chest tube is usually not indicated if the visceral pleura is intact.

5. A chest tube is indicated following repair if the visceral pleura has been disrupted or the patient has a hemothorax.

6. If the diaphragm has been avulsed from the chest wall, it may be approximated to a rib with pericostal sutures.

XIII. **Thoracoabdominal Wounds** A thoracoabdominal wound is due to a penetration of the diaphragm, which may cause damage to structures within the chest or abdomen. A penetrating wound at or below the nipple is likely to enter the chest, pierce the diaphragm, and enter the abdominal cavity.

A. **Manifestations**

1. Respiratory distress

2. Hemothorax

3. Pneumothorax

4. Shock

5. Peritonitis

6. "Asymptomatic"

7. Stab or gunshot wound to the chest or abdomen

B. **Diagnosis**

1. Chest x-ray may reveal
   a. Hemothorax
   b. Pneumothorax

      c. Pulmonary contusion

      d. Negative result

    2. The missile path may have **obviously** traversed the diaphragm, based on clinical and radiographic evidence.

    3. Bile may exit a chest tube placed in the right hemithorax.

  C. Treatment

    1. A chest tube should be inserted into the affected hemithorax.

    2. A thoracotomy is performed for the same indications described below.

    3. A laparotomy is indicated if the left lower chest is penetrated, to exclude an abdominal injury.

    4. If the lower right chest is penetrated, a peritoneal lavage is performed. If the peritoneal lavage is positive, a laparotomy is performed. If the lavage is negative, the patient is observed.

    5. If it is apparent that the abdomen has been entered, based upon physical and/or radiographic evaluation, a laparotomy is indicated.

    6. The diaphragmatic defect should be debrided and closed in two layers with "0" nonabsorbable sutures.

    7. If the patient is unstable, the clinician must rapidly diagnose cardiac tamponade, tension pneumothorax, hemothorax, or hemoperitoneum.

XIV. Thoracic Duct Disruption of the thoracic duct may occur secondary to blunt or penetrating trauma, but this is rare. The manifestations and treatment are as described on p. 140 for "Reexploratory Thoracotomy."

XV. Indications for Thoracotomy Following Chest Trauma

  A. Thoracic aorta control

  B. Massive or persistent bleeding from the chest (see p. 111)

  C. Cardiac tamponade

  D. Cardiac arrest

  E. Hemodynamic deterioration ("pre-arrest")

  F. Major intrathoracic vascular injury on angiography

G. Uncontrolled air leak

H. Esophageal injury

I. Ruptured diaphragm $(+/-)$

J. "Sucking" chest wound

K. Large, clotted hemothorax

L. Transbronchial aspiration of blood with progressive hypoxia

If an emergency thoracotomy must be performed as a result of hemodynamic deterioration, an anterolateral thoracotomy is performed on the side of the penetrating wound or where the breath sounds are significantly impaired. If there is no lateralization, a left thoracotomy is performed. If necessary, the incision is taken across the sternum into the opposite hemithorax. Pressure is applied to control bleeding. Extension of the incision is undertaken, if necessary, to gain proximal and distal vascular control.

XVI. **Mediastinal Emphysema**   See p. 332.

A. Alveolar rupture (intraparenchymal)

B. Tracheal tear

C. Bronchial tear

D. Esophageal tear

XVII. **Prophylactic Antibiotics**   See p. 410 for the policies that relate to the use of prophylactic antibiotics in penetrating chest trauma.

XVIII. **Reexploratory Thoracotomy**   Reexploratory thoracotomy in the trauma patient is not a rare occurrence. A second exploration may be required for
   —Bleeding
   —Suture line disruption
   —Complications of cardiac injury or surgery
   —Stenosis after repair of the trachea, bronchus, or vascular structures
   —Bronchopleural fistula
   —Empyema

A. Vascular

1. **Aorta and great vessels**
   a. **Postoperative bleeding**
      (1) This may be due to a leaking anastomosis, but it is most likely due to failure to ligate a severed vascular structure or a pulmonary laceration.
      (2) **Treatment** Exploration is usually required if one of the following develops:
      (a) Sudden bleeding of > 500 cc
      (b) > 200 cc/hr for 4–6 consecutive hr
      (c) > 150 cc/hr for 3 consecutive hr in a patient over 50 years of age or in an unstable patient.
      (d) Close observation, correction of coagulopathy, etc., are required in the stable patient who is bleeding 50–100 cc/hr. A red blood cell (RBC) count on the drainage may be helpful in assessing the degree of hemorrhage.
   b. **Graft infection** A vascular prosthesis may become infected secondary to contamination at the time of surgery, by hematogenous seeding or from postoperative contamination, e.g., chest tubes.
      (1) **Manifestations**
      (a) Bacteremia
      (b) Fever and leukocytosis
      (c) Bleeding secondary to suture line disruption
      (d) Graft thrombosis
      (2) **Diagnosis**
      (a) High index of suspicion
      (b) Arteriography
      (c) Radionuclide scan (tagged white blood cells)
      (d) A positive blood culture
      (3) **Treatment**
      (a) Removal of graft
      (b) Extra-anatomical bypass
         (See p. 426.)
   c. **Postoperative stenosis** Usually, a technical operative failure or infection can result in stenosis.
      (1) **Manifestations**
      (a) Aortic stenosis
         i. Upper extremity hypertension
         ii. Left ventricular failure
      (b) Great vessel stenosis
         i. Cerebral ischemia
         ii. Upper extremity ischemia
      (2) **Diagnosis** is determined by an arteriogram.
      (3) **Treatment** Usually graft replacement is required. However, thrombectomy occasionally is all that is needed.

2. Heart
    a. **Intracardiac injuries**   Injuries that involve the septae, valves, and/or conduction system may not be appreciated at the initial operative procedure, or it may be decided to address these lesions at a later time. During the postoperative period, the patient may become symptomatic and require operative intervention.
        (1) **Manifestations**
            (a) Murmurs
            (b) Thrills
            (c) Arrhythmias
            (d) Conduction defects
            (e) Congestive heart failure
            (f) Cardiogenic shock
        (2) **Diagnosis**
            (a) Angiocardiography
            (b) Echocardiogram
            (c) Chest x-ray may reveal pulmonary congestion and/or cardiomegaly.
            (d) EKG may reveal ventricular hypertrophy or arrhythmias.
            (e) Electrocardiographic "mapping" may reveal a focus of myocardium which is creating an arrhythmogenic area.
        (3) **Treatment**
            (a) If a septal defect results in a greater than 3:1 shunt or the patient is symptomatic despite medical therapy, surgery is recommended.
            (b) Patients with valvular disease should first be treated with a medical regimen for congestive heart failure. However, if this fails, surgery is required.
            (c) Conducting defects may warrant a pacemaker.
    b. **Pericardial effusion or tamponade**   The following may be causes of pericardial effusion or tamponade:
        —Pericardial edges may bleed.
        —Bleeding from heart muscle at a suture site
        —Coronary arterial bleeding
        —The development of an effusion from previous hemopericardium or postpericardiotomy syndrome
        (1) **Manifestations**
            (a) Hypotension
            (b) Oliguria
            (c) Quiet heart tones
            (d) Widening of the mediastinum
            (e) Neck vein distention
            (f) Paradoxical pulse
        (2) **Diagnosis**
            (a) Echocardiogram will reveal pericardial fluid.

(b) Electrocardiogram may reveal decreased voltage and/or electrical alternans.

(c) The central venous pressure is elevated.

(d) Swan-Ganz catheterization may reveal a low cardiac output; equalization of diastolic pressures and a right ventricular diastolic:right ventricular systolic pressure >1:3. These findings are highly suggestive of pericardial tamponade.

(3) Treatment

    (a) **Acute hemorrhagic tamponade** A thoracotomy is required for the postoperative patient who is hemorrhaging into the pericardial space. Preoperative means to restore hemodynamic stability include

        i. Volume infusion

        ii. Administration of dopamine (Intropin) or dobutamine (Dobutrex)

        iii. Pericardiocentesis

    (b) **Subacute tamponade (effusion)** Pericardiocentesis may be attempted and the patient may be treated on a medical regimen. However, if this fails, a pericardial window draining into the subxyphoid or the pleural space or a pericardiectomy may be required.

c. **Constrictive pericarditis** Constrictive pericarditis is the development of a constricting peel around the heart, which fails to allow the heart to fill adequately during diastole. This peel occurs secondary to blood and/or infection in the pericardium.

(1) **Manifestations**

    (a) Ascites

    (b) Peripheral edema

    (c) Hepatomegaly

    (d) Findings are as described for pericardial effusion or tamponade (p. 120).

(2) **Diagnosis** The diagnostic findings are as described for pericardial effusion or tamponade (p. 121).

(3) **Treatment** If the patient has hemodynamic instability, an anterior pericardiectomy is recommended.

d. **Cardiac herniation** The heart may herniate through the pericardial incision.

(1) **Manifestations**

    (a) A patient developing hemodynamic instability following a procedure which requires a pericardial incision should be suspected of cardiac herniation.

    (b) Chest x-ray may reveal cardiac displacement and/or cardiomegaly.

(2) **Treatment** If cardiac herniation is suspected, reoperation and reduction are necessary.

e. **Ventricular aneurysm** Transmural ischemia may develop secondary to ligation of a coronary artery or suture of a ventricular laceration and result in an aneurysm.

    (1) **Manifestations**
        (a) Congestive heart failure
        (b) Peripheral emboli
        (c) Arrhythmia
        (d) Systolic murmur

    (2) **Diagnosis**
        (a) Chest x-ray may reveal an abnormal cardiac silhouette.
        (b) Echocardiogram
        (c) Angiocardiography

    (3) **Treatment** Aneurysmectomy is required if the above symptoms are present.

f. **Coronary artery injury** Usually a distal coronary artery has been ligated during an operative procedure for a lacerated vessel; the patient subsequently develops ischemia.

    (1) **Manifestations**
        (a) Angina
        (b) Ventricular failure

    (2) **Diagnosis**
        (a) EKG may reveal ischemic changes.
        (b) Thallium-201 scan or technetium pyrophosphate scan may reveal an ischemic area of myocardium.
        (c) Coronary arteriography will reveal the precise coronary arterial anatomy.

    (3) **Treatment** Coronary artery bypass is required if there is a significant decrease of coronary flow and angina is unable to be managed medically. If the patient has been previously healthy and develops ventricular failure subsequent to coronary arterial ligation, coronary revascularization is recommended, if medical therapy fails.

B. Pulmonary

1. Tracheobronchial tree

a. **Stenosis** A patient who has been explored for a tracheal or bronchial injury for which the lesion has been repaired may subsequently develop a symptomatic stenosis.

    (1) **Manifestations**
        (a) Recurrent atelectasis
        (b) Recurrent pneumonia
        (c) Lung abscess
        (d) Intercostal retractions and acute respiratory distress

    (2) **Diagnosis**
        (a) Bronchography

          (b) Bronchoscopy

          (c) Tracheal xeroradiograms

    (3) **Treatment** If tracheal or bronchial dilatation fails, revision or resection of the previous repair will be required.

  b. **Air leak** A tracheal or bronchial injury which has been repaired may subsequently leak.

    (1) **Manifestations**

          (a) Pneumothorax

          (b) Persistent air leak through chest tubes

          (c) Pneumomediastinum

          (d) Mediastinitis

          (e) Empyema

    (2) **Diagnosis (bronchoscopy)**

    (3) **Treatment**

          (a) **Tracheal air leak** If the patient develops significant pneumomediastinum while **on a ventilator,** the cuff of the tube is advanced below the leak, if possible. The airway pressure is minimized, if possible, to allow for spontaneous closure of the leak. If the patient develops progressive emphysema despite these measures, the patient should be taken to the operating room and the tracheal leak should be repaired to prevent mediastinitis. If the patient develops a tracheal air leak and has been **spontaneously ventilating,** he or she is intubated and the tube cuff is advanced below the leak. The patient should be placed only on continuous positive airway pressure (CPAP), if possible, to minimize airway pressure. If the patient continues to develop emphysema or the cuff cannot be advanced below the leak, he or she should be taken to the operating room for repair.

          (b) **Bronchial leak** If the patient requires ventilatory support, manipulation should be performed to decrease the airway pressure. If the patient's lung is expanded and the patient can be weaned from the ventilator, extubation should be performed since the lower airway pressures associated with spontaneous breathing may result in closure of the leak. Operative repair of the bronchial leak is usually required in the following cases:

            i. Inability to expand the lung

           ii. Inability to ventilate the patient, i.e., to prevent respiratory acidosis or to maintain PEEP

          iii. If the patient has an empyema and a significant air leak

          iv. If the patient is spontaneously breathing and the bronchopleural air leak has not decreased after 10–14 days

2. **Lung injury** Reexploration of the chest may be required following pneumonectomy, lobectomy, segmentectomy, or suturing of the lung following trauma.

a. **Bleeding** Surgery is usually indicated if there is bleeding at a rate of >300 cc/hr for 3 consecutive hr.

b. **Bronchopleural fistula**

(1) **Manifestations** There is persistent air leak.

(2) **Treatment** See p. 138.

3. **Empyema** may develop following thoracotomy secondary to: contamination at the time of the original injury or thoracotomy; a subsequent bronchial or esophageal repair that has leaked; an unevacuated hemothorax and/or chest tube contamination of the pleural space (see p. 419).

4. **Fibrothorax** A hemothorax or empyema may develop following thoracotomy. If this is inadequately drained with chest tubes, a fibrous peel may develop around the lung.

a. **Manifestations** Shortness of breath develops.

b. **Diagnosis**

(1) Chest x-ray reveals pleural thickening.

(2) Decreased lung volumes (extrinsic, restrictive pulmonary disease)

c. **Treatment** Decortication to remove the pleural peel and expand the lung may be required if the pleural thickening is not resolving after 4–6 weeks or earlier if the patient is symptomatic.

C. **Esophagus** Suture line disruption may occur following repair of an esophageal injury.

1. **Manifestations**

a. Mediastinitis (sepsis)

b. Hydropneumothorax

c. Empyema

2. **Treatment**

a. Repair the esophageal leak, if possible.

b. The esophageal disruption should be drained by mediastinal and/or pleural tubes.

c. If the wound is large and/or will not hold sutures, a cervical esophagostomy and ligation of the abdominal esophagus should be performed to prevent contamination of the esophagus with saliva and gastric reflux.

D. **Chest wall incision**

1. **Bleeding**

a. **Manifestations**

(1) Hematoma (early)

(2) Seroma (later)

b. **Treatment**

(1) If a significant hematoma develops in the early postoperative period, the wound should be opened and the bleeding points controlled.

        (2)   The seroma is usually aspirated and a compression bandage is applied or a continuous vacuum drainage system is placed within the wound.

    2. **Infection**
      a. **Manifestations**
          (1)   Fever
          (2)   Leukocytosis
          (3)   Local tenderness
          (4)   Suppurative drainage
          (5)   Erythema and induration
      b. **Treatment**
          (1)   Remove skin and subcutaneous sutures.
          (2)   If the patient is toxic, administer parenteral antibiotics.
          (3)   Irrigate the wound and follow this with frequent dressing changes.
          (4)   If the sternum is separated or air or pus is emanating from the sternum, it must be opened. Otherwise, the infection is treated as a superficial, soft tissue infection.
              (a)   Open the sternum and debride nonviable tissue, bone wax, etc.
              (b)   Irrigate the mediastinum with an antibiotic solution.
              (c)   Insert irrigation tubes into the mediastinum; close the sternum with wires passed around it; close the fascia and sternal muscle with wire.
              (d)   Perform intermittent irrigation with saline following closure of the sternal wound.

    3. **Dehiscence**   A thoracotomy or sternotomy dehiscence should be closed following debridement. Wire is the recommended suture of choice.

E. **Thoracic duct**   The thoracic duct may be injured at or prior to thoracotomy and not recognized at initial exploration, but subsequently may be diagnosed. The injury may be found at surgery, repaired, and followed by recurrence.

    1. **Manifestations**
      a. If a chest tube is not in place, a pleural effusion will develop.
      b. If a chest tube is in place, the drainage has the following characteristics:
          (1)   Milky appearance
          (2)   High lymphocyte count
          (3)   High fat content
          (4)   4–5 gm % of protein
          (5)   Fat globules on microscopic examination
      c. Lymphangiography will reveal a thoracic duct leak.

    2. **Treatment**   A chest tube is inserted to expand the lung and drainage is monitored on a daily basis. The patient should be made NPO and initially

treated with parenteral hyperalimentation followed with a medium chain triglyceride diet. If this regimen fails to terminate the leak, a lymphangiogram is performed to specifically locate the leak, and the thoracic duct is ligated at surgery.

F. **Mediastinum**   This may become infected from
   —A leak from a previous repair of the tracheobronchial tree
   —A leak from an esophageal repair
   —Contamination during surgery for a mediastinal injury
   —Hematogenous seeding of a hematoma within the mediastinum

   1. **Manifestations**
      a. Sepsis (chills, fever, shock)
      b. Empyema
      c. Hamman's crunch

   2. **Diagnosis**   Chest x-ray may reveal
      a. Pneumomediastinum
      b. Widened mediastinum
      c. Pleural effusion
      d. Empyema
      e. Air-fluid level

   3. **Treatment**
      a. Parenteral antibiotics
      b. Correction of primary pathology
      c. Surgical drainage by way of mediastinal and/or pleural tubes
      d. Betadine irrigation via mediastinal or pleural tubes
      e. Cardiovascular support, if unstable
      f. Nutritional support

G. **Diaphragm**   Diaphragmatic rupture is uncommon after repair, yet not rare.

   1. **Manifestations**   See p. 130.

   2. **Treatment**   A transthoracic approach should be performed to repair the diaphragm, if abdominal pathology is not suspected.

11
ABDOMINAL AND PELVIC INJURIES

Blunt or penetrating trauma may cause injury to the parietes or vascular-visceral structures within the confines of the abdomen and pelvis. The patient must be evaluated for the presence of a surgical abdominal or pelvic injury any time the torso has been subjected to blunt or penetrating trauma. Injury to the spleen, pancreas, liver, kidney, or tributaries of the aorta, vena cava, portal vein, or hepatic veins may cause variable degrees of hemorrhage. Depending on the extent of hemorrhage, hemodynamic instability may be minimal or profound. If hollow or solid viscera are disrupted, peritonitis may result. The peritonitis is usually negligible if the contamination is minimal and the defect is controlled early. If abdominal contamination is significant and/or control of the disruption is delayed, the patient is likely to develop generalized peritonitis or an intra-abdominal abscess. The common sequel to an abdominal abscess or peritonitis is systemic sepsis and multiple systems failure.

The key to the successful management of abdominal and pelvic injuries is rapid detection of the presence of a vascular or visceral injury and control of the hemorrhage and abdominal contamination. The surgeon's diagnostic armamentarium includes physical examination, radiographic examination, and peritoneal lavage. If these investigative modes are equivocal, diagnostic laparotomy is a valuable method for assessing the abdomen.

I. **Management of Blunt Abdominal Trauma** When the patient sustains blunt trauma, significant abdominal pathology, which requires surgical intervention, must be identified. The abdomen is difficult to evaluate by physical examination when the patient has incurred blunt trauma. This is particularly true if extra-abdominal pain distracts the physician and patient from the abdomen. The presence of a head injury and/or drug abuse (usually alcohol) renders the abdominal examination of little value. The presence or absence of torso marks or tenderness frequently does not correlate with the presence and degree of intra-abdominal injury. The principal question confronting the trauma surgeon is "who needs a laparotomy?" The patient is assessed by peritoneal lavage, physical examination, or both. Peritoneal lavage is frequently the only reliable method for evaluating the abdomen, especially during the first 4–6 hr. All patients should have a physical examination, since findings may be present which mandate laparotomy. A negative physical examination is a reliable indicator for conservative treatment in a select group of patients.

A. Peritoneal lavage

  1. **Absolute indications**
      a. Abdominal pain and/or abdominal tenderness
      b. Altered sensorium due to a head injury and/or drugs

    c. Hypotension; falling Hct
    d. Paraplegia or quadriplegia
    e. Thoracic or lumbar spine fractures
    f. Pelvic fracture
    g. History or evidence of lower thoracic cage trauma

2. The need for prolonged anesthesia for treatment of extra-abdominal injuries may be considered a **relative indication.**

Perspective

If a patient demonstrates deteriorating signs from a traumatic intra-cranial lesion without evidence of shock, the peritoneal lavage should be deferred until a CAT scan or carotid angiogram is performed. If a craniotomy is indicated, the lavage is performed in the operating room during the neurosurgical procedure.

---

3. **Method of lavage** An open or a semi-open method for performing a diagnostic peritoneal lavage is used. With the open technique, the lavage catheter is introduced into the abdominal cavity under direct vision after the peritoneum has been opened. In the semi-open method, the peritoneum is not opened. This technique is faster and is almost as safe as the open method.

4. **Technique** A Foley catheter and nasogastric tube are inserted to decompress the urinary bladder and stomach. The patient is in the supine position. The lower abdomen is shaved, scrubbed, and painted with povidone-iodine (Betadine) solution. Sterile drapes are applied. This procedure is performed while a surgical cap, mask, and gloves are worn. Local anesthesia containing epinephrine is used. The uncooperative or combative patient is sedated after neurologic evaluation.

    a. Open technique
        (1) One percent lidocaine (Xylocaine) with epinephrine is infiltrated into the skin and subcutaneous tissues for a distance of about 3–5 cm below the umbilicus. The length of incision depends on the amount of body fat. In the case of a previous midline surgical scar, a left lower quadrant muscle splitting approach is employed (a right lower quadrant incision may later be confused with the performance of an appendectomy). In the presence of a known or suspected major pelvic fracture, a supraumbilical approach of the open variety is recommended. This maneuver is performed in an attempt to avoid transversing an abdominal hematoma, which could result in a false positive lavage (see p. 196).

(2) A longitudinal incision down to the linea alba is made; subcutaneous bleeders are ligated with gut suture. Retracting the skin and subcutaneous tissue with a self-retaining retractor is helpful.

(3) Just to the right of the linea alba, the fascia is opened the length of the incision and the rectus muscle is retracted laterally.

(4) The transversalis fascia is opened and the preperitoneal fat is gently cleaned off the underlying peritoneum.

(5) The peritoneum is picked up with two hemostats and a small opening is made between them.

(6) A dialysis catheter is gently introduced through the peritoneal opening, advanced along the anterior abdominal wall, and directed toward the pelvis.

(7) A purse-string suture of 2-0 absorbable material is placed through the peritoneum around the catheter and tied firmly to create a water-tight seal.

(8) Gentle aspiration of the catheter is performed. The return of gross blood (10–15 cc) is considered an indication for laparotomy and negates the performance of a lavage.

(9) Using an intravenous set with a vent, 1,000 cc of crystalloid fluid is instilled into the abdominal cavity (20 cc/kg is recommended in children).

(10) The patient is placed in the head-down position (if neurologically allowable) for a few minutes and then returned to the neutral supine position. To maintain a continuous fluid column, which allows for siphonage of the lavage fluid, the lavage tubing is clamped just as the infusion bottle empties.

(11) The bottle is placed on the floor and the infusion apparatus is forced into the air vent dislodging the tube connected to this hole. The tubing is unclamped and the lavage is drained. Closure or manipulation of the lavage incision is not recommended during infusion or drainage of the fluid. During lavage and drainage, the wound is covered with a sterile drape.

(12) If the lavage is negative, the fascia is closed with a nonabsorbable suture of 0 gauge. The subcutaneous tissue is irrigated with normal saline. The skin is then closed.

b. **Semi-open method**   The patient is prepared in the manner similar to the open method.

(1) An infraumbilical incision down to the rectus fascia is made. The semi-open method requires a shorter incision than the open method.

(2) Hemostasis is obtained using gut ligatures.

(3) A 0 silk traction suture is placed through the linea alba; the linea alba is then incised with a No. 11 blade just cephalad to the traction suture.

(4) The traction is pulled forward and the dialysis catheter trocar assembly is pushed through the incised linea alba into the abdominal cavity. This gentle firm push is made at an angle of 30–40°

toward the pelvis. A "give" indicates penetration of the peritoneum, after which the catheter is advanced over the trocar assembly, which is then withdrawn.

(5) The rest of the semi-open method is similar to the open method. Only one or no suture is required to close the fascial defect.

(6) Another popular approach is by a left paraumbilical incision. There is minimal to absent preperitoneal fat between the posterior rectus sheath and peritoneum at this point.

| Note | —**Length of incision** When the open method is employed, a generous incision may be needed in heavier patients to facilitate dissection down to and identification of the peritoneum. A short incision in such patients creates a time-consuming and difficult procedure often with poor hemostasis, which may result in a false positive return.

—**Difficult retrieval of fluid** If little or no lavage fluid returns, several techniques can be employed.

With aseptic technique, gently manipulate the catheter, e.g., twist, withdraw, or advance.

Place the patient in a slight head-up position.

Infuse an additional 500–1,000 cc of the lavage fluid. This procedure is particularly helpful in large adults in whom the intraabdominal fluid level has not reached the tip of the dialysis

—To avoid a **false positive result,** it is important to use meticulous hemostatic technique during catheter insertion. If blood leaks into the abdominal cavity, infusion of 500 cc to 1 liter of fluid after drainage of the first lavage will usually reveal a clearer effluent.

5. **Interpretation of results**
   a. **Qualitative analysis of the dialysate** Inspection of the dialysate return in the bottle or the plastic tubing is performed. A bloody return in the bottle or the inability to read newsprint through the lavage tube is usually a positive result mandating laparotomy.
   b. **Quantitative analysis of the dialysate** The following are considered positive:
      (1) An erythrocyte count of greater than $100,000/mm^3$
      (2) A leukocyte count greater than $500/mm^3$
      (3) The presence of gastrointestinal contents, including vegetable fibers, bile, and bacteria (via Gram stain)
      (4) An elevated amylase suggests a small bowel injury.

| Note | An erythrocyte count is the most frequent factor that determines the positivity or negativity of a lavage. A count of $50,000–100,000/mm^3$ produces a red dialysate and is a dilemma. If the patient is stable, the

catheter is left in place for 1–2 hr and the lavage is repeated. If the patient is not explored, all other dialysate parameters must be negative. Whenever a questionable result is obtained, the decision to perform laparotomy must be determined by viewing the entire patient and the other injuries. If the patient is going to require heavy sedation and/or has multiple extra-abdominal injuries that can cause significant blood loss and/or has a decreased level of consciousness, it is best to explore the abdominal cavity. The patient who is awake and has few other injuries may be followed with serial complete blood counts, physical examination, and repeat lavage.

6. **Repeat lavage and delayed lavage** In some patients, a repeat or initial lavage may be necessary a day or more after admission. Indications for repeat or delayed diagnostic lavage include:
   a. Unexplained blood loss and transfusion requirements
   b. The appearance of abnormal abdominal signs and/or symptoms
   c. In some cases, unexplained fever or leukocytosis

7. **Pitfalls of peritoneal lavage** All diagnostic tests have limitations. To effectively and safely use peritoneal lavage, a knowledge of its pitfalls is necessary. Generally, the amount of blood in the return reflects the degree of intra-abdominal pathology. However, significant life-threatening injuries may be associated with a clear or minimally blood-tinged return. These include:
   a. Gastrointestinal perforations
   b. Ruptures of the diaphragm
   c. Injured retroperitoneal organs (pancreas, duodenum, kidney, urinary bladder, and ureter)

Fortunately, the pancreas and/or duodenum are rarely injured without an associated intra-abdominal injury, giving rise to a bloody lavage return. Injury of these structures can often be diagnosed by employing a high index of suspicion. Radiologic evaluation includes an upper GI series to rule out a ruptured diaphragm or duodenal perforation, a cystogram to detect a bladder perforation, and an intravenous pyelogram (IVP) to identify renal and ureteral injuries. A CAT scan may be useful in identifying a pancreatic injury (see p. 172).

Perspective

We strongly advocate the use of peritoneal lavage in all patients who have sustained blunt trauma. If peritoneal lavage is not performed, the clinician should mentally list those reasons. Physical examination of the abdomen after blunt trauma is very deceptive. The more systems traumatized, the greater the difficulty in excluding abdominal pathology without peritoneal lavage.

B. **Physical evaluation**

1. **Physical findings mandating laparotomy** There may be findings in the alert patient or in a patient with a depressed level of consciousness that re-

quire laparotomy. Laparotomy is indicated for the following:

    a. Free abdominal air seen on the upright chest x-ray

    b. Peritonitis (exclude tenderness from abdominal wall contusion or rib or pelvic fractures)

    c. Abdominal distention and hemodynamic instability (exclude gastric distention from face mask ventilation)

    d. Disrupted abdominal wall

2. **Physical findings mandating conservative management** When the patient has no indication for peritoneal lavage, the abdomen is observed if

    a. Bowel sounds are active

    b. The abdominal wall is intact

    c. The abdomen is soft

    d. The abdomen is not distended

    e. The abdomen is not tender

    Conservative management involves NPO (nothing by mouth), **minimal** pain medication, serial Hct and WBC determinations, serial amylase values, and a repeat physical examination. If the patient develops evidence of blood loss or abdominal tenderness, peritoneal lavage should be performed.

Perspective

The principal challenge with blunt abdominal trauma is "who needs a laparotomy?" Despite peritoneal lavage and physical evaluation, there may yet be uncertainty as to whether the patient needs a laparotomy. In these cases, it is usually best to perform a laparotomy to exclude major pathology. An occasional "unnecessary laparotomy" in these unconscious or multiply injured patients is better than a "delayed laparotomy" in the patient who develops a major complication from a missed injury.

C. **Laparotomy**

1. **Timing of laparotomy** When the need for laparotomy is ascertained, it should be promptly carried out. Deterioration from a severe intracranial injury, such as an epidural hematoma, or intrathoracic injury, such as a ruptured aorta, takes precedence over laparotomy. Generally, intracranial and abdominal surgery can be performed simultaneously. Despite the presence of severe extra-abdominal injuries requiring surgery, if there is evidence of severe intra-abdominal hemorrhage, laparotomy should be performed first. In the presence of a distending abdomen and hypotension, a left thoracotomy with compression of the aorta should be considered before abdominal exploration if cardiac dysrhythmias develop.

2. **Preoperative preparation** Prior to laparotomy a nasogastric tube and Foley catheter should be inserted. Sufficient intravenous lines should be inserted, with lines above and below the diaphragm.

3. **Antibiotics** If peritonitis is suspected, preoperative antibiotics (clindamycin and gentamicin, or cefoxitin) should be given.

4. **Skin preparation** The shaved, prepped, and draped operative field should include the area from the sternal notch to the pubic symphysis and groin, in case the chest must be entered or a vein must be harvested.

5. **The incision** The abdomen may be explored through a long midline incision or an upper transverse abdominal incision. In the absence of a pelvic fracture, over 90% of blunt trauma involves the upper abdomen. A mid-epigastric transverse incision allows ready access to the entire upper abdomen. Splenic and hepatic surgery is usually easier through a transverse incision rather than a vertical incision. The midline incision is less bloody and generally a little faster to open. The needs of the patient determine the type of incision used.

   The fascia should be closed in layers with interrupted wire or prolene. The subcutaneous tissue should be irrigated with saline. The skin should be closed, unless there has been abdominal contamination.

6. **Planned second look** There are situations during laparotomy when the surgeon feels that optimal management cannot be performed at the initial procedure or that the evaluation or repair of the pathology is questionable. Therefore, a second-look procedure should be strongly considered when coagulopathy, tenuous mesenteric vascular supply, or "questionable" small bowel anastomosis is present. A coagulopathy associated with a liver or splenic injury will usually result in an abdominal hematoma that cannot be adequately removed by a drain. A reoperation may be useful to remove this "culture medium." If there are multiple mesenteric hematomas, with or without bowel resection, or ligation of a segment of the portal system, consideration for a second-look procedure should be entertained to assess bowel viability. If a small bowel anastomosis has been performed under less than ideal circumstances, a second-look procedure should be considered. The second-look procedure is a valuable concept when used in the appropriate setting.

II. **Management of Penetrating Abdominal Trauma** There is controversy regarding the appropriate management of penetrating abdominal trauma. Guidelines are established to manage the patient most efficiently, depending on the likelihood of intraperitoneal pathology and the ability of the staff to sequentially evaluate the patient. It should be considered that penetrating wounds to the chest at or below the nipple have entered the abdomen. Wounds may be classified as gunshot, shotgun, stab, and miscellaneous, e.g., flying glass, shrapnel, or stakes. Management of each is discussed separately.

A. **Gunshot wounds**

1. Intravenous access above the diaphragm is obtained.

2. Cardiovascular and respiratory stabilization is obtained.

3. Type and crossmatch and baseline laboratory data are obtained.

4. A preoperative chest x-ray and AP and lateral x-ray of the abdomen are obtained; an IVP is obtained, if the patient is stable, whether hematuria is present or not.

5. If the lower thorax is in the proximity of injury, a chest tube is inserted on the side of injury to avoid intraoperative pneumothorax.

6. Preoperative antibiotics (clindamycin and gentamicin or cefoxitin) are administered and tetanus immunization is evaluated.

7. A nasogastric (NG) tube and Foley catheter are inserted.

8. A patient with a gunshot wound to the abdomen (flank and back wounds included) needs a formal laparotomy.

9. The patient is prepped from chin to mid-thigh.

10. A midline abdominal incision is performed, but a midepigastric transverse incision may be used if the wound is confined to the upper abdomen.

11. Intra-abdominal pathology is dealt with, as necessary.

12. Entrance and exit sites are debrided.

13. Slugs and missile fragments must be saved for the Medical Examiner.

B. **Shotgun wounds**

1. These require the same general management as for gunshot wounds.

2. If the wound was at close range, the surgeon must remove all wadding, clothing, and other foreign material from the wound to prevent suppuration, and a laparotomy must be performed.

3. Wounds sustained at a distance produce widely scattered pellet tracks over the body surface with varying degrees of penetration, usually in the subcutaneous tissues but possibly deeper. These are considered low velocity injuries and the decision to operate is based on clinical evaluation, i.e., blood loss or peritonitis.

    |Note| Pellet wounds may be difficult to find intraoperatively. All pellet injuries to the bowel should be sought and oversewn or resected.

C. **Stab wounds**

1. Absolute indications for immediate laparotomy include shock, signs of peritonitis, gastrointestinal bleeding, free air in the peritoneal cavity, evisceration, and massive hematuria.

2. If the patient is asymptomatic, yet peritoneal penetration has taken place, a laparotomy is performed.

3. If there is a question of peritoneal penetration, local wound exploration is performed to determine if penetration has occurred.

4. If a stab wound has been inflicted to the left lower chest, laparotomy is performed.

5. If a stab wound to the right lower chest has been inflicted and the abdomen is asymptomatic and the patient is stable, observation of the abdomen is indicated.

6. Preoperative and operative management is the same as described for gunshot wounds (above).

Note An impaled object should not be removed until the part is exposed at surgery.

D. **Miscellaneous injuries**   Treatment must be individualized using a combination of criteria previously stated for gunshot and stab wounds.

III. **Spleen**   The spleen, a highly vascular organ with poorly developed structural substance, lies in the left upper quadrant of the abdomen. The spleen may be damaged secondary to blunt or penetrating trauma. The spleen is considered important in conferring immunity, but its specific role is unknown. There is information available in the infant and child to support the observation that there is an increased incidence of infection in later life in post-splenectomy trauma patients compared to patients with a healthy spleen. Not only is the incidence of infection higher, but once a bacteremia is established, the mortality is quite high. It is not certain whether the same risk following splenectomy for trauma is present if the spleen is removed in the later decades of life. The present issue is, at what age is it safe to remove the post-traumatized "normal" spleen without increasing the risk of infection to the patient in subsequent life? There is a tendency at the present time to conserve the total spleen or at least half the spleen, if possible.

A. **Manifestations**   The signs and symptoms of splenic trauma are related to peritoneal irritation and/or hemorrhage. Manifestations secondary to hemorrhage cover a spectrum that varies from severe shock to minimal or absent findings.

1. **Symptoms**
   a. Abdominal pain that is frequently localized to the left upper quadrant
   b. Complaint of pain in the left shoulder or neck, which is produced by placing the patient in the Trendelenburg position.

2. **Signs**
   a. There may be guarding upon palpation of the left upper quadrant.
   b. With significant hemorrhage, the abdomen may become distended, the patient may be hypotensive, tachycardia may be present, and/or the patient may show pallor.
   c. There is a frequent association of left lower rib fractures.

d. A gunshot wound or stab wound to the abdomen, chest, back, or flank may involve the spleen.

3. Laboratory data The hematocrit may be low secondary to significant hemorrhage.

B. Diagnosis

1. Peritoneal lavage is positive for blood when there is disruption of the splenic capsule.

2. An abdominal x-ray may reveal medial displacement of the stomach or downward displacement of the splenic flexure of the colon with intrasplenic hematoma or left upper quadrant hematoma.

3. If peritoneal lavage is negative and there is a fall in the hematocrit and/or the presence of left upper quadrant pain, an intrasplenic hematoma may be present. In this situation, the following diagnostic aides may be helpful:
   a. Liver/spleen scan
   b. CAT scan
   c. Angiogram

C. "Delayed" splenic rupture This clinical entity usually manifests as shock following an undiagnosed splenic injury from 1 to 2 weeks after trauma and is secondary to one of the two following explanations:

1. The patient sustains a splenic fracture which was not diagnosed because a peritoneal lavage was not performed; the clot dissolves over the next several days resulting in intraperitoneal hemorrhage.

2. The patient had an intrasplenic hematoma which resulted in a negative peritoneal lavage; several days later, expansion of the subcapsular hematoma causes disruption of the splenic capsule and hemorrhage into the peritoneal cavity.

   The end result is a patient who presents 7–14 days following trauma with left upper quadrant pain (precapsular rupture) and/or shock from acute blood loss.

Perspective
These are almost always missed diagnoses. The patient usually manifests with some evidence of splenic trauma, but the findings are not pursued with peritoneal lavage and/or splenic scan. This is not a common event for the astute clinician.

D. Treatment The management of splenic injuries generally consists of splenectomy, splenorrhaphy, or nonoperative management. The spleen may be approached via a transverse or vertical abdominal incision. It has been found that in the absence of pelvic fractures, over 90% of significant intra-abdominal pathology following blunt trauma lies within the upper abdomen. The spleen is frequently difficult to approach from a vertical incision. There are advantages and disadvantages to both incisions; however, we feel that the transverse incision provides optimal exposure for splenectomy or splenorrhaphy.

1. **Splenectomy**
    a. **Indications**
        (1) Multiple fractures of the spleen
        (2) A patient with a coagulopathy or likelihood of developing a coagulopathy
        (3) Multiply injured patient (should the hematocrit continue to fall in the postoperative period, the surgeon would not be certain whether the fall in hematocrit was secondary to other injuries or to bleeding from the spleen if a splenorrhaphy was performed)
        (4) It would be advisable to remove the spleen in an unstable patient since it takes at least 30 additional min to perform a splenorrhaphy as opposed to a splenectomy.
        (5) Inability to gain complete hemostasis with splenorraphy

---

Perspective
Following removal of the spleen, meticulous hemostasis should be obtained, and the splenic flexure of the colon, the greater curvature of the stomach, and the tail of the pancreas should be visualized for associated injuries that may have occurred during the splenectomy. These precautions are necessary to minimize postoperative complications. We do not advocate routine drainage following splenectomy. Drainage may be beneficial in the patient with a coagulopathy and who is oozing blood from the operative site. The drain should be removed as soon as the drainage slows. (See **Planned second look**, p. 149.)

---

   b. **Pneumovax** This polyvalent pneumococcal vaccine is administered to the post-splenectomy patient in hopes of minimizing post-splenectomy pneumococcal septicemia. However, the effectiveness of this vaccine is questionable at the present time. The length of effectiveness of the vaccine is unknown; therefore, the frequency with which repeated injections must be administered during the subsequent years of the patient's life is also unknown.
   c. **Prophylactic antibiotics** Daily administration of penicillin has been suggested to minimize post-splenectomy sepsis, but this has not met with great success because of lack of patient compliance. There are no studies available to prove that this practice is efficacious in mitigating post-splenectomy infectious complications.

2. **Splenorrhaphy**
    a. **Indications**
        (1) Capsular laceration

(2) Superficial parenchymal lacerations

(3) Damage to the superior or inferior pole, not involving the hilum.

  b. Technique The spleen should be completely mobilized so that it may be delivered into the incision for adequate exposure; i.e., the splenic attachments to the splenic flexure of the colon, diaphragm, and kidney should be freed.

    (1) Suture technique Sutures are used to control bleeding from the edge of the splenic laceration.

      (a) Sutures that are placed through splenic parenchyma parallel to the edge of a laceration may control bleeding from the laceration.

      (b) Simple or horizontal mattress sutures may be applied with or without Teflon pledgets to coapt the edges of the laceration to control hemorrhage.

      (c) Segmental arterial ligation may be performed to minimize hemorrhage from the splenic parenchyma.

    (2) Splenic arterial ligation If there are multiple superficial lacerations of the spleen, splenic arterial ligation may control the hemorrhage, yet not impair splenic viability.

    (3) Partial resection A superior or inferior "polectomy" may be performed for fractures or intrasplenic hematomas which involve the inferior or superior pole of the spleen. Simple sutures may be placed parallel to the resection line, with or without the use of Teflon pledgets. The sutures are usually inserted prior to transection of the splenic parenchyma.

    (4) Avitene (microcrystalline collagen) may be applied to the surface of the spleen in addition to using the suture technique. If the capsule is partially stripped from the surface of the spleen, Avitene may control oozing.

Perspective
The exact incidence of post-splenectomy sepsis in the adult is unknown. The stressed trauma patient should not be placed at further risk, i.e., of losing blood, by an attempt to save an irreparable spleen.

---

  c. Follow-up

    (1) The patient is followed with serial hematocrit determinations in the immediate postoperative period.

    (2) Splenic scans are indicated on a weekly basis for the first 3 weeks.

    (3) If the patient remains hemodynamically stable and is stable according to the spleen scan, the patient is discharged during or at the end of the 3rd week following splenic repair.

3. Nonoperative management A patient who presents with a negative peritoneal tap, yet has a falling hematocrit and/or left upper quadrant pain, may suggest the presence of an intrasplenic hematoma. The patient should be evaluated by a CAT scan, spleen scan, and/or angiography. If these studies reveal an intrasplenic hematoma, operative versus nonoperative management must be considered. The latter may be considered using the following criteria:

a. Easy i.v. access for resuscitation

b. A young patient who could tolerate a cardiovascular insult, i.e., hypotension

c. A thin patient who would be easily and rapidly approached surgically should he or she become unstable

d. A setting in which the patient may be frequently examined

e. A small intraparenchymal or subcapsular hematoma

Patients managed in a nonoperative fashion should be followed by frequent clinical examination, serial hematocrit determinations, and frequent spleen scans. Coagulation tests should be normal during observation. If a patient has remained stable for a period of time between 2½–3 weeks postinjury, that patient may be discharged and followed on an outpatient basis.

E. **Complications of splenectomy or splenorrhaphy**

1. Post-splenectomy sepsis

2. Subdiaphragmatic abscess

3. Gastric fistula

4. Pancreatic fistula

5. Colonic fistula

6. Hemorrhage after splenorrhaphy

7. Left lower lobe atelectasis

8. Post-splenectomy thrombocytosis

9. Wound infection

10. Postoperative hemorrhage following splenectomy secondary to poor hemostatic technique and/or coagulopathy

IV. **Gastrointestinal Tract**   Abdominal trauma resulting in injury to the gastrointestinal tract presents one of the most challenging problems, diagnostically and therapeutically, in the management of the multiply injured patient. A specific approach to injuries of the stomach, duodenum, small intestine, colon, and rectum is presented in the following discussion. Certain principles are relevant to the management of these injuries.

A. Gastric decompression is advised in any patient suspected of having intra-abdominal injury. An awake patient will usually tolerate a nasogastric tube better than an oral gastric tube. However, the latter is preferable in patients who will need prolonged decompression, since the oral route seems to diminish the development of sinusitis. Gastric decompression is continued postoperatively until peristalsis resumes.

B. Patients with penetrating abdominal trauma receive gentamicin and clindamycin or cefoxitin, preoperatively. If a colon injury is found, the antibiotics are continued for 3–5 days, postoperatively. If a penetrating upper gastrointestinal injury is found, clindamycin or cefoxitin is continued for two additional doses. Patients with blunt trauma, but a suspicion of perforated viscus, are likewise managed with this regime, preoperatively. Upper gastrointestinal tract injuries may be treated with antibiotics for 3–5 days if contamination is gross and there has been a lengthy delay in operative intervention.

C. Since nutritional needs are a major factor in convalescence, consideration is given to needle catheter jejunostomy during abdominal procedures. Obviously, this will not be necessary in all patients, but may be particularly useful in patients with severe maxillofacial injuries, head injuries, or those in whom prolonged ventilatory support is anticipated.

D. Irrigation of the peritoneal cavity prior to closure is routinely employed. The temperature of the irrigant is adjusted to the needs of a hypothermic or febrile patient. Saline irrigation is used to clear residual intestinal material, blood, or clot.

E. Complications following gastrointestinal injuries may include hemorrhage, fistulization, obstruction, or abscess formation (see p. 184).

V. **Stomach** The stomach is frequently injured with penetrating abdominal trauma, but is infrequently injured with blunt trauma. A nasogastric (orogastric) tube should be placed after stabilization.
    —**Diagnostic** Blood in aspirate may suggest a penetrating gastric wound.
    —**Therapeutic** Decompression may lessen peritoneal soilage if a gastric wound is present.

    Note In blunt trauma, the gastric tube should not be passed until a cervical spine injury has been excluded. If a cervical spine injury is identified, a hard collar should be applied. In this case, the patient may be log-rolled, if necessary, for vomiting, which may occur as the gastric tube is passed.

    A. **Penetrating gastric injuries**

        1. **Manifestations**
            a. Abdominal pain and evidence of peritoneal irritation may be present; this is unreliable in an obtunded or head-injured patient.
            b. Blood in the gastric aspirate may be associated with a penetrating gastric wound or may represent swallowed blood in the multiply injured

patient. Ongoing fresh bleeding in a supine patient suggests a gastric source.

    c. Peritoneal penetration mandates celiotomy and exploration.

2. **Diagnosis** Upright chest x-ray or lateral decubitus abdominal x-ray may reveal pneumoperitoneum secondary to gastric perforation.

3. **Treatment** Surgical goals are to decrease further contamination, debride devitalized tissue, and close the defect.

    a. **Exploration** The entire stomach is inspected for defects. If an anterior wall penetration is encountered, the posterior gastric wall is evaluated by entering the lesser sac via the gastrocolic ligament.

    b. **Debridement** Devitalized tissue must be resected. High velocity missiles create wounds requiring wider debridement than low velocity missiles.

    c. **Closure** The gastric defect is closed in two layers. A full thickness inner layer of 2-0 or 3-0 running Dexon is imbricated by an outer row of interrupted 3-0 silk. Drainage is usually not indicated. In selected instances, an anterior gastric defect may be converted to a gastrostomy.

       Despite the relative absence of gastric flora, copious irrigation of the peritoneal cavity is indicated with perforation of the stomach.

    d. **Postoperative care**

      (1) With penetrating abdominal trauma, broad-spectrum antibiotics are administered preoperatively. Gentamicin and clindamycin or cefoxitin usually provide appropriate coverage. Continuation of antibiotics, as well as dose and frequency, are dictated by operative findings, extent of contamination, and renal function. Antibiotics are not indicated for an isolated gastric injury unless significant contamination has occurred.

      (2) Gastric decompression is continued until effective peristalsis resumes.

B. **Blunt gastric injuries** The stomach rarely receives sufficient blunt force to cause penetration of the muscular layers.

1. **Manifestations**

    a. If there is significant blood loss, the patient may be hemodynamically unstable.

    b. Full thickness gastric injury may result in local or general peritonitis.

    c. The patient may be asymptomatic.

    d. Gastric aspirate may be positive for blood.

2. **Diagnosis**

    a. Upright chest x-ray or lateral decubitus abdominal x-ray may reveal pneumoperitoneum.

    b. Peritoneal lavage may be positive for RBC, WBC, bile, or amylase.

3. **Treatment** Management is similar to that described for penetrating gastric wounds.
    a. Occasionally, the distal stomach is so destroyed that an antrectomy is required.
    b. Transection of the body or antrum can usually be debrided and closed in two layers.
    c. If a hematoma is encountered at the attachment of the greater or lesser omentum, the hematoma is evacuated and the gastric wall between the omental leaves is inspected.
    d. If a large area of omentum not adjacent to the stomach is contused, local omentectomy is performed.
    e. Bleeding from the omentum can usually be controlled by simple ligation.

VI. **Duodenum** Duodenal injuries may result from either penetrating or blunt abdominal trauma. A significant mortality and morbidity is related both to the severity of these injuries and the number of associated injuries.

  A. **Penetrating duodenal injuries** The extent and severity of penetrating duodenal trauma varies according to the type of injury, e.g., stab, gunshot, or shotgun wound.
    1. **Manifestations**
        a. **Abdominal tenderness**, particularly in the right upper quadrant, may be present in the conscious patient. **Vomiting** may be a prominent symptom. The abdominal pain and tenderness from duodenal perforation may be very severe, but a confined retroperitoneal injury may manifest initially with **few signs or symptoms.**
        b. Fever often rises within a short time (hours) after injury.

    2. **Diagnosis**
        a. If there is peritoneal penetration, celiotomy is performed and the definitive diagnosis is made.
        b. Plain x-rays may reveal pneumoperitoneum if there is free rupture, or right upper quadrant gas bubbles and loss of psoas shadow if there has been retroperitoneal rupture.
        c. Serum amylase may be elevated if there is an associated pancreatic injury, but this is not a consistent or reliable index.

    3. **Treatment**
        a. **Preoperative preparation**
            (1) A nasogastric tube should be placed prior to operation.
            (2) With any penetrating abdominal injury, preoperative antibiotics, gentamicin and clindamycin or cefoxitin, are administered to cover anaerobic and aerobic enteric organisms.
        b. **Surgery**
            (1) If a penetrating duodenal injury is suspected or found, exposure should include a Kocher maneuver as well as lesser sac explora-

tion. Exploration of the third and fourth portions of the duodenum may be obtained by incising the right peritoneal attachment of the colon and reflecting it upward with its mesentery.

(2) Specific management of a duodenal wound depends on the size of the defect. The primary operative principle is to obtain closure of the defect without compromising the duodenal lumen.

(3) Following debridement, a small duodenal defect is closed in two layers. The inner layer is a full thickness 3-0 synthetic absorbable polyester suture, such as Vicryl or Dexon. The outer layer is a seromuscular closure of 3-0 or 4-0 silk.

(4) If a direct two-layer repair will not suffice because of integrity of the closure, size of the defect, or stenosis of the duodenal lumen, another technique is utilized:

(a) A segment of jejunum is "patched" to the duodenal defect. This is a retrocolic approach via the right transverse mesocolon. An inner layer of absorbable suture is used for the duodenal edge and seromuscular layer of jejunum. The outer layer consists of nonabsorbable suture as a seromuscular closure to both jejunum and duodenum.

(b) A Roux-en-Y technique may be used, anastomosing a defunctionalized segment of jejunum to the duodenal defect.

(c) A duodenal diverticulization procedure can be performed for a duodenal injury associated with a major pancreatic injury. This includes: repair of the duodenal perforation, periduodenal drainage, tube duodenostomy, truncal vagotomy, hemigastrectomy, and gastrojejunostomy.

(d) A pancreatico-duodenectomy is only indicated for devascularization of the duodenum or head of the pancreas.

(5) Drainage of duodenal wounds is accomplished by Penrose drains adjacent to but not in direct contact with suture lines.

(6) Operative management of duodenal injuries includes inspection to evaluate any associated biliary injury.

(7) The presence of a penetrating duodenal injury mandates a thorough evaluation of the pancreas.

(8) Duodenal decompression is important to allow the wound to heal. The following are modes of "duodenal decompression":

(a) Decompression with a gastrostomy or orogastric tube
(b) Transpyloric (antegrade) duodenal decompression
(c) Transduodenal Foley catheter
(d) Retrograde jejunostomy

c. **Postoperative management**

(1) Duodenal decompression is usually continued for at least 5–7 days postoperatively. We recommend the insertion of a feeding catheter jejunostomy at the time of surgery. Elemental feedings may be started via the jejunostomy while duodenal decompression continues.

(2) The need for postoperative antibiotics is guided by the extent of contamination at operation and the interval between injury and operation. (See p. 156.)

B. **Blunt duodenal injuries**   Blunt trauma to the abdomen may result in duodenal injury ranging from intramural hematoma to rupture of the duodenum. We have seen rupture of the duodenum resulting from both vehicular and personal trauma.

1. **Manifestations**
   a. Abdominal **pain and tenderness** in the right upper quadrant may be seen. **Vomiting** may be a prominent symptom with duodenal injury. If there has been free rupture into the peritoneal cavity, early signs of **peritonitis** may be evident, whereas a retroperitoneal rupture may manifest in a much more **subtle clinical picture**. Pain referred to the right groin and testicle should raise the suspicion of a duodenal injury.
   b. **Fever** may rise within a short interval following duodenal rupture.
   c. Extensive third space loss from peritoneal soilage may result in **hemodynamic instability**, if significant time has elapsed since injury.
   d. Because the clinical picture is so variable, and the consequences of a delayed diagnosis so severe, any patient with right upper quadrant pain and tenderness following blunt abdominal trauma should be suspected of having a duodenal injury.

2. **Diagnosis**
   a. A flat abdominal x-ray and an upright chest x-ray are obtained prior to peritoneal lavage. The intent of this sequence is to prevent confusion regarding the finding of a pneumoperitoneum, i.e., to decide whether this is extraluminal bowel gas or air introduced during lavage. Pneumoperitoneum may be seen with duodenal rupture, but its absence does not exclude injury. Radiographic evidence of duodenal rupture includes air bubbles in the right upper quadrant, particularly along the upper pole of the right kidney, and loss of the psoas shadow. Large bowel ileus may be an early finding.
   b. Contrast radiography with water-soluble medium is useful in demonstrating a duodenal injury. If fluoroscopy is not available, a right lateral decubitus x-ray is obtained after the instillation of 200–300 cc of Gastrografin via the nasogastric tube. A secure airway must be ensured prior to this procedure, since aspiration of Gastrografin can result in severe bronchospasm and pulmonary edema. Demonstration of contrast outside the duodenum is diagnostic and mandates exploration. Gastric outlet obstruction may be identified secondary to an intramural duodenal hematoma.
   c. Peritoneal lavage may demonstrate the presence of bile or elevated amylase if there has been intraperitoneal duodenal rupture. If the rupture is retroperitoneal, peritoneal lavage can be entirely normal.

d. Duodenal injury may be identified at the time of laparotomy for another injury.

e. Initially, the abdomen may be asymptomatic on examination and by peritoneal lavage. The later development of a symptomatic abdomen will usually lead to evaluation by contrast study or laparotomy, at which time the diagnosis is secured.

f. Leukocytosis and elevation of serum amylase may occur, but neither is specific or diagnostic.

3. Treatment

a. **Nonoperative management**   If an intramural hematoma of the duodenum is diagnosed by contrast radiography, nonoperative management including prolonged gastric suction and intravenous alimentation may be elected. This choice implies that the patient is stable, can be monitored closely, and has no other indication for abdominal exploration.

b. **Operative management**

(1) If a duodenal injury has not been suspected preoperatively, a Kocher maneuver and lesser sac exploration is performed if

(a) There is evidence of a bile leak

(b) Bubbles, gas, or a glassy appearance is noted in the retroperitoneum or right colic gutter

(c) There is a hematoma near the duodenum

(2) Once the duodenum has been exposed, it may be difficult to identify a small duodenal rupture. If this is the case, the nasogastric tube can be advanced into the duodenum, the distal duodenum occluded by finger pressure, and saline or methylene blue instilled into the tube. Egress of saline or methylene blue will then demonstrate a duodenal rupture that otherwise might not be detected.

(3) An intramural duodenal hematoma found at operation is explored, evacuated, and evaluated to ensure that the mucosa is intact. The serosa is then closed with interrupted nonabsorbable suture.

(4) The specific operative management of blunt duodenal injuries resulting in rupture is the same as outlined for the management of penetrating duodenal wounds.

VII. **Small Intestine**   Small bowel injuries may result from blunt or penetrating trauma.

A. **Penetrating small intestinal injuries**

1. **Manifestations**   Abdominal pain and evidence of peritoneal irritation in a patient with penetrating abdominal trauma commonly reflects the presence of a small bowel injury. A significant small bowel leak may lead to pain with local or generalized **peritonitis**. There may be **shock** from injury to a major mesenteric vessel or third space loss. The patient may be relatively **asymptomatic,** in which case the lesion is identified at laparotomy, when the bowel is carefully examined.

2. **Diagnosis** Upright and decubitus x-rays of the chest and abdomen may or may not reveal pneumoperitoneum. Small bowel ileus may be seen on x-ray, if there has been a significant lapse in time.

3. **Treatment**
   a. **Preoperative preparation** This includes gastric decompression and the intravenous administration of gentamicin and clindamycin or cefoxitin.
   b. **Surgery**
      (1) Low velocity small bowel injuries are managed by debridement and two-layer closure, using an inner layer of chromic and an outer layer of silk. Multiple injuries in a segment of bowel are better treated by resection and anastomosis than by multiple closures.
      (2) High velocity injuries require wider resection.
      (3) When direct closure of a defect would compromise the bowel lumen, resection and anastomosis are performed.
      (4) Drainage is usually not indicated.
      (5) Mesenteric defects are closed to prevent internal herniation.
      (6) For a discussion of peritoneal irrigation, see p. 156.
      (7) If there has been gross ileal contamination, especially if surgery has been delayed, delayed primary wound closure is advisable.
   c. **Postoperative care**
      (1) Antibiotics are continued for 3–5 days if the lesion involves the distal ileum, if there is a significant degree of contamination, or if there has been a significant lapse in time since the injury.
      (2) Gastric decompression is continued until peristalsis resumes.

B. **Blunt small intestinal injuries**

1. **Manifestations** Except for the history of the injury, the presentation of a patient with small bowel injury secondary to blunt abdominal trauma is essentially like that of a patient with a penetrating small bowel injury. The clinical picture can range from **peritonitis** or **shock** to a patient who is **asymptomatic.**

2. **Diagnosis**
   a. Abdominal radiographs and upright chest x-ray may reveal pneumoperitoneum.
   b. Peritoneal lavage may reveal amylase or bile if free rupture has occurred, or hemoperitoneum if there has been significant associated injury. Elevation of leukocyte count in the lavage reflects an inflammatory response. Lavage may be "normal" early in the course of a blunt small bowel injury.

   Note If the abdomen is cleared initially, yet peritonitis eventuates, laparotomy is indicated. If "abdominal findings" short of peritonitis develop, re-lavage is indicated.

3. **Treatment** See p. 162.
   a. **Surgery**
      (1) Full perforation of the small intestine by blunt injury should be managed by resection and two-layer anastomosis.
      (2) An isolated serosal lesion is treated by primary closure.
      (3) Small bowel contusion poses a hazard, since there is a risk of necrosis with subsequent perforation. The actual injury may be larger than is initially apparent. Small contusions (1 cm or less) can be imbricated with silk or left alone. Resection is indicated for larger areas of contusion.
      (4) Mesenteric defects are closed to prevent internal herniation.
      (5) Mesenteric hematomas require evacuation and exploration if they are major, expanding, or compromising the bowel blood supply.
      (6) Distal ileal injuries (within 12 inches of the ileocecal valve) should usually be managed by a right hemicolectomy, since suture line disruption of an ileo-ileal anastomosis is likely to occur.
   b. **Postoperative care**
      (1) Gastric decompression is continued until effective peristalsis resumes.
      (2) Antibiotic considerations are discussed on p. 156.

Perspective
If the patient develops any instability following a small bowel anastomosis, the abdominal wound should be opened and/or the peritoneal cavity should be explored in order to exclude an abscess and/or anastomotic disruption. A delay in detecting these complications is highly lethal.

VIII. **Colon** Colon injuries are associated with a relatively high morbidity and mortality because of the bacterial content of the large bowel. The prevention of septic sequelae related to colonic injuries mandates early diagnosis and treatment. Colonic injuries may occur secondary to penetrating or blunt trauma.

A. **Penetrating colon injuries**

1. **Manifestations**
   a. **Abdominal pain** and evidence of **peritoneal irritation** may be present, depending on the patient's sensorium and extent of peritoneal contamination.
   b. Initially, the abdomen may be **asymptomatic**; the lesion is identified during laparotomy for a wound that penetrates the peritoneum.

2. **Diagnosis** Pneumoperitoneum may be evident radiographically, but lack of this sign does not rule out colonic injury.

3. **Treatment**
   a. **Preoperative** preparation of a patient with a penetrating abdominal wound includes antibiotic administration to cover anaerobic and aerobic organisms. Our choice is gentamicin and clindamycin or cefoxitin.
   b. **Surgery**
      (1) There are several operative **options** and no single correct answer for the management of all penetrating colonic wounds.
         (a) Primary closure of the wound or resection and anastomosis (least conservative)
         (b) Closure of the colonic wound and exteriorization, with return of the sutured colon to the peritoneal cavity in 5–7 days
         (c) Exteriorization of the wound as a loop colostomy, or resection of involved bowel with proximal end colostomy and distal mucous fistula or Hartmann's pouch (most conservative)
      (2) The choice of operation cannot be dictated in advance and must be judged individually. Some factors that increase the likelihood of septic complications are
         (a) Shock which has been present or is continuing
         (b) Significant time lapse from the time of injury to operation
         (c) Gunshot or shotgun wounds as opposed to knife or ice pick wounds
         (d) Gross contamination
         (e) The presence of other intra-abdominal injuries
         (f) The presence of multisystem injuries which require urgent intervention
         (g) Patients over 50 years of age are more susceptible to complications related to colon injuries.
         The higher the number of risk factors, the more conservative the therapy.
      (3) In making the operative decision, it should be remembered that although a colostomy is a form of disability, a temporary colostomy is far better tolerated than gangrenous injured bowel or an anastomotic leak with the subsequent development of intra-abdominal sepsis.
      (4) A severe ileocecal injury may be better managed by resection and ileotransverse anastomosis, as opposed to an ileostomy.
      (5) In all cases of colonic injury, the peritoneum should be cleared of all gross contamination, and irrigated with saline.
      (6) Mesenteric defects should be closed to prevent internal herniation.
      (7) Mesenteric hematomas are discussed on p. 184.
      (8) If there is gross peritoneal contamination, delayed primary wound closure is advisable.

c. **Postoperative care**
  (1) Antibiotics should be continued for 3–5 days, depending on the extent of injury and contamination.
  (2) Gastric decompression should continue until peristalsis resumes.
  (3) The patient should be closely observed for evidence of sepsis (see pp. 185 and 369).

B. **Blunt colon injuries** Complete perforation of the colon from blunt trauma is rare. Serosal tears, often of the cecum, are less unusual.

  1. **Manifestations** **Abdominal pain** and **peritoneal signs** may be present. A serosal tear is not uncommonly an incidental finding during celiotomy for another indication.

  2. **Diagnosis** Peritoneal lavage may demonstrate hemoperitoneum associated with colonic wall damage. Bacteria, an elevated leukocyte count, or vegetable fiber may be identified in the lavage if there has been full thickness disruption. Peritoneal lavage may be positive because of other lesions, and the colonic injury may be found incidentally.

  3. **Treatment**
    a. **Surgery**
      (1) Uncomplicated serosal tears are repaired primarily.
      (2) Mesenteric defects should be closed to prevent internal herniation.
      (3) Severe colon contusion or mesenteric disruption associated with colonic ischemia should prompt resection.
      (4) Principles of operative management are the same as those described for penetrating colonic injuries.
    b. **Postoperative care** is the same as described for penetrating wounds.

IX. **Rectum** Rectal injuries may result from penetrating or blunt trauma. Early recognition and management are necessary to minimize septic sequelae.

A. **Penetrating rectal injuries**

  1. **Manifestations**
    a. Because of the unpredictability of a missile path, a rectal injury should be considered with any lower abdominal or pelvic penetrating wound. **Abdominal pain** and **generalized tenderness** may or may not be present, depending on the level of injury in relation to the peritoneal reflection, the extent of contamination, and associated injuries. **Rectal tenderness** and the finding of **blood on rectal examination** should raise the suspicion of injury.
    b. **Laboratory data** Leukocytosis may be present, but obviously is not specific for a rectal injury.

2. **Diagnosis**
   a. Radiographic evaluation may be helpful in suggesting that the path of a missile transversed the rectum.
   b. Proctosigmoidoscopy defines the anatomy of the rectal injury.
   c. Celiotomy is indicated for a penetrating wound of the peritoneum and/or a known diagnosis of rectal injury. The pathology is better delineated at the time of celiotomy.

3. **Treatment**
   a. **Preoperative** preparation of a patient suspected of having a rectal injury includes the administration of antibiotics (gentamicin and clindamycin or cefoxitin) to cover aerobic and anaerobic organisms.
   b. **Operative** management of a penetrating rectal wound includes the following:
      (1) A proximal diverting end colostomy is made.
      (2) A distal mucous fistula or Hartmann's pouch is formed.
      (3) The abdominal wound is closed and dressed.
      (4) The colostomy and mucous fistula are matured.
      (5) The rectum is thoroughly irrigated to remove fecal content.
      (6) The rectal wound is closed, if this is feasible.
      (7) If the wound is large, it is drained through the perineum.
   c. **Postoperative care**
      (1) Gastric decompression is continued until effective peristalsis resumes.
      (2) Clindamycin and gentamicin or cefoxitin are continued for 3–5 days.

B. **Blunt rectal injuries**

1. **Manifestations** Patients with severe pelvic fractures may suffer rectal injuries, which are **overlooked** unless specifically sought. A rectal examination should be performed in all patients with blunt trauma, especially if a pelvic fracture is present. Rectal examination may reveal **blood in the rectum**, frank disruption of the rectal wall and communication with the bony pelvis, or the presence of a urinary catheter within the rectum.

2. **Diagnosis**
   a. Proctosigmoidoscopy should be performed in patients when blood is identified during rectal examination. Whether or not blood is found on rectal examination, endoscopy should be considered in all patients with a severe pelvic fracture.
   b. Contrast enema may be indicated in selected cases.
   c. Peritoneal lavage may be positive (WBC, bacteria, vegetable fibers, RBC) if the injury extends above the level of the peritoneal reflection.

3. **Treatment** The treatment of blunt trauma to the rectum is the same as that outlined for penetrating rectal trauma.
   a. Perineal wounds should be widely debrided and closed in a delayed manner.

b. Occasionally, rectal trauma is so severe that a proctectomy must be performed.

(See p. 194.)

X. Liver This section is a guideline for the methodical intraoperative management of hepatic trauma. There are two major concerns with liver injuries:

—Control of bleeding
—Prevention of intra-abdominal abscess formation

The primary cause of death related to hepatic injuries is exsanguinating hemorrhage. The second major cause of death is intra- or extra-abdominal sepsis. In approximately 10–15% of liver injuries, the trauma is severe and the mortality rate extraordinary. The key to managing most liver trauma is selectivity of therapy based on the entities involved: hepatic veins, retrohepatic vena cava, hepatic arterial tributaries, portal venous tributaries, biliary radicles, and hepatic parenchymal damage.

General principles of traumatic liver surgery are as follows:

—Incision which allows adequate exposure
—Control of hemorrhage
—Debridement of devitalized tissue
—Control of biliary ductal leakage
—Evacuation of blood, bile, and parenchymal slough in the postoperative period, if necessary.

This discussion is concerned primarily with blunt liver trauma, but the principles relating to penetrating hepatic trauma are, in general, the same.

A. Classification of liver injuries

1. Depth
    a. Superficial
    b. Deep

2. Configuration
    a. Linear
    b. Fracture
    c. Bursting

3. Location
    a. Peripheral
    b. Central

4. Hemorrhage
    a. None
    b. Moderate
    c. Severe

[Note] In general, under each category above, **a** indicates the least degree of injury.

B. Intraoperative management

1. Incisions (exposure is of utmost importance)
   a. **Midline abdominal**
      (1) Extended into right chest
      (2) Extended into median sternotomy
   b. **Epigastric transverse**
      (1) Extended laterally
      (2) Extended into a median sternotomy

2. Control of hemorrhage
   a. **Temporary packing** for 10–15 min is often sufficient to gain hemostasis.
   b. **Manual compression of the liver** is the initial step to control bleeding.
   c. **Control of portal triad** will control bleeding from hepatic arterial or portal venous sources.
      (1) **Digital control**
      (2) Vascular clamp
      (3) Romel tourniquet
   d. **Liver clamp** will control bleeding from peripheral branches of the hepatic veins, portal veins, and/or hepatic arteries.
   e. **Suture control**
      (1) Individual ligation of bleeding vessel (ideal hemostatic measure)
      (2) Sutures parallel to wound for vascular compression (less ideal than individual ligation, but may be necessary if the vessels cannot be seen)
   f. **Hemostatic agents** to control minimal oozing
   g. **Fulguration**
   h. **Ligation of the left or right hepatic artery** is performed if its compression slows the bleeding and **other techniques are not successful.**
   i. **Hemoclips** for control of individual bleeding points
   j. Prevent or treat **coagulopathy** early with component therapy and rapid obtainment of hemostasis.
   k. Prevent or treat **hypothermia** early.
   l. **Incision adjacent to the hepatic wound** to locate and control hidden, deep hemorrhage
   m. Vascular isolation with **intracaval shunt** (see p. 169)

3. Debridement of devitalized tissue
   a. **Finger fracture technique is performed adjacent to the wound (non-anatomical resection).**
   b. **Formal lobectomy** is seldom indicated unless
      (1) There is massive hemorrhage from the left or right lobe
      (2) There is massive destruction of the left or right lobe
      (3) Access to the retrohepatic vena cava is necessary.

4. Control of biliary ductal leakage
   a. **T-tube drainage** of the common bile duct is not indicated.

b. **Direct ligation** of biliary radicles

c. **Perihepatic drainage**

5. **Postoperative drainage of blood, bile, and parenchymal slough**

   a. Need for **selectivity**   We tend to drain only the moderate to severe injuries.

   b. **Passive drains** (Penrose)

   c. Soft, active **sump drains** preferred

   d. **Second-look operation**   This is used when the surgeon is not satisfied that nonviable tissue was resected or that hemostasis was well controlled. (See p. 149.)

   e. **Twelfth rib resection with drains**   This is usually reserved for a second-look procedure.

C. **Ancillary considerations**

1. **Vascular access**   Due to "kinking" of the inferior vena cava during surgery, blood return to the right heart may be decreased. We suggest using supradiaphragmatic lines; large bore catheters (Swan-Ganz **introducer sheaths** in each subclavian or internal jugular vein).

2. **Exposure**   This should be attained very early during the operation and should be optimal. A BUMP under the right torso usually improves exposure. Take down the liver completely by incising the triangular, falciform, and/or coronary ligaments.

3. **One member of the team** should direct the conduct of the operation (the senior surgeon). One surgeon should be solely responsible for controlling hemorrhage from the liver wound.

4. **Anesthesia support**   Before attempting to control the liver pathology definitively, give the anesthesia staff time to replace the blood loss each time there is a major drop in pressure. Use autotransfused blood and liberal amounts of fresh frozen plasma (FFP) and platelets.

5. **Intracaval shunts**   Caval shunts are indicated only if the hepatic veins or retrohepatic cava are torn. Injury to the retrohepatic cava and/or central hepatic veins is suspected when compression of the porta hepatis fails to control hemorrhage; this assessment should be made early during the exploration. The shunt, which is rarely successful, can be homemade or purchased. We recommend placement via a median sternotomy through the right atrial appendage. Hemorrhage must be controlled by manual compression **before** shunt insertion is attempted. We have had very little success with managing these injuries even with the intracaval shunt.

6. **Devascularization procedures**   If compressing the portal triad controls bleeding, selective ligation of the left or right hepatic artery or portal vein may be used to control bleeding. The liver has usually suffered an ischemic insult due to shock. Ligation of a major portal venous or hepatic arterial

branch will lead to a second ischemic insult. If **other techniques** of hemostasis are unsuccessful, central ligation of the offending vessel is performed. **Remember**, hepatic bleeding comes from three main sources:

a. Hepatic artery
b. Portal vein
c. Retrograde from the hepatic veins or vena cava.

Ligation of the left or right hepatic artery will not stop bleeding from the cava or portal vein.

7. **Subcapsular hematomas** Avoid the temptation to unroof these hematomas. If the hematoma is unroofed, you may have to selectively ligate the hepatic arterial branch to control bleeding. Postoperative arteriography and embolic tamponade are usually safer than the surgical approach.

8. **Major resections** The remaining hepatic segment must have intact hepatic venous and biliary drainage.

9. **Avoid iatrogenesis** Do not probe a nonbleeding wound. Do not use hepatostomy tubes. Sutures are not necessary in the normotensive patient who is not bleeding from a liver injury.

10. **Equipment** A liver pack should be previously assembled and contain shunts, liver clamps, special sutures, Romel tourniquets, etc.

| Note | Frequently, patients are hypotensive on admission, but stabilize after volume infusion. Aggressive clot removal or mobilization and rough handling of the liver may be associated with torrential hemorrhage.

D. **Postoperative complications**

1. **Hemorrhage**
   a. Arteriography with embolic tamponade
   b. Laparotomy

2. **Hemobilia**
   a. Arteriography for anatomic localization and possible embolic tamponade
   b. Laparotomy with resection or selective arterial ligation

3. **Sepsis**
   a. Identify abdominal versus extra-abdominal source
   b. Inflammation versus infection (see p. 369)
   c. Antibiotics to control systemic instability
   d. Liver scan to detect a hepatic defect
   e. CAT scan with needle aspiration to assess intra- and extrahepatic fluid collections
   f. Drainage of abscess
   (See p. 185.)

4. **Hepatic dysfunction**
   a. Prevent hypoxia.
   b. "Moderate" nutritional support. (Total parenteral nutrition is a metabolic stress to liver.)
   c. Stabilize cardiovascular function.
   d. Serial coagulation, glucose and albumin determinations; supplement the patient, if necessary.
   e. Classic liver failure is uncommon unless a major resection has been performed (see p. 359).

5. **Multiple systems failure**   See p. 369.

XI. **Extrahepatic Biliary System**   Injury to the extrahepatic biliary tree may occur secondary to blunt or penetrating trauma. The clinical management entails
   —Making the diagnosis
   —Correcting the anatomic injury
   —Treating associated injuries

A. **Structures involved**

   1. Gallbladder

   2. Cystic duct

   3. Hepatic ducts

   4. Common hepatic duct

   5. Common bile duct

B. **Diagnosis** may be made by incidental finding during laparotomy for another injury, peritoneal lavage positive for bile, or delayed diagnosis.

   1. **Early posttraumatic period**   During laparotomy, the diagnosis is suspected or confirmed by
      a. Bile staining in the region of the porta hepatis
      b. Direct inspection of the biliary structures
      c. Intraoperative cholangiogram

   2. **Late posttraumatic period**   The patient may not have had a laparotomy initially or the injury may have been missed at surgery. The patient may present with
      a. Jaundice
      b. Sepsis
      c. Peritonitis
      d. Ascites
      e. Acholic stools
      f. A leak or stricture of the extrahepatic ducts, as revealed by a cholangiogram or hepatobiliary scanning.
      The specific diagnosis may be made preoperatively or during laparotomy.

C. **Intraoperative management** There are many surgical techniques available, and that technique should be used that best suits the surgeon's experience.

1. **Gallbladder** The injured gallbladder should be removed unless it is needed for an associated ductal injury.

2. **Common bile duct** Biliary-enteric drainage should be reconstituted.
   a. Direct repair or anastomosis of the ductal system is preferred, when possible. A major repair is usually stented by passing one arm of a T-tube through the duodenum and into the common duct.
   b. Bypass procedures
      (1) Cholecystojejunostomy (preferred)
      (2) Choledochojejunostomy via Roux-en-Y or with an enteroenterostomy
      (3) Choledochoduodenostomy

3. **Hepatic duct**
   a. The hepatic duct is repaired and stented, if possible.
   b. The duct may be anastomosed to a loop of jejunum.
   c. If the duct cannot be repaired, it may be ligated. After the ducts dilate, they may be decompressed via percutaneous catheterization.

Perspective

The common bile duct is usually stented after primary repair of a major injury or the performance of a choledochoenteric anastomosis. The stent should not be removed until the tube is clamped for 72 hr and
   —The patient is afebrile.
   —The patient is eating and has no postprandial pain.
   —Cholangiography reveals biliary decompression.

Short-term antibiotics may be beneficial with biliary tract injuries.

D. **Complications**

1. Suture line disruption

2. Ductal stricture
   a. Ascending cholangitis
   b. Biliary cirrhosis

XII. **Pancreas** The pancreas may be injured secondary to blunt or penetrating trauma. Pancreatic injuries, in general, are uncommon following blunt trauma. In reviewing 600 consecutive cases of exploratory laparotomy for blunt trauma, only one case of pancreatic injury was identified. Since we explore all penetrating peritoneal injuries, the diagnosis of pancreatic injury in this situation is made early. On the other hand, pancreatic injury secondary to blunt trauma may be very deceptive in the early hours following injury due to its retroperitoneal location and paucity of early symptoms.

A. Manifestations

1. **Penetrating injuries** There are usually no specific manifestations following penetrating injury to the pancreas. The patient with penetrating abdominal trauma may present without major symptoms or signs, or may present with variable manifestations of peritonitis and/or shock. In our institution, penetrating peritoneal wounds mandate celiotomy.

2. **Blunt injuries**
   a. **Early** In the first couple of hours following blunt abdominal trauma, the patient may be totally **asymptomatic**. On the other hand, the patient may present with upper **abdominal pain and/or tenderness**, but this is relatively unusual. The patient may have a symptomatic abdomen secondary to **intraperitoneal visceral or vascular injury**. If the patient is unconscious, it is virtually impossible to identify isolated pancreatic trauma secondary to blunt injury in the early hours following trauma.
   b. **Late** The patient may develop symptoms or signs in 12–36 hr following injury. Manifestations of pancreatic injury at this time may consist of **epigastric pain, tenderness, or guarding**. Later, the patient may develop manifestations of **ileus, cardiovascular instability, respiratory insufficiency, and/or sepsis**. If the patient is unconscious, a longer period of time may pass before manifestations of pancreatic injury are detected.

B. Diagnosis

1. **Serum amylase** If a patient has an elevated serum amylase and abdominal tenderness, celiotomy is recommended. An isolated elevation of the serum amylase without associated abdominal symptomatology is not an indication for celiotomy. If the initial amylase value is normal or elevated and subsequent values approximately 6 hr later are rising or persistently elevated, celiotomy should be strongly considered, especially if there is associated abdominal pain.

2. **Peritoneal lavage** The peritoneal lavage is usually negative if the patient has isolated pancreatic injury. If there is significant intraperitoneal pathology, the peritoneal lavage is positive.

3. **Manifestations of upper abdominal trauma** A high index of suspicion for associated pancreatic injury should be maintained in patients who have manifestations of upper abdominal trauma. Manifestations of upper abdominal trauma are
   a. Ecchymosis of the upper abdomen or flanks
   b. A spinal fracture at the T_{11}/L_2 level
   c. Lower rib fractures

4. **X-ray** There are no early, specific radiographic manifestations of isolated pancreatic trauma. Later, abdominal radiography may reveal manifestations of ileus and/or extraluminal gas formation if a phlegmon is developing in the region of the pancreas.

C. **Management** Principles in the management of pancreatic trauma are
   —Prompt operative intervention
   —Resection of devitalized tissue
   —Adequate external drainage
   —Control of hemorrhage

Almost all pancreatic injuries can be managed by control of hemorrhage with sutures and external drainage. In general, all pancreatic injuries should be drained with the exception of minor contusions.

If the patient is explored and a pancreatic injury is suspected, the pancreas should be visualized by entering the lesser sac. Routine mobilization of the pancreas is not advisable. We advise mobilization of the pancreas only when there is obvious parenchymal disruption. If there is a peripancreatic hematoma and the parenchyma is grossly intact, the peritoneal surface over the pancreas should be incised and the pancreas externally drained.

1. **Body and tail** Minor wounds of the body or tail of the pancreas are best managed by obtaining hemostasis and external drainage. Major wounds of the body or tail of the pancreas, i.e., parenchymal disruption, are best managed by distal pancreatectomy. When a distal pancreatectomy is performed, the major pancreatic duct should be identified and ligated. External drainage should be performed following resection.

2. **Head** Almost all injuries to the head of the pancreas may be managed by controlling hemorrhage with suture ligatures and securing external drainage. A pancreaticoduodenectomy is rarely indicated for injuries to the head of the pancreas, but should be reserved for injuries which result in devitalization and devascularization of the head of the pancreas or duodenum.

   Note Small penetrating knife wounds may be closed with sutures and drained externally.

3. **Drainage** We recommend the use of Penrose and soft sump drains for the drainage of pancreatic injuries. The sump vent should have a bacterial filter. We suggest bringing the sump and Penrose drains out of the same stab wound. The Penrose drain and sump drain should be individually secured to tissue adjacent to the pancreas with a 5-0 chromic suture. Suturing the sump drain prevents dislodgment of the tube from the pancreas and prevents erosion into adjacent structures. Suturing the Penrose drain will prevent dislodgment from its appropriate position. If the patient develops pancreatic drainage through the sump tube, the tube should be left in position until drainage terminates. If the patient develops drainage along the Penrose drain and not through the sump, the sump drain should be withdrawn.

If there is no drainage along the Penrose drain or through the sump drain, the drains are removed at 5–7 days. Allowing the drains to remain in site for a longer period of time may result in bacterial colonization of the abdominal cavity.

D. **Complications**   The most common complications following pancreatic injury are

1. Fistula

2. Pseudocyst

3. Delayed hemorrhage

4. Abscess formation

Pancreatic fistulization is a relatively common sequel when major pancreatic injuries are drained. Most fistulae will close spontaneously in a period of about 6 weeks. During this time the skin should be protected against excoriation, and electrolyte and fluid losses must be replaced. A persistent, high-output fistula may require pancreaticojejunostomy. Nutritional support should be maintained by feeding catheter jejunostomy or total parenteral nutrition.

A pseudocyst may occur after pancreatic trauma. If the patient develops abdominal pain and/or an abdominal mass, an ultrasound evaluation should be performed. If the patient develops a pseudocyst, internal drainage is usually required.

A pancreatic abscess may develop following pancreatic injury; the clinical result is an unstable postoperative course. The patient may develop fever, leukocytosis, and evidence of systemic stress and/or multiple systems failure. Abdominal x-rays may reveal air fluid levels and/or gas in the retroperitoneal tissues. Ultrasonography and CAT scanning may assist in the diagnosis. Generally, the patient's septic appearance, in the setting of previous pancreatic injury, will suggest the diagnosis and lead to celiotomy. External drainage, broad-spectrum antibiotic therapy, and cardiovascular and pulmonary support are necessary.

Perspective
We emphasize that blunt pancreatic injury is a relatively rare entity. In the majority of cases, pancreatic injuries are managed by adequate debridement, hemostasis, and external drainage. Distal pancreatectomy is the procedure of choice in major pancreatic injuries involving the body and tail of the pancreas. Pancreaticoduodenectomy has a limited role in the management of pancreatic trauma.

XIII. **Urinary Tract**   Most urologic injuries should be recognized soon after admission or early in the hospital course, if one maintains a high index of suspicion for them. The mode of injury, certain symptoms, physical findings, and roentgenographic evidence should arouse suspicion.

Any patient sustaining blunt trauma from a fall, motor vehicular crash, a crush, or other significant traumatic insult is suspect. Particular attention should be focused on patients sustaining trauma to the torso (especially in the back and flanks) and the pelvis. Any penetrating injury could conceivably involve the urinary tract. Any patient suffering a straddle injury may have a urologic injury.

A. **Manifestations**

    1. **Symptoms**
       a. Abdominal pain
       b. Back and/or flank pain
       c. Inability to void

    2. **Signs**
       a. Hypotension, tachycardia, i.e., signs of shock
       b. Evidence of torso and/or pelvic trauma (particularly an open or unstable pelvic fracture)
       c. Abdominal tenderness with or without distention
       d. Flank tenderness with or without flank discoloration and/or a mass
       e. Evidence of perineal trauma, including ecchymosis, lacerations, and hematoma
       f. Signs of a dislocated hip
       g. Hematuria
       h. Blood at the urethral meatus
       i. A rectal examination revealing a palpable, boggy prostatic mass or a "high riding" or "absent" prostate
       j. Absence of urine output after catheterization of the urinary bladder
       k. Difficulty in passing a urethral catheter

    3. **Simple roentgenogram findings suggesting urologic trauma**
       a. Abdominal flat plate
          (1) Absent renal outline (this may be a normal finding)
          (2) Obliteration of psoas shadows. They will be absent in about 7.5% of normal patients. If a psoas shadow is absent and the lower pole of the kidney on the same side is not seen, a hematoma is likely.
          (3) Fracture of the lower ribs
          (4) Fracture of the lumbar vertebrae and/or transverse processes of L_1 or L_2
       b. A pelvis roentgenogram showing a fracture, particularly of the pubic symphysis or a Malgaigne's fracture (a disruption of both anterior and posterior elements of the pelvic ring)

    4. **Specific findings and their augmented roentgenographic investigation** A host of the preceding symptoms, signs, and simple x-ray findings are nonspecific and may or may not be associated with urologic trauma; however,

certain factors have a high incidence of association with urinary tract injury and must be evaluated. These include

a. **Hematuria** Although hematuria is usually associated with urinary tract injury, in 2–20% of cases even microscopic hematuria may not be present, including one-half to one-third of pedicle injuries. The degree of hematuria may not correlate with the degree of injury. In general, hematuria should be evaluated with an intravenous pyelogram (IVP) and cystogram. The IVP should be done first because extravasation from a cystogram may obscure a lower ureteral injury.

(1) **Intravenous pyelography** Ideally, IVP should be performed in the x-ray suite with the assistance of tomographic technique. Unless the patient is completely stable and not endangered by transport, an IVP should be performed in the Admitting Area. Generally, an IVP of poor quality or without visualization will be obtained in the shock patient; however, if a pressure of at least 70 mm Hg systolic is obtained, a urogram may be obtained. Emergency IVP may reveal

(a) Normal renal shadows

(b) Absent unilateral renal shadow
  i.   May be congenital
  ii. May represent a pedicle injury
  iii. May represent major renal destruction

(c) Partial visualization of a renal shadow, i.e., avascular segment of kidney

(d) Nonvisualization, bilateral, usually due to shock

(e) Dye extravasation
  i.   Major
  ii. Minor
  For technique, see p. 32.

(2) **Cystogram** A cystogram is usually indicated as part of the evaluation of hematuria and/or a major pelvic fracture. If the patient is awake and complains of pain during gentle injection, stop and obtain an x-ray to check for extravasation (see p. 32).

(3) **Indications for renal arteriography**

(a) Absent or poor unilateral visualization on IVP

(b) Renal injury is suspected and the patient requires other angiography such as for diagnosis of a ruptured aorta

(c) Uncertainty regarding the need to explore the kidney

b. **A bloody meatal discharge or inability to void** Meatal blood or inability to void is highly suggestive of a urethral injury. In either case, a urinary bladder catheter **should not** be placed until a urethrogram is obtained. Other factors suggestive of a urethral injury include bleeding around a previously placed urinary bladder catheter, poor function of such a catheter, history of a straddle injury, or perineal ecchymosis.

One of two **urethrographic techniques** is used. Without previous bladder catheterization, 15 cc of one-half strength diatrizoate sodium

(Renografin) mixed with either normal saline or sterile lubricant is slowly injected and a roentgenogram is obtained. Ideally, the patient should be placed in an oblique position. Alternatively, leave the urinary bladder catheter in place and inject contrast material within the urethra next to the catheter.

> **Note** In the patient without evidence of urethral injury in whom difficulty is encountered passing a urinary bladder catheter, obtain a urethrogram and urologic consultation.

5. **Peritoneal lavage and urinary tract injury** Peritoneal lavage should be liberally used in diagnosing intra-abdominal injury. Certain injuries defy detection by lavage, particularly those located extraperitoneally such as injury to the kidneys, ureter, and bladder. Unless associated intra-abdominal injury results in a positive lavage, negative results may be obtained despite the presence of a significant urinary tract injury. With intra-abdominal ruptures of the urinary bladder, a sudden increase in the urinary output may be noted during peritoneal lavage. Confirmation of such a communication can be obtained by adding a small amount of sterile methylene blue to an additional amount of lavage solution and observing for its drainage from the urethral catheter.

B. **Specific urinary tract injuries: Diagnosis and management**

1. **Kidney** Injury to the kidney is usually confirmed by roentgenographic techniques during the evaluation of hematuria and/or flank signs and symptoms. Less often, diagnosis is first made at exploratory laparotomy.
   a. **Classification of renal injuries**
      (1) **Class 1**
          (a) Renal pedicle injury
          (b) Renal pelvis laceration (major dye extravasation)
          (c) Massive bleeding from a parenchymal laceration (hemodynamic instability)
          (d) An expanding hematoma at laparotomy
      (2) **Class 2**
          (a) Transcortical lacerations (minor dye extravasation)
          (b) Selected patients with subcapsular hematomas
          (c) Selected patients developing hypertension after injury
      (3) **Class 3**
          (a) Renal contusion
          (b) Cortical lacerations without dye extravasation
          (c) Intrarenal laceration without evidence of disruption of the renal capsule
   b. **Treatment of renal injuries**
      (1) **Conservative management** Class 3 injuries, of which the great majority are contusions, are treated conservatively. A patient

with microscopic hematuria should be kept at bed rest. The patient should be monitored for signs of blood loss and infection. An IVP prior to discharge should be obtained.

(2) **Surgical considerations** All Class 1 patients require immediate exploration. Penetrating wounds require surgery. If a small non-expanding retroperitoneal hematoma is encountered, it should be left alone. An expanding hematoma should be explored. Gerota's fascia is opened, **after** proximal control of the renal pedicle is obtained. All pulsatile hematomas should be explored regardless of size, after gaining proximal control. Unless life-threatening hemorrhage is encountered and/or the patient is unstable from other injuries, attempts should be directed at preservation of renal parenchyma, including techniques of partial nephrectomy. Surgical principles include

(a) Debridement of devitalized tissue

(b) Suture ligation for hemostasis

(c) Watertight closure of the collecting system with absorbable sutures

(d) Closure of the renal capsule with absorbable sutures, if possible

(e) Cover defects of the parenchyma with either renal capsule, peritoneal grafts or omental pedicle grafts, if possible.

(f) Posterior retroperitoneal drainage should accompany all partial or complete renal resections and closure of renal or calyceal defects.

(3) **Conservative surgical management** Whereas the management of Class 1 and Class 3 injuries is well defined, controversy surrounds the management of Class 2 injuries. Generally, if such injuries are surgically approached as an elective delayed procedure (3–5 days after admission), there is a greater salvage of renal tissue.

(4) **Follow-up care** All patients sustaining any degree of renal trauma should be followed after discharge for the development of infection, renovascular hypertension, A-V fistulas, urinomas, and ureteral obstruction.

2. **Ureter**

   a. **Diagnosis** Ureteral injuries which may occur as a result of blunt or penetrating trauma are uncommon. An expanding flank mass may be the only suggestive sign. Hematuria is variable. Diagnosis is usually confirmed with an IVP or at laparotomy.

   b. **Treatment of ureteral lacerations** After debridement and spatulation of the ends, an end-to-end repair with an absorbable suture should be performed primarily, when possible. With caudad mobilization of the kidney, and/or mobilization of the ureter, defects of 6 cm can be primarily repaired. Ureteral stents are employed if anastomotic tension, potential infection, or a pancreatic injury is present. Stents are brought out through a nephrostomy or suprapubic cystostomy. Distal ureteral injuries may be implanted into the bladder wall.

3. **Bladder**
   a. **Diagnosis** of bladder injury is generally made in patients investigated for hematuria and/or pelvic trauma, particularly those suffering pubic rami, protruding acetubular, or Malgaigne fractures. Bladder perforations must be recognized early in their course to decrease morbidity and mortality. Perforations are confirmed by cystography using adequate amounts of contrast material, i.e., 250–400 cc. Perforations may be intra- or extraperitoneal. The former are commonly seen in the drinking patient with a full bladder who sustains blunt steering wheel trauma. With intraperitoneal rupture, cystography reveals contrast material extravasating into each pelvic gutter producing a "Mickey Mouse" appearance. Extraperitoneal bladder ruptures are more frequently associated with pelvic fractures, particularly anterior fractures. Isolated extraperitoneal perforations may result in a negative peritoneal lavage, unless intraperitoneal diapedesis of red cells has occurred. With extraperitoneal ruptures, cystography reveals a "sunset" appearance.

   b. **Treatment**   Bladder contusions are treated conservatively with urinary catheter decompression and removal of clots, as necessary, with irrigation. Bladder perforations should be debrided and treated with a three-layered closure, with absorbable sutures. In the male patient, suprapubic cystostomy should usually complement Foley catheter drainage. In female patients, repair and Foley drainage is sufficient. Bladder ruptures require repair, decompression of the bladder, and drainage of the perivesical space of Retzius with a Penrose drain. **Small extraperitoneal ruptures** may be treated simply by drainage of the bladder. Bladder decompression is discontinued in about 10 days if the urine is clear.

4. **Urethra**
   a. **Posterior urethra**
      (1) **Diagnosis**   Lacerations of the posterior urethra (superior to the urogenital diaphragm) should be suspect in any patient with a pelvic fracture, particularly when the bladder is noted to be elevated on cystography, or in the male patient in which rectal examination reveals a boggy, "high-riding," or "absent" prostate. One should note that in 8–17% of cases of prostatomembranous perforations, associated bladder perforations are present. Urethrography confirms the diagnosis of urethral disruption (see p. 177).
      (2) **Treatment**   There is controversy concerning immediate versus delayed repair of posterior urethral lacerations. In the severely injured patient, a suprapubic cystostomy should be the only surgery performed for this injury. In stable patients, some physicians

recommend suprapubic cystostomy and urethral catheterization with or without a primary urethral repair. We suggest a suprapubic cystostomy followed by urethral repair 3–4 months post-injury, when pelvic hematomas have resolved and the bladder has descended, allowing for easier reconstruction of the urethra. **Certainly, in the multiply injured patient or when urologic consultation cannot be obtained, conservative suprapubic drainage alone should be employed.** A urethral catheter should be passed after the bladder is opened, if possible. Do not explore the urethra to pass the catheter or uncontrollable hemorrhage may develop. If large bony fragments are evident which will impede bladder descent, these fragments may be resected days later when the patient is more stable.

    b. **Anterior urethra**
       (1) **Diagnosis** Lacerations of the anterior urethra, distal to the urogenital diaphragm, should be particularly suspect in patients sustaining straddle injuries. These patients **should not** be asked to void. Such attempts will result in massive urinary extravasation. Extravasation of urine from anterior urethral injuries may be contained within Buck's fascia or result in large perineal or scrotal collections. Anterior urethral injuries are confirmed by urethrography (see p. 177).
       (2) **Treatment** For small uncomplicated lacerations, primary repair with urethral stenting with a Foley catheter for 24–48 hr with complementary periurethral space drainage is ideal. In other patients, where primary repair cannot be accomplished, or may be compromised, a suprapubic cystostomy is indicated.

XIV. **Retroperitoneal Hematoma** Management of bleeding into the retroperitoneal space differs according to the area and the mechanism of injury. In our unit, 90% of abdominal trauma is blunt and 10% is penetrating. Retroperitoneal hematomas can be **abdominal** (those above the pelvic brim) or **pelvic** (those originating within the confines of the true pelvis). The abdominal variety can be divided into midline and flank hematomas. Flank hematomas may be further subdivided into those in the renal area and those in the extraperitoneal space lateral to the colon and extending into the anterior abdominal wall. Pelvic hematomas may be anterior or posterior. The posterior hematoma can exist on one or both sides.

  A. **Penetrating injury** For practical purposes, bleeding into the retroperitoneum secondary to penetrating injuries is discovered at operation. This finding mandates that the trajectory of the injury be explored.
     A **midline hematoma** following penetrating trauma is an injury to the vena cava or aorta, until proved otherwise. Aortic control must be obtained proximal to the hematoma, usually at the level of the diaphragmatic crus, before exploration is attempted. This is most safely accomplished by compression, until

the nature of the injury clearly demonstrates the need for application of a vascular clamp. An aortic injury may be closed with sutures or patched, if the lesion is small. Larger aortic injuries usually require replacement with a prosthesis.

Penetrating trauma to the vena cava causing a retroperitoneal hematoma should be approached with great respect. Mobilization and the use of clamps for proximal and distal control should be done with extreme caution. In general, adequate control by compression can be obtained. Unless venorrhaphy can be accomplished with comfort and dispatch, ligation should be considered as an acceptable alternative. The suprarenal vena cava should be repaired, if at all possible.

Active **perinephric bleeding** should be explored after aortic or unilateral renal pedicle control is established. The ability of Gerota's fascia to tamponade bleeding is well recognized with blunt trauma. With penetrating trauma, the integrity of Gerota's fascia may be destroyed and will no longer tamponade the hemorrhage. Injury to the kidney from penetrating wounds usually demands exploration and hemostasis.

In **pericolic hematomas,** the colon should be mobilized to exclude a colonic wound.

A **pelvic hematoma** which has developed following a penetrating wound should be explored to exclude damage to major vascular structures, the bladder, ureters, uterus, and rectum.

In all cases of penetrating trauma to the retroperitoneum, careful evaluation of the organs in the extraperitoneal space must be performed.

B. **Blunt injury**   Blunt injury causing a retroperitoneal hematoma can occur in patients who may or may not otherwise require exploratory celiotomy, and treatment will vary accordingly. Diagnostic techniques, e.g., CAT scan, angiography, sonography, etc., can assist in establishing the diagnosis in nonoperated patients.

A **midline hematoma** must be presumed to be due to disruption of a major retroperitoneal vessel. Aortic control at the crus is necessary. A tape should be passed around the aorta before the hematoma is explored. It must be emphasized that vena caval and aortic wounds following blunt trauma are uncommon, but occur with enough frequency to mandate that all posterior retroperitoneal midline bleeding be explored for that possibility.

Pericolic hematomas secondary to blunt trauma should be treated expectantly, if not actively expanding.

A **perinephric hematoma** discovered at operation requires careful evaluation and judgment. Gerota's fascia is a firm fibrous structure which will contain and tamponade renal parenchymal bleeding. When bleeding is confined within Gerota's fascia, exploration is not warranted. If the hematoma has expanded beyond Gerota's fascia into the hilar area, obtain aortic or, preferably, renal pedicle control and visualize the kidney. Once Gerota's fascia has been breached, it can no longer serve to obtund bleeding. If a perinephric hematoma is not expanding or pulsating, it should not be explored.

Significant extraperitoneal bleeding in the pelvis is usually associated with pelvic fractures. Bleeding in the **anterior portion of the pelvis** is a signal for the possibility of bladder or uretheral injury and a cystourethrogram is mandatory, if this has not been accomplished preoperatively. Unless injury to these organs is demonstrated, observation only is required.

Posterior pelvic bleeding discovered at operation represents the second most common cause of intraoperative mortality in our unit and presents a difficult and controversial problem. If the patient has been stabilized during the resuscitation and remains reasonably stable during the operation, the hematoma should not be opened. If it becomes apparent that the bleeding is uncontrolled by the tissue tamponade, exploration by opening the retroperitoneum over the common and external iliac arteries and veins to exclude their injury is the first step. If bleeding continues to be profuse, the next step is to embolize and ligate the internal iliac arteries bilaterally. Surgically there is little more that can be done. Packing as a means of control is a consideration. Hemipelvectomy may be a life-saving desperate consideration (see p. 198).

Perspective

Most retroperitoneal hematomas should be explored, except nonpulsating or nonexpanding perihepatic, perinephric, and pelvic hematomas associated with blunt trauma.

XV. **Abdominal Vasculature**   Injury to vessels of the abdomen comprises slightly less than 3% of the total vascular experience in our unit. The immediate mortality exceeds 50%. The major vessels of the abdomen are in the retroperitoneum. Management of these is discussed on p. 181.

A most significant vascular injury sustained in the abdomen is injury to the **"root" of the mesentery,** which is usually inflicted when an automobile steering column impinges the mesentery against the vertebral column. This type of injury has infinite variation and no single surgical technique will suffice. Arterial and venous injury is almost always present. Control by hemostatic clamping is dangerous and should only be used with caution after definitive assessment and identification of the injury are made. Point compression, best applied by the senior surgeon, is the sine qua non for controlling hemorrhage. The superior mesenteric vein integrity must be maintained to avoid infarction of the bowel, but tributaries may be ligated. Arterial injury at the root of the mesentery should be repaired by suture or grafting, as indicated.

Portal vein injury should be repaired when possible. If the portal vein cannot be repaired, it should be ligated. A second-look operation is then indicated within 24 hr to determine bowel viability. A portosystemic shunt is indicated if there is ischemic bowel or if the patient develops manifestations of portal hypertension.

Elsewhere in the abdomen, the rich vascular anastomosis between major vessels of the mesentery allow ligation to control bleeding without danger. Other clinicians advocate the use of antibiotics and heparin or dextran 40 in these injuries. However, our experience is minimal in the use of these therapeutic modalities.

Note The majority of patients, in our experience, who sustain major disruption at the root of the mesentery exsanguinate due to an inability to obtain vascular control.

Mesenteric injuries may present as a hematoma or tear. If a **mesenteric hematoma** is small and there is no evidence of ischemia, no therapy is indicated. If a mesenteric hematoma is large, it should be opened and the severed vessels should be ligated. If bowel ischemia develops following ligation of these vessels, resection of the ischemic bowel is indicated. Failure to explore the mesenteric hematoma may result in subsequent expansion and impairment of local bowel circulation, which may progress to infarction.

A **mesenteric tear** which produces bowel ischemia requires resection. The more closely the mesenteric tear approaches the bowel, the more likely the subsequent development of ischemia. A mesenteric tear adjacent to a loop of bowel may not reveal obvious ischemia; however, there may be relative ischemia with a subsequent production of intestinal stenosis. Judgment is required regarding the necessity of bowel resection when frank ischemia is not present. Mesenteric defects need to be closed to prevent internal bowel herniation. **Shearing of the mesentery** from the intestine virtually always results in ischemic bowel, which should be resected.

XVI. **Reexploratory Laparotomy** If, after laparotomy for repair of intra-abdominal trauma, a patient fails to pursue the anticipated normal postoperative course, a high index of suspicion should be maintained for a major complication. The most common indications for reoperation are intra-abdominal abscess, bleeding, and small bowel obstruction. Other sequelae are fistula formation, wound dehiscence and evisceration, and stress gastrointestinal ulceration.

A. **Bleeding** is usually secondary to a surgical lesion and/or a coagulopathy. Surgical bleeding, in general, is amenable to suture ligation control, whereas bleeding secondary to a coagulopathy is usually from a "raw" surface. In general, the more profound the manifestations of intraperitoneal bleeding, the more likely that the bleeding is secondary to a surgical lesion. The manifestations of continued intraperitoneal bleeding usually become evident within the first 24 hr, postoperatively.

1. **Manifestations**
    a. Falling hematocrit, despite transfusion
    b. Hypotension
    c. Abnormal PT, PTT, platelets
    d. Abdominal distention
    e. Decreased pulmonary compliance secondary to abdominal distention
    f. Positive peritoneal lavage
    g. Bleeding through a drain and/or wound
    h. Low wedge and/or CVP
      Gross abdominal distention and/or arterial blood from the wound and/or drain tract implies a surgical bleeder.

2. **Treatment** Surgical intervention is usually required despite a coagulopathy, when the patient develops gross abdominal distention, decreased pulmonary compliance, persistent hypotension, and/or arterial bleeding from the wound and/or drain sites.
    a. Coagulation factors should be vigorously replaced (FFP and platelets).
    b. Suture surgical bleeding points.
    c. Apply pressure to raw surface areas.
    d. Apply Avitene to raw bleeding surfaces.

B. **Infection** Abdominal infection usually presents as visceral infections, intraperitoneal abscess, infected hematomas, or peritonitis. Visceral infections are intrahepatic abscess, intrasplenic abscess, and acalculous cholecystitis. Occasionally, ischemic bowel leads to a diffuse peritonitis.

1. **Manifestations**
    a. Leukocytosis
    b. Temperature elevation
    c. Multiple systems failure (see p. 369)
    d. Physical examination may reveal an abdominal or rectal mass or an ileus.

2. **Diagnosis**
    a. **Chest x-ray**
        (1) Pleural effusion
        (2) Atelectasis
        (3) "Elevated" diaphragm
    b. **Abdominal x-ray**
        (1) Extraluminal air
        (2) Displaced abdominal viscera
        (3) Ileus pattern
    c. **Fluoroscopy** may reveal an immobile hemidiaphragm.
    d. **The CAT scan, gallium scan, and ultrasonogram** have failed to be highly accurate ($\sim$60%) in the determination of postoperative intraabdominal abscess formation. We have found the CAT scan to be the most reliable evaluation. If an intraperitoneal fluid collection is identified, a needle may be inserted under CAT scan direction and the material aspirated to evaluate for the presence of infection.
    e. **Hepatobiliary scan** If the biliary tree and duodenum visualize and the gallbladder fails to visualize with this scan, it is likely that the patient has cystic duct obstruction, which would imply cholecystitis if the patient has other manifestations of infection (see p. 425).

3. **Surgical intervention** The diagnosis of intraperitoneal postoperative infection remains very much a clinical diagnosis. The above-mentioned physical examination, clinical evaluation, and diagnostic aids are complementary in assisting the surgeon in making a decision to reexplore the patient. We consider the organ(s) involved at the original trauma and the above-mentioned evaluation in deciding to reexplore the patient for

abdominal infection. Manifestations of organ system dysfunction (see p. 369) force the clinician's hand toward abdominal exploration. If the patient only has temperature elevation and leukocytosis but his organ systems are stable, we are less likely to reexplore the patient at that point. If there are no extra-abdominal foci of infection, the abdomen is more likely to be incriminated as the source of fever. The following bacteremias make one concerned with the possibility of intra-abdominal infection:

— *Bacteroides fragilis*
— Persistent bacteremia despite antibiotic therapy
— Biliary tract organisms (klebsiella, E. coli, enterococcus, enterobacter)

4. **Laparotomy for abdominal infection**
   — Preoperative antibiotic coverage (penicillin, clindamycin, and gentamicin)
   — Preexploratory steroid administration (2 gm of methylprednisolone)˜
   — Adequate intravascular volume resuscitation
   — Postoperative ventilatory support until stable
   — Local versus generalized laparotomy   If a solitary large abscess can be localized, we generally prefer to drain this septic focus, with the intention of performing a generalized laparotomy should the patient not improve within 36–48 hr.

C. **Fistulization**   Any injured abdominal visceral structure may leak its contents into the peritoneal cavity. A controlled fistula adequately drains the visceral leak to the outside and there is no sepsis. An uncontrolled fistula is inadequately drained and is accompanied by sepsis. Causes of fistulization are:
   — Breakdown of repair of visceral trauma
   — Missed injury
   — Technical error, e.g., strangulation of a portion of the splenic flexure of the colon and/or greater curvature of the stomach with a ligature while performing a splenectomy
   — A suture that perforates the bowel as the abdominal wound is closed
   — An intraperitoneal retention suture that saws through the wall of the small bowel
   — A sump drain that erodes an intra-abdominal viscera

1. **Manifestations**
   a. **Controlled fistula**   A controlled fistula manifests as external drainage via the abdominal incision and/or drain tract without the presence of sepsis.
      (1) Bile leak   The drainage is positive for bilirubin without amylase.
      (2) Stomach
         (a) Positive contrast study (Gastrografin)
         (b) External drainage of charcoal that has been instilled into the stomach

  (3) Duodenum
    (a) Positive contrast study (Gastrografin)
    (b) External drainage of charcoal that has been instilled into the stomach
    (c) Positive for bilirubin
    (d) Positive for amylase
  (4) Small bowel Same as for duodenum
  (5) Colon
    (a) Positive hypaque enema examination
    (b) Feculent drainage (positive Gram stain)
  (6) Pancreas
    (a) High amylase content
    (b) Absence of bilirubin
    (c) Absence of charcoal drainage after enteric instillation

b. **Uncontrolled fistula** A poorly controlled fistula may show no external drainage of visceral content or may reveal external drainage via the drain tract or wound. In either case the drainage is inadequate, resulting in a septic process.
  (1) If there is external drainage, the characteristics of the drainage will be as described for controlled fistula.
  (2) There is usually leukocytosis and fever.
  (3) There may be manifestations of organ dysfunction if the systemic, stress response is severe.
  (4) X-ray
    (a) Air fluid level
    (b) Visceral effacement
    (c) Ileus
  (5) CAT scan may reveal an intra-abdominal fluid accumulation.

2. **Surgical intervention**
 a. **Controlled fistula** If the patient has had fistulous drainage for more than 4–6 weeks and the drainage is not slowing, this is usually an indication for operative intervention.
  (1) The optimal treatment is resection and primary anastomosis, if possible, or
  (2) Defunctionalize (bypass)
    (a) Side-to-side anastomosis
    (b) End-to-side anastomosis, or
  (3) Debride and close the defect. This is associated with a moderately high failure rate.
  (4) Treat distal obstruction.
 b. **Uncontrolled fistula**
  (1) Provide adequate external drainage.
  (2) Treat the patient with antibiotics until the systemic septic manifestations are controlled and an external tract has formed.
  (3) After the fistula is controlled, the guidelines under management of controlled fistula pertain.

D. **Dehiscence—evisceration** Wound dehiscence is partial or complete separation of the abdominal wound occurring in the early postoperative period. Evisceration is extrusion of the bowel from the peritoneal cavity through a dehisced wound. Evisceration usually occurs in a dehisced wound following removal of the skin closure.

1. **Manifestations** The presenting sign is usually a serosanguineous drainage from the wound, and if this occurs subsequent to the first 24 postoperative hr, it is virtually pathognomonic.
   a. Wound dehiscence may not become manifest until the skin sutures are removed and evisceration takes place.
   b. Wound dehiscence may initially manifest as total wound disruption and evisceration.
   c. Wound dehiscence may present as a postoperative ventral hernia.

2. **Treatment** Immediate versus delayed closure depends on the general status of the patient.
   a. **Wound dehiscence without evisceration**
      *(1) Close the wound with retention sutures, if stable.
      (2) If unstable, treat the defect with an abdominal binder.
   b. **Evisceration**
      *(1) Following intraperitoneal exploration, close the wound with retention sutures, if possible.
      (2) If an intraperitoneal septic process has caused the evisceration, explore the peritoneal cavity.
         (a) Close the wound and drain the process if localized.
         (b) If there is generalized peritonitis, the wound may be closed with retention sutures or left open and closed as a delayed primary or secondary closure.
      (3) If there is profound hemodynamic and/or pulmonary instability, the wound may be closed in a delayed primary or secondary fashion.

E. **Bowel obstruction** may follow posttraumatic abdominal exploration secondary to
   —Adhesions
   —Internal hernia (mesenteric defect, etc.)
   —Bowel that is trapped within the wound closure

Bowel obstruction must be differentiated from adynamic ileus which occurs much more commonly than intestinal obstruction. Radiographically, adynamic ileus usually reveals small bowel and colonic distention as opposed to intestinal obstruction which reveals dilated small bowel without colonic distention.

---

*We favor abdominal wound closure (fascial), if at all possible.

1. **Manifestations**
   a. Nasogastric output greater than 1,000 cc
   b. Abdominal distention
   c. Absence of bowel movements
   d. Absence of flatus
   e. X-ray revealing absent distal bowel gas (usually absence of colonic gas)
   f. Presence of air fluid levels on upright x-ray
   g. Cramping abdominal pain
   h. Vomiting
   i. Peristaltic rushes or hypoactive bowel sounds

2. **Treatment**   The greatest concern in the patient with intestinal obstruction is intestinal strangulation. In general, aggressive surgical intervention is dictated to prevent intestinal strangulation.
   a. If the patient has partial obstruction, a brief attempt at intestinal decompression may be tried. If tube decompression fails to resolve the obstruction, surgical intervention is indicated.
   b. Complete obstruction dictates prompt surgical intervention. Surgical intervention should be performed as soon as the diagnosis of bowel obstruction is made and the patient is rapidly and adequately intravascular volume-expanded.

F. **Stress gastrointestinal ulceration**   See p. 365.

XVII. **Abdominal Drains**   The specific indications and management of drains are controversial. There are certain concepts generally accepted, which should predicate the use of abdominal drains in situations that the trauma surgeon will encounter.

A. **Indications**   Drains are used for **prophylaxis** to prevent accumulation of fluids within the abdominal cavity and for **therapy** to evacuate fluid that has accumulated within the abdominal cavity.

1. **Prophylactic drains**
   a. **An expected leak**   Whenever there is damage to a solid organ such as the liver or pancreas, drains are **considered** in order to prevent abdominal accumulation of the organ's excreta.
   b. **Coagulopathy**   If the patient has developed a coagulopathy during the operative procedure and bleeding from the operative site cannot be completely controlled by surgical means, a drain may be indicated to decrease the accumulation of blood within the abdomen. The drain may also serve as a sentinel, which will be important if there is a large amount of blood flowing along the drain. The absence of bleeding along the drain, however, does not exclude significant intra-abdominal hemorrhage. The drain cannot completely evacuate blood that has oozed into the peritoneal cavity. If there is a major coagulopathy, reexploration after stabilization to evacuate the clot is advisable.

2. **Therapeutic drains** The following are indications for the use of a therapeutic drain:
   a. Abscess
   b. A large, liquified hematoma
   c. Biloma
   d. Poorly drained fistula
   e. Urinoma

B. **Complications**

1. The incidence of anastomic leaks may be higher if the drain is placed on the suture line. We do not advocate the use of drains at intestinal suture lines. The drain should not be a substitute for good surgical technique.

2. Nonpliable drains may erode into an adjacent organ.

3. With time, bacteria will colonize the drain and enter the peritoneal cavity. Colonization of the drain may lead to an infected abdominal focus. Drains inserted for the purpose of prophylaxis should be removed as soon as there is minimal drainage. If a drain was inserted for a therapeutic reason or an infection develops along a prophylactic drain, the drain should be withdrawn over a period of several days; otherwise, a drain tract abscess may form.

C. **Drainage systems**

1. **Closed vacuum drainage** This system is suitable for the relatively "dry" abdomen. The apparatus should only be emptied when suction is lost or when the container is full. This system tends to "clot off" early and is generally useful for 24–48 hr.

2. **Soft sump drain** This drain system should incorporate a bacterial filter at the sump port. The tube should be relatively soft, yet rigid enough to allow maintenance of the lumen during suction. On occasion, the attending physician may elect to gently irrigate the sump drain while using aseptic technique. These drains have a relatively limited duration of usefulness before they become blocked with tissue, debris, or clot.

3. **Penrose drains** These drains act primarily by delaying surface wound closure and promoting capillary action. Since these are passive drains, they allow stagnation of abdominal secretions, unless the drain exits through a dependent portion of the abdominal wall. Since this is not a closed system, bacteria are more likely to enter the abdominal cavity. Soft rubber drains are useful in maintaining already established drain sites, but are seldom useful in establishing reliable drainage from an injured organ such as the pancreas or liver.

D. **Drain care** It is important for the attending or senior surgeon to be responsible for supervising the management of the drain. The surgeon should discuss with the primary nurse the plan for the daily evaluation and management of the drain site. The drain site should be inspected for the presence of erythema, foul odor, purulent or fecal drainage, and security of the sutures holding the drain in place.

Perspective

—Drains should not be routinely used since the incidence of complications in this situation will outweigh the potential benefit.

—Drains that are inserted for the purpose of prophylaxis should consist primarily of a sump or closed vacuum system. If it is expected that the drainage may become long-term, the addition of a Penrose drain should be considered.

—If a drain is inserted for a therapeutic purpose, a Penrose drain should be used so that it may be advanced over time after the drainage has terminated. A sump drain may also be advisable if the wound is not drained in a dependent manner.

—Prophylactic drains should be removed as soon as possible to prevent colonization of the abdomen, which may eventuate into an abdominal abscess.

—A small gauge, absorbable suture is recommended for securing drains to maintain proper position and avoid erosion into a vital structure.

—Attempts at general drainage of the abdomen are futile.

—Drainage of anastomotic sites is discouraged.

—The abdominal drain should not pass through the surgical wound since it may increase the incidence of dehiscence, incisional hernia, and wound infection.

—Drains should be placed in the most dependent position possible.

(See pp. 151, 167, 171, 172, and 175.)

XVIII. **Abdominal Wound Management** The genesis of most wound complications is a break in intraoperative technique or faulty judgment in terms of intraoperative wound management. Poor attention to postoperative wound care may also contribute to wound complications.

Important intraoperative principles to be followed include

—A wide field should be prepped with the surgical scrub solution, followed by a bactericidal solution, well beyond the areas of the incision itself (at least 4 cm). Ideally, the bactericidal solution should be allowed to dry on the skin and not be wiped off.

—Excessive or prolonged wound retraction should be avoided. Such retraction results in edema and subsequent hypoxia of wound margins with increased potential for wound infections/dehiscence.

—Wound dessication should be avoided; wound edges should be periodically bathed with saline solution.

—Careful attention should be given to copious peritoneal and wound irrigation prior to closure.

—Meticulous wound hemostasis must be observed.

—Contaminated wounds should not be closed primarily. Wound packing with delayed primary closure or secondary closure is recommended and the use of retention sutures is encouraged.

Until healing is well established (i.e., fibrin seal occurs in 24 hr in an uncomplicated wound), sterile technique should be used during wound observation on rounds and during dressing changes. Specifically:
—The hands should be washed before and after every dressing change.
—Bare hands should never touch the wound or drains.
    The individual performing the dressing changes should use sterile gloves for each wound, or,
    The dressings and drains should be handled with sterile instruments.
—Wounds should be probed only by means of sterile instruments or a gloved hand.
—If there is a series of dressing changes, clean wounds without drains should always be changed first, then clean wounds with drains, and, finally, dirty or contaminated wounds.
—Where possible, patients with clean uninfected postoperative wounds should not be placed in the same room as patients with infected wounds.

A. Management of clean wounds

1. Clean wounds should be covered for the first 24 hr with a sterile dressing. Topical agents (antibiotic ointments, Betadine, etc.) may be used at the discretion of the surgeon.

2. After 24 hr, clean wounds may be dressed or left open at the discretion of the surgeon.

3. Suture removal shall be at the discretion of the surgeon.

B. Management of contaminated or dirty wounds

1. Inspection and dressing changes on contaminated or dirty wounds should be performed at least once a day or more frequently, as indicated.

2. Aggressive surgical debridement of necrotic tissue and drainage of any residual abscess should be carried out.

3. All purulent material should be cultured and Gram-stained and the results recorded on the chart.

4. Wounds should be dressed so as to isolate the contaminated wound from any adjacent clean wounds.

5. Wound irrigation, continuous or intermittent, has been found to be of limited use.

6. Open contaminated wounds should be packed. The general principle involved in packing is to keep the skin edges apart while allowing the wound to granulate from the base up. The type of packing utilized shall be at the

discretion of the surgeon. However, it should be remembered that Betadine and hydrogen peroxide are cytotoxic; therefore, normal saline is the solution of choice for irrigation and packing of wounds, although in a more purulent or contaminated wound, one may choose to use Betadine or hydrogen peroxide for the initial 24–48 hr.

C. **Potentially contaminated wounds** Wounds in this category may be treated initially as clean wounds, but must be carefully observed for signs of infection. Questionable areas in the wounds should be locally probed with surgical instruments. If infection develops, the principle of contaminated wound management should apply.

XIX. **Pelvis** The presence of a pelvic fracture should be entertained in any trauma patient, particularly one sustaining multiple injuries. Pelvic fractures may be simple and nondisplaced with little consequence to the patient, except some discomfort, or be associated with significant hemorrhage and other systems injuries, particularly of the lower urologic tract, the vagina, the rectum, the sacral roots, and the sciatic nerve. Generally, the severity of pelvic injury parallels the number of associated injuries and the amount of blood loss. The trauma surgeon must be able to quickly recognize and treat the spectrum of injury and hemorrhage associated with pelvic fractures. Multidisciplinary input is often required for successful patient management.

A. **Pelvic fractures**

1. **Classification**
   a. **Type I** Comminuted (crush) fracture: most serious type of injury (highest mortality and morbidity)
   b. **Type II** Unstable fracture: two or more points of pelvic ring disruption constitute an unstable fracture. Points of disruption are
      (1) Pubic symphysis
      (2) Bony pelvis
      (3) Sacroiliac (SI) joint
      (4) Sacrum
   c. **Type III** Stable fracture
   d. **Open or closed** Higher mortality and morbidity are associated with open fractures.

2. **Manifestations**
   a. **Symptoms** Pain in the region of the pelvis is the primary symptom.
   b. **Signs**
      (1) Obvious rotary malalignment of an entire lower extremity
      (2) Ecchymosis and/or fullness of the perineum, scrotum, abdominal wall, or buttocks
      (3) Bony crepitus elicited by palpation over the iliac crest, the pubic symphysis, and behind the sacroiliac joints. Observation of unusual motion on palpation of these areas (particularly on compres-

sion of the iliac crests) should substantially increase the index of suspicion for the presence of a pelvic fracture.

3. **Diagnosis**
    a. **Roentgenographic evaluation of the pelvis**
       (1) **An AP roentgenograph** which includes both hips and sacroiliac joints

       > Note | Since many multiple trauma patients have a depressed level of consciousness and cannot complain of pain, this is considered a standard screening roentgenograph for our trauma patients.

       (2) **Pelvic inlet roentgenograph** This roentgenograph is taken if the AP projection reveals a major pelvic fracture. It delineates the amount of pelvic ring disruption and displacement of the SI joints. It is taken by directing the x-ray tube positioned over the patient's head toward the pelvis, making an angle of 60° with the patient's supine body.
    b. **Laboratory data**
       (1) Admission and serial hemoglobin and hematocrit determinations are necessary to monitor blood loss.
       (2) Admission and serial coagulation profiles should be followed.

4. **Orthopedic management of pelvic fractures** Orthopedic consultation should be obtained in all cases of pelvic fracture to outline the therapeutic modalities and recommendations for patient management and activity. Severely disruptive or displaced fractures should be appropriately reduced and stabilized as soon as possible. Methods available to achieve these ends include
    a. MAST
    b. External skeletal fixator (Hoffman device)
    c. Skeletal traction
    Many nondisplaced pelvic fractures require only short periods of bed rest or no bed rest.

5. **Open pelvic fractures** Open pelvic fractures are associated with a high morbidity and mortality. The major causes of morbidity and mortality are related to hemorrhage and sepsis. The major complication seen early after injury is exsanguination. The late sequela of poorly controlled hemorrhage is multiple organ failure. If hemorrhage is initially controlled, the most common cause of morbidity and mortality is sepsis. The initial priority in dealing with open pelvic fractures is to obtain hemostasis as rapidly as possible.

    To minimize subsequent septic complications, the following maneuvers should be considered:
    a. Colostomy for rectal injuries and/or wounds that are likely to be soiled by feces (see p. 166)

b. Repair of bladder injuries and urinary diversion by suprapubic cystostomy, if there is a urethral injury

c. Proper management of vaginal injuries (see p. 200)

d. Adequate initial debridement of the wound and aggressive subsequent debridement of necrotic tissue

e. Short-term prophylactic antibiotics with clindamycin and gentamicin or cefoxitin for 3–5 days may be helpful.

f. Evaluate the need for tetanus prophylaxis.

6. **Infection**   Hematomas associated with pelvic fractures may become infected. Hematoma infection associated with pelvic fractures is more likely to occur with open fractures, but may occur with closed fractures. The diagnosis of an infected hematoma is difficult and is made by exclusion, i.e., by ruling out other sources of sepsis. The CAT scan may be helpful in identifying significant pelvic hematomas. It also **may** reveal evidence of superimposed infection. Attempt at aspiration of the hematoma may be performed under CAT scan direction for appropriate bacteriologic studies. Therapy consists of appropriate antibiotic coverage and surgical drainage.

> **Note**   The diagnosis of an infected hematoma associated with a pelvic fracture requires a high index of suspicion and follow-up with the above-mentioned diagnostic evaluation.

B. **Associated Injuries**

1. **Neurologic**   Injury to the sacral roots secondary to pelvic fracture is uncommon, but should be ruled out if a sacral fracture is seen. Sciatic nerve injuries most commonly occur with hip dislocations.

   a. **Symptoms**
      (1) Pain radiating down the posterior aspect of the buttock, thigh, and lower leg
      (2) Weakness or paralysis of muscles of the lower leg
      (3) Inability to void

   b. **Signs**
      (1) Absent ankle jerk
      (2) Weak dorsiflexion and eversion of the foot (common peroneal nerve)
      (3) Weak plantarflexion and inversion of the foot (tibial nerve)
      (4) Absent rectal tone and perianal and posterior leg hypesthesia (sacral nerves)

   c. **Treatment**   Most injuries are secondary to traction or stretch which leaves the nerve in continuity. In the pelvis, operation on the lumbosacral plexus is fruitless. Injuries of the sciatic nerve at the hip rarely call for exploration because the length of nerve disruption precludes a functional result.

2. **Urologic**   The presence of a urologic injury should be entertained in any patient suffering a pelvic fracture. Urologic injuries associated with a pelvic

fracture most often involve the bladder and/or the prostatomembranous urethra. The ureters and kidneys are rarely involved.

The presence of the urologic injury is usually heralded by hematuria, urethral meatal blood, or difficulty in passing a urethral catheter.

a. **Symptoms**   Inability to void
b. **Signs**
   (1) Hematuria
   (2) A bloody urethral meatal discharge
   (3) Blood draining around a previously placed urinary bladder catheter
   (4) Inability to pass a urinary bladder catheter or poor urine drainage through a previously placed catheter, i.e., the catheter tip is extraurethral
   (5) Signs of trauma in the area of the perineum
   (6) A boggy mass, "high-riding," or "absent" prostate on rectal examination
c. **Diagnosis and treatment**   It is important to emphasize that the complete evaluation for a suspected urologic injury (usually because of hematuria and/or meatal bleeding) consists of urethrography, cystography, and intravenous pyelography (see p. 177).

3. **Intra-abdominal injuries and diagnostic peritoneal lavage**   The more severe a pelvic fracture, the greater the chance of an associated intra-abdominal injury. The best test to detect intra-abdominal injury is diagnostic peritoneal lavage. If there is a known severe pelvic fracture and/or there is evidence of an abdominal wall hematoma, the procedure should be performed above the umbilicus in an open manner. In such injuries, a large retroperitoneal hematoma occupying much of the pelvis may be inadvertently entered by a catheter placed by the infraumbilical technique. If there is a minor pelvic fracture without clinical evidence of an abdominal wall hematoma, the procedure may be performed in an open fashion infraumbilically. If an abdominal wall hematoma is encountered, one should cease and perform a supraumbilical, open technique. Generally, extraperitoneal injuries, e.g., a disrupted urethra or lacerated bladder, are not detectable by lavage; however, by maintaining a high index of suspicion and performing cystography and urethrography, such injuries will be diagnosed. In some cases, particularly involving severe pelvic fractures, false positive results may be obtained because blood is leaking through holes in the peritoneum or because of diapedesis of red blood cells across an intact peritoneum; however, this cannot be determined without laparotomy.

4. **Rectal-vaginal injuries**   These injuries are usually associated with motorcycle accidents. They should be suspected when
   a. There is a severe disruptive pelvic fracture, particularly an open fracture associated with a deep perineal laceration. Rectal injuries are most commonly associated with ischial fractures.

b. Blood appears spontaneously through the rectum or vagina or is obtained on digital examination

c. A bony spicule is palpated on digital examination

For a more detailed discussion of the treatment of these injuries, see pp. 166 and 200.

C. **Pelvic hemorrhage**   The pelvic basin is richly supplied by the anterior and posterior divisions of the hypogastric arteries and drained by a complex venous system. Multiple arterial and venous collaterals exist. Like the arteries, the veins are valveless and capable of bidirectional flow. Because of its vasculature, pelvic fractures are usually associated with hemorrhage. Generally, the more severe the injury, the greater the blood loss.

The control of bleeding associated with pelvic fractures may be very difficult. When associated injuries are present, it may be difficult to ascertain how much blood loss is due to the pelvic fracture and how much is due to associated injuries.

The following guidelines are suggested in the management of pelvic fracture bleeding:

1. **Transfusion and expectancy**   If the fracture is minor, and vital signs are stable, transfusion therapy alone will suffice.

2. **Military Anti-Shock Trousers (MAST)**   If there is a severe pelvic fracture and/or the systolic blood pressure is less than 100 mm Hg with a less severe fracture, apply MAST. Initially, the trousers may be maximally inflated for 2 hr. After 2 hr and appropriate infusion of fluid and blood, efforts to lower the abdominal and leg compartment pressures to 40 and 50 mm Hg, respectively, should be made. With the lower pressure, the MAST can be left in place for 48 hr with little fear of skin necrosis.

3. **Angiography and transcatheter embolic tamponade**
   a. With MAST in place, if transfusion requirements continue despite the infusion of approximately 10 units of blood, angiography and transcatheter embolic tamponade should be considered.
   b. If angiography reveals bleeding from the common or external iliac artery, laparotomy is mandatory with repair of the vessel. To perform a laparotomy, the abdominal portion of the MAST must be deflated.
   c. If angiography reveals arterial bleeding from sites other than the common or external iliac artery, embolic tamponade should be performed.

4. **External skeletal stabilization**   For severely displaced and/or unstable fractures, reduction and stabilization with external fixators of the Hoffman variety may be useful if MAST compression and angiography and embolic tamponade are ineffective in controlling hemorrhage. During placement of the Hoffman device, the abdominal section of the MAST must be deflated. If the systolic pressure drops below 80 mm Hg and is unresponsive to volume infusion, the abdominal part of the trousers is reinflated and the application of the Hoffman device is abandoned.

5. **Vaginal packing** Vaginal packing may assist in providing tamponade to control pelvic hematoma formation.

6. **Surgery for pelvic fracture hemorrhage** Surgical intervention for hemorrhage associated with pelvic fractures **must be considered** in the following circumstances:
   a. Persistent hypotension despite the use of MAST, embolic tamponade, and/or application of the Hoffman device
   b. Hypotension which is nonresponsive to massive volume infusion
   c. A pelvic hematoma which is identified during exploratory laparotomy
   If the patient remains hemodynamically unstable despite the use of MAST, embolic tamponade, or application of the Hoffman device, surgical intervention must be strongly considered. If a patient has hemorrhage that is associated with a pelvic fracture and the patient cannot be initially stabilized with massive volume infusion and MAST, laparotomy must be considered for control of the pelvic bleeding. It is likely in this situation that there is an injury to the iliac artery and/or vein. A laparotomy may be indicated for a positive peritoneal lavage and a pelvic hematoma may be found. Exploration of the hematoma is not indicated if it is nonpulsatile or nonexpanding. If there is moderate expansion and pulsation of the hematoma, yet the patient is hemodynamically stable, closure and postoperative arteriography with embolic tamponade are indicated. If the pelvic hematoma is massive, pulsatile, and rapidly expanding, exploration of the hematoma is indicated.

   If an iliac arterial injury is found on arteriography, and the patient is hemodynamically unstable, exploration and repair of the lesion are indicated. If arteriography reveals an iliac arterial injury, yet the patient is hemodynamically stable and there is no evidence of limb ischemia, delayed repair is indicated.

   If surgery for pelvic bleeding is indicated, the following options are available:
   —Ligation of bleeding vessels
   —Intraoperative embolic tamponade of the hypogastric arteries **and** ligation
   —If ligation and embolic tamponade fail to terminate the bleeding, the pelvis may be temporarily packed.
   —Hemipelvectomy may be a life-saving procedure if there is uncontrollable hemorrhage.

   Patients who need massive blood replacement due to hemorrhage from pelvic fractures require close monitoring of the volume status and cardiopulmonary function. The following are employed:
   —An arterial line
   —A Swan-Ganz catheter which allows for the evaluation of arterial and mixed venous gases and determination of cardiac output
   —Frequent monitoring of coagulation

To control pelvic fracture hemorrhage effectively, more than one modality of therapy may be necessary. The following flowchart is a suggested plan of management for the patient with hemorrhage that is associated with a pelvic fracture.

Flowchart for the management of hemorrhage associated with pelvic fractures

(1) **Hemodynamically stable**—expectant treatment (CV monitoring, serial Hct/Hb, and serial coagulation profile)

(2) **Hemodynamically unstable**→MAST trousers→Stable——→(1)

    Unstable→No pelvic instability

(1)   Pelvic instability   Arteriogram

Stable←Hoffman device→Unstable

            Iliac* lesion   Non-iliac lesion
              Surgery   Embolize

(3) **(a)** **Persistent hemodynamic instability** despite **(2)**, **or**
    (b) Patient with **"nonresuscitatable shock,"** i.e., cannot control shock with massive volume infusion → **laparotomy** (rapidly expanding hematoma):
        —Embolize **and** ligate hypogastrics
        —Pack the pelvis
        —Repair major arterial injury
        —Hemipelvectomy

(4) **Pelvic hematoma found at laparotomy**
    (a) Nonexpanding or pulsatile—(1)
    (b) Modest expansion and/or pulsatile—Close the abdomen and perform an arteriogram (embolic tamponade)
    (c) If rapidly expanding—(3)

*Iliac—common or external

XX. Gynecologic Tract

A. **Hematoma of the vulva and perineum** Blunt trauma between the legs frequently results in a "straddle injury." The cause may be a fall astride a fence or a railing or sliding along the fuel tank of a motorcycle.

1. **Manifestations**
    a. **Symptoms**
        (1) Severe perineal pain
        (2) Marked swelling
        (3) Anxiety

b. **Signs**
   (1) Local swelling; may be marked and progressive
   (2) Discoloration—bluish mottling of skin
   (3) Occasional rupture of skin or mucosa with bleeding
c. **Laboratory data** Falling hemoglobin and hematocrit in extreme cases

2. **Diagnosis**
   a. Consider cystography and proctoscopy for the diagnosis of bladder and rectal injury.
   b. Consider vaginal, rectal, and abdominopelvic examinations to fully assess the trauma.

3. **Surgical treatment**
   a. Direct pressure with large pad and "T" binder
   b. Incision and evacuation
   c. Ligate or suture bleeding sites in the cavity.
   d. Place a drain and apply a pressure dressing.

4. **Complications**
   a. Overlooked associated injury
   b. Extension of hematoma
   c. Infection with abscess formation

B. **Vulvovaginal laceration** Vaginal laceration is the result of either accidental or intentional trauma. The circumstances are nearly always presented by the patient or another person. Occasionally, an unconscious patient may have unsuspected genital trauma in association with other more conspicuous injury. This is particularly likely in the victims of the more violent sexual assaults (see p. 203).

1. **Manifestations**
   a. **Symptoms**
      (1) Moderate to profuse vaginal bleeding
      (2) Surprisingly mild pain
   b. **Signs**
      (1) Visible laceration demonstrated by speculum or vaginal retractor
      (2) Presence of other genital injuries
      (3) Tachycardia and hypotension in proportion to blood loss. If the degree of shock is more severe, search for deep pelvic or abdominal injury. A large amount of blood may have been lost at the scene and/or en route to the hospital.
   c. **Laboratory data** Falling hemoglobin and hematocrit (variable)

2. **Diagnosis**
   a. Cystography or urethrography may be indicated.
   b. Proctoscopy should be performed.
   c. Vaginal and abdominopelvic examination should be performed.

| Note | These examinations may need to be performed under anesthesia.

3. **Surgical treatment** Anesthesia, adequate lighting, and two assistants with right angle retractors are necessary to inspect the entire vaginal canal. Debridement and generous irrigation of the wound are indicated. If there is bleeding deeper than the vaginal mucosa, control is obtained by ligature or figure-of-8 sutures. Do not close mucosa over active bleeding or a hematoma will result. Suture the laceration with absorbable continuous suture beginning at furthest point. If the top of the laceration is difficult to reach, place interrupted sutures where access is easier and leave them long for mild traction. Continuous locking suture should control mucosal edge bleeding.

If the laceration reaches the upper angles (fornices) of the vagina, suspect penetration of the pelvis with possible injury of pelvic vessels and ureter. Soft tissue injuries of the perineum should be debrided, irrigated, and closed in layers. If the damage is extensive and adequate debridement is questionable, or the wound is greater than 12 hr old, the wound should be irrigated, drained, and left open. A colostomy should be strongly considered for extensive perineal wounds. Sharp penetrating wounds of the anal sphincter or wounds that create a rectovaginal or vesicovaginal fistula should be repaired if minimal time has elapsed since injury. A 3- to 5-day course of clindamycin and gentamicin or cefoxitin may be beneficial. See pp. 165 and 181.

4. **Complications**
   a. Overlooking associated injuries
   b. Hematoma
   c. Infection; abscess (rare)
   d. Fistula formation to bladder or rectum

C. **Wounds of the genital organs** The internal reproductive organs are not as frequently injured as the abdominal viscera, unless advanced pregnancy is present. In the nongravid patient, the bony protection of the pelvis is effective. Stab and gunshot wounds of these structures can occur. Occasionally, a fall on a sharp object will penetrate the pelvis. Blunt injuries in the nongravid patient are rare.

1. **Uterus**
   a. **Penetrating trauma**
      (1) **Manifestations** Simple perforations of the vagina or uterus are not usually serious if bleeding and infection are controlled. Injury to the vascular supply lateral to the uterus such as in the broad ligament and pelvic wall (internal iliac, uterine, and ovarian vessels), on the other hand, leads to massive hemorrhage with hemoperitoneum and often progressive retroperitoneal hematoma. As in any wound penetrating the abdominal cavity, there is a possibility of visceral injury.
         (a) **History and symptoms** The nature of the injury is usually evident or known.
            i. Pain may be out of proportion to the visible injury, with severe pain in the pelvis and lower abdomen.

ii. External bleeding
- (b) **Signs**
  - i. Puncture wound or laceration
  - ii. Lower abdominal tenderness, rebound, or rigidity
  - iii. Tachycardia and hypotension unexplained by visible blood loss
  - iv. Palpable vaginal, pelvic, or abdominal hematoma
  - v. Vaginal bleeding
- (c) **Laboratory data** Eventual falling hemoglobin and hematocrit, if hemorrhage is significant.

(2) **Diagnosis**
- (a) X-ray (abdominal, cystogram, IVP)
- (b) Penetrating trauma of the pelvic or peritoneal cavity mandates celiotomy.

(3) **Surgical treatment** If possible, the surgical team should consist of persons experienced in bowel and urologic as well as gynecologic surgery. When retroperitoneal hematoma is massive, considerable distortion of anatomical features will be encountered. When specific bleeding vessels can be identified and ligated, the team is indeed fortunate. Uterus, fallopian tubes, and even ovaries may be sacrificed, if necessary, to obtain exposure for hemostasis. Hypogastric (internal iliac) artery ligation may control broad ligament pelvic hemorrhage/hematoma. This must be done bilaterally because of extensive anastomoses. Ligated arteries should not be severed.

If there is minimal damage to the uterus, the wounds are debrided and closed with figure-of-8 chromic sutures. If the injury is extensive in a young female and it can be reconstructed, it should be repaired. If the uterus cannot be reconstructed, it should be removed. Repair of the lower uterus is likely to be followed by cervical canal stenosis; therefore, a hysterectomy should be considered. After laparotomy, vaginal and rectal examination should be done to detect pelvic hematomas or abscess. Tight vaginal packing after laparotomy will help to minimize pelvic hematoma formation. If a hysterectomy is performed, the vaginal cuff should be left partially open and drained because of the likelihood of abscess formation.

b. **Blunt trauma** This injury is rare in the nongravid patient.
(1) **Manifestations** A pelvic fracture is likely to be present. A pelvic hematoma associated with a pelvic fracture is not specific for a uterine injury. Bleeding from the vagina in the absence of a vaginal laceration is suggestive of a uterine injury.
(2) **Treatment** Massive hemorrhage will require laparotomy and repair, if feasible, or hysterectomy. Conservatism is advised, if possible. Observation for a pelvic abscess is warranted if conservative therapy is followed (see p. 195).

2. **Ovarian and adnexal injuries** The adnexa are small and protected by the pelvis. They are rarely involved in injuries of either pregnant or nonpregnant women. Occasionally, the presence of ovarian cysts, tumors, or pyosalpinx will predispose the ovary or salpinx to play a role in the evaluation and treatment of an injured woman. The specific injury is usually not suspected before surgery. The lesion will be identified at laparotomy. Laparotomy is indicated for the following reasons:

—In blunt trauma, the patient will have a positive peritoneal lavage or will be explored for peritoneal irritation without the necessity for lavage.

—Celiotomy is mandated for penetrating wounds of the peritoneal or pelvic cavity.

The following lesions may be found:

—**Rupture of ovarian cyst** Trim the redundant cyst wall. Suture the ovarian tissue to secure hemostasis. Use absorbable sutures.

—**Torn and bleeding infundibulopelvic ligament** (contains ovarian artery) Ligate the vessels and remove the ovary because the blood supply is seriously damaged.

—**Simple laceration of ovary** Suture the ovary with locked, continuous absorbable suture. The ovary will tolerate a lot of suture. Handle gently because it fragments under tension. If the blood supply is good and hemostasis is secured, the result of conservation should be excellent, even if the organ is bristling with sutures. Severe lesions are managed by oophorectomy.

—**Torsion of ovary** This is usually the consequence of a twisting motion plus the presence of tumor. The most common tumor is a dermoid cyst. If cyanotic ovarian structures are present, **do not unwind the pedicle,** since this results in embolization. The pedicle should be clamped and all distal structures removed.

| Note | Always consider the need for tetanus prophylaxis and the possibility of subsequent development of gas gangrene in patients with uterine or vaginal trauma. The uterus is usually sterile; therefore, we would suggest a pre-, intra-, and postoperative dose of clindamycin and gentamicin or cefoxitin if there is an isolated uterine injury. We suggest a 3-to 5-day course of antibiotics if the vagina has been breached.

D. **Sexual assault**

1. **Manifestations**
   a. **Symptoms** History or other injuries from assault may suggest sexual assault. Usually gynecologic injuries are absent or insignificant compared to other wounds.
   b. **Signs**
      (1) Vulvar abrasion, laceration, discoloration, or ecchymosis
      (2) Vaginal tears or bleeding

  c. **Laboratory data**
   (1) Baseline hematology
   (2) Culture for gonorrhea
   (3) Serology for syphilis

 2. **Diagnosis**
  a. Vaginal fluid should be examined microscopically for sperm.
  b. Vaginal swabs and acid phosphatase should be obtained.

 3. **Treatment**
  a. **Surgery** Pressure and vaginal packing may be used temporarily to reduce blood loss. Lacerations should be repaired as soon as possible. In children, injury to the rectum or bladder may require surgical repair.
  b. **Medications**
   (1) Analgesics
   (2) Prophylactic antibiotics for venereal disease or wound contamination; procaine penicillin, 4.8 million units i.m. with probenicid (Benemid)
   (3) Tetanus prophylaxis

 4. **Complications**
  a. Infection
  b. Fistula
  c. Psychologic trauma

Perspective

Sexual assault and rape victims are not usually seen at MIEMSS, unless associated injuries are severe.

 There is no specific time factor regarding the examination for rape victims. The policy is to rectify any life-threatening problems first, as well as complete any necessary radiologic evaluations, etc., and then contact the OB-GYN Department regarding the proper examinations of these victims.

 Shaving and other necessary preparations of the perineal area are not contraindicated in these patients. If the patient is shaved, a dry shave should be performed and the hairs collected and presented to the police. The pubic hairs should be combed and collected before shaving.

 Ideally, the examination should take place in the Admitting Area prior to the patient's departure to the floor. The OB-GYN Department is ready and willing to perform these examinations. From a legal standpoint, it is preferable that members of the OB-GYN staff perform these examinations.

 If the patient's condition makes complete sexual assault work-up inadvisable, cotton swabs taken of material in the vagina or other orifices should be placed in **unsealed** paper envelopes, because of the fact that anaerobes will otherwise destroy the material. These should be labeled for patient identification and source, and marked "for police laboratory—acid phosphatase."

XXI. **Injuries in Pregnancy** Whenever a female is injured, the possibility of pregnancy must be considered. In general, what is best for the injured mother is also best for her fetus, but when a gestation is known to be present it may influence many of the decisions and techniques of study and treatment. In most situations, the diagnosis of pregnancy may be made immediately by palpating the enlarged uterus. When the individual is not noticeably pregnant, the question should be specifically asked in all cases. When the patient is not conscious, a relative may be able to answer. When the uterus is at or above the umbilicus, the fetal heart tones may be auscultated. If the fetus is significantly hypoxic, fetal bradycardia will occur. This can be defined as a rate of 100 beats/min or less. A rate of < 120 is cause for concern. Care should be taken to distinguish the maternal pulse from the fetal heart rate.

A. **Generalizations**

1. **Vena cava syndrome** The enlarged uterus will compress the vena cava when the patient is supine. The uninjured gravida will avoid the supine position because it is uncomfortable and she becomes restless. When forced to remain flat, there is a marked lowering of venous return and cardiac output with these important undesirable results:
    a. Fetal hypoxia due to diminished uterine blood flow
    b. Maternal hypotension which may cause inappropriate treatment
    Vena cava compression is avoided by keeping the patient on her left side or by manually pressing the uterine bulk gently to the left.

2. **Danger to other structures because of pregnancy** The large uterus may transmit forces that increase the likelihood of splenic or hepatic injury and even rupture of the diaphragm. Diaphragmatic ruptures which have been repaired during pregnancy may break down during labor. If the patient is near term, consideration should be given to performing a cesarean section at the time of diaphragmatic repair. If the patient is not near term, cesarean section at a later time should be considered.

3. Pregnant women acquire a 30% **increase in blood volume.** This is associated with a physiologic ability to selectively reduce uterine blood flow. Therefore, pulse rate and blood pressure signs of hypovolemia may not occur until late.

4. **X-rays** The more advanced the gestational age, the less harmful are x-rays. When needed for maternal study, x-rays should be done with shielding of the fetus, if possible. It is the more vulnerable early, unknown pregnancy that needs shielding the most. **At no time should needed x-rays of the pregnant female be withheld.** Limited x-rays are relatively safe during the last trimester. The earlier the female is in her pregnancy, the more the clinician needs to question the benefit of the study to the patient.

B. **Blunt trauma to the pregnant uterus** The enlarged uterus is vulnerable to external force. Injury to the uterus may transmit force and cause injury to the spleen, liver, etc. Automobile crashes or assault with a blunt weapon are common sources of gravid uterine injury.

1. **Manifestations**   When injury to the uterus is severe, the picture will be that of uterine rupture, placental separation, or both. Uterine rupture will produce hemorrhage into the abdominal cavity with or without vaginal bleeding. The fetus is frequently living unless the mother's condition produces anoxia.

   a. **Symptoms**   Severe abdominal pain is the most notable symptom.

   b. **Signs**

      (1) Marked tenderness over the uterus

      (2) The signs of hemorrhage are usually present and progressive.

      (3) Uterine contractions may be present.

      (4) Abdominal distention may be present.

      (5) A hard uterus and absent fetal heart in advanced pregnancy mean abruption of the placenta (see p. 210).

      (6) Vaginal bleeding may be present.

      (7) Gravid uterus is palpable.

2. **Diagnosis**

   a. Place indwelling bladder catheter for possible cystogram and evaluation of bladder.

   b. If there is a question regarding the presence of abdominal pathology, a peritoneal lavage is performed.

3. **Treatment**

   a. **Surgery**   The evidence of intra-abdominal catastrophe is usually marked and exploratory laparotomy should not be delayed. Avoid the vena cava syndrome.

      (1) If the uterus is above the umbilicus, try to include neonatology standby, but do not wait for this help. Provide appropriate cardiovascular support.

      (2) Begin exploratory laparotomy as soon as possible.

      (3) At abdominal exploration, secure hemostasis. If the uterus interferes with hemostasis, empty the uterus through a midline "classical" incision.

          The placenta must usually be separated manually. If the fetus is living, clamp and cut the cord. Hand the infant to the nurses or neonatologist. Intravenous oxytocics will reduce uterine bleeding and greatly reduce the size of the uterus. If uterine rupture is the principal injury, empty the uterus. Extend the laceration, if needed, but be sure to extend it vertically near the midline. Do not extend the laceration laterally to the broad ligament. Usually, apposition of the rupture with debridement and continuous locked suture with 00 chromic suture is suitable for repair. Often a second layer and additional figure-of-8 sutures are needed to secure hemostasis. If hemostasis is unsatisfactory, consider the possibility of a coagulopathy. If the situation is still uncontrolled, either hysterectomy or bilateral hypogastric ligation must be done. It is wise to use blunt pressure if a coagulopathy is present, until clotting ability is restored.

    b. **Medications**

        (1) **Oxytocics** should be given only after fetus and placenta are removed.

            (a) **Methergine** (0.2 mgm) (one-half i.v. and one-half i.m.), or

            (b) **Pitocin** (20 units in 1,000 ml as a drip) will provide appropriate uterine contraction.

           These dosages given before delivery will produce uterine rupture.

        (2) Prophylactic antibiotics (clindamycin and gentamicin or cefoxitin) should be given before and during surgery. Do not continue the antibiotics more than 24 hr without bacteriologic information.

4. **Complications**

    a. Postoperative hemorrhage and hematoma formation

    b. Infection producing an abdominopelvic abscess

C. **Penetrating trauma to the pregnant uterus** In advanced pregnancy there is a greater likelihood that the enlarged uterus will be penetrated by intentional or unintentional sharp trauma. The gravid uterus is of some protection to the mother. Near-term gunshot and stab injuries often do not produce serious maternal consequences. The fetus, on the other hand, is quite likely to receive serious or fatal injury.

    1. **Gunshot wounds** If the entrance wound is not in the upper abdomen, the uterus may be the only maternal organ significantly injured. Upper abdominal gunshot wounds will characteristically result in multiple organ perforation with serious maternal consequences.

        a. **Symptoms**

            (1) Pain (mild to severe)

            (2) Anxiety

        b. **Signs**

            (1) Tenderness which may be minimal to marked

            (2) Guarding which may be absent

            (3) Tachycardia which may be a late sign

            (4) Hypotension may be a late sign. Be sure uterine compression of vena cava is not a factor.

            (5) Slowing of the fetal heart rate suggests distress (slower than 110). Make certain it is not the maternal pulse. This sign indicates fetal injury or hypoxia from the maternal response to injury.

            (6) Absent fetal heart tones

        c. **Laboratory data** Hct/Hb may be low

d. Diagnosis

(1) If fetal heart rate is present, it should be monitored constantly; a portable Doppler device is excellent and a fetoscope or stethoscope may be adequate in advanced pregnancy.

(2) Ultrasound can detect fetal life when other methods are inadequate, as in early gestation with a small fetus.

(3) Amniocentesis can establish the presence of fetal bleeding. Ultrasound direction of needle can help avoid false positives by aspirating placental blood.

e. Treatment Gunshot wounds to the abdomen or pelvis of a pregnant female mandate celiotomy. Hypotension is a "late" finding in the gravid mother; therefore, its presence requires urgent intervention. Slowing of the fetal heart rate requires urgent intervention. If fetal heart tones are absent, care of the mother becomes the only consideration.

(1) **Surgery**

(a) If the uterus is found uninjured with a live fetus, treat the injuries and leave the uterus alone. Pregnancy can be expected to continue. If necessary for treatment of the mother, the fetus and/or uterus may be sacrificed to secure surgical exposure for hemostasis.

(b) If the uterus is unwounded, but the fetus is dead, treat the major injuries. Leave the uterus and fetus for later management.

(c) Often the projectile is stopped by the fetus or the amniotic fluid in the uterine cavity. In this case, there is no exit wound. If the uterus is penetrated by a small wound

   i. Suture the entrance wound and leave the dead fetus for later vaginal delivery.

   ii. If the fetus is alive, an immediate cesarean section is indicated. Try to have a neonatal surgeon available to treat fetal wounds.

   iii. If the uterus is in tetanic contraction, with living or dead fetus, do a cesarean section.

(d) Extensive uterine damage and/or damage to the broad ligament may result in hemorrhage. In this case, cesarean section is performed and followed by hysterectomy, because of difficult hemostasis. Bilateral hypogastric artery ligation may be necessary.

(2) **Medications**

(a) Do not use oxytocics unless the uterus is empty of fetus and placenta.

(b) Tetanus prophylaxis should be given.

(c) A dose of clindamycin and gentamicin or cefoxitin should be given pre-, intra-, and postoperatively. If the bowel or vagina is involved, a 3- to 5-day antibiotic course may be helpful.

f. **Complications**
 (1) Inadequate hemostasis
 (2) Infection—possible peritonitis and abscess formation
 (3) Fetal death with retention of dead fetus for weeks leading to dead fetus syndrome and disseminated intravascular coagulopathy (DIC).

2. **Stab wounds** The prognosis for both mother and infant is better for stab wounds than for gunshot wounds. In late pregnancy, the uterus is most often penetrated by stab wounds and it tends to protect other viscera of the mother. Stab wounds of the upper abdomen are serious since the uterus concentrates the mother's viscera in this region.
 a. **Symptoms**
  (1) Pain at the site of wound
  (2) Abdominal pain (variable)
 b. **Signs**
  (1) Visible wound and hemorrhage
  (2) Abdominal tenderness
  (3) Rebound (may be diminished in pregnancy)
  (4) Uterine tenderness
  (5) Tachycardia (a late sign in pregnancy)
  (6) Hypotension (a late sign in pregnancy)
  (7) Fetal heart rate changes
  (8) Absent fetal heart tones
 c. **Laboratory data** Hct/Hb may or may not be low.
 d. **Diagnosis**
  (1) Local wound exploration may rule in or out the presence of peritoneal or pelvic penetration.
  (2) Peritoneal lavage In advanced pregnancy a stab wound of the lower abdomen may penetrate the uterus only. Peritoneal lavage may help decide if exploratory laparotomy is necessary.
  (3) Amniocentesis If amniotic fluid is free of blood, the cord and fetus are not significantly bleeding. Retroplacental bleeding will not be revealed by this procedure.
  (4) IVP and cystogram will exclude ureteral and bladder injury.
  (5) Fetal heart rate Fetal bradycardia below 110 may indicate distress due to fetal injury or retroplacental bleeding.
  (6) Proctoscopy may rule out the presence of rectal lesions.
 e. **Treatment** Occasionally, stab wounds penetrating the **lower abdomen** may be managed expectantly. This becomes a reasonable choice under the following conditions:
   —Peritoneal lavage does not indicate severe bleeding.
   —There is no evidence of fetal distress.
   —Amniocentesis does not suggest fetal bleeding.
   —Vital signs are monitored closely and are never a cause of concern.
   —The Hct/Hb is stable.

Stab wounds above the umbilicus are associated with multiple visceral perforations and occasionally laceration of the diaphragm. Since vital sign changes are late in the pregnant woman, immediate exploration is required in upper abdominal stab wounds.

(1) **Surgery** The maternal injuries must be effectively treated. If reduction of uterine size is necessary for exposure or hemostasis, cesarean section is performed followed by oxytocics, regardless of fetal outcome. If further exposure is demanded, hysterectomy may be required. Supracervical hysterectomy may save time, reduce blood loss, and reduce the hazard of ureteral injury.

  (a) If the uterus is penetrated with the gestational age beyond 36 weeks and a live fetus, cesarean section should be done.

  (b) If the uterus is penetrated, the fetus is alive, in no distress, and the gestational age is less than 36 weeks, the wound may be repaired and pregnancy allowed to continue if the following conditions prevail:

    i. Small wound

    ii. Amniocentesis free of blood

    iii. No evidence of fetal distress

    iv. Continuous monitoring of fetus and mother postoperatively

  (c) If the uterus is penetrated and the fetus is dead, the wound may be repaired and delivery vaginally induced later.

  (d) When uterine damage is extensive or broad ligament damage is associated with uncontrollable hemorrhage, cesarean section should be done followed by hysterectomy, if necessary, to gain exposure in order to control bleeding. Bilateral hypogastric artery ligation may be helpful to secure hemostasis and occasionally permits conservation of the uterus.

(2) **Medications** Oxytocic drugs should not be administered until the fetus and placenta have been removed (see p. 207).

  f. **Complications**

    (1) Hemorrhage

    (2) Sepsis

    (3) Fetal death

Perspective

At all times, especially when the fetal welfare is considered, avoid compression of the maternal vena cava by an enlarged uterus. In other words, use the left lateral position during procedures; during surgery when the patient has to be flat, designate someone to displace the uterus until it is empty or the patient can be moved.

D. **Premature separation of placenta** Special consideration must be given to the possibility of placental separation when the pregnant uterus is subjected to trauma. Premature placental separation, abruptio placentae, may lead to high mortality for both mother and fetus, secondary to hemorrhage. It is a feared obstetric complication. Because the separation is a matter of degree, the picture varies from the obvious dramatic case to a subtle situation which may present a golden moment to save the fetus. The two extremes are outlined separately.

1. **Abruption of the placenta, severe form**
   a. **Manifestations**
      (1) **Symptoms**
         (a) Uterine pain, moderate to severe
         (b) Vaginal bleeding; **often there is no visible bleeding.**
      (2) **Signs**
         (a) Tense, often tetanic uterus
         (b) Fetal heart tones absent or severely depressed (less than 90 beats/min).
         (c) Maternal tachycardia and hypotension may be present to a degree beyond that explained by visible blood loss.
         (d) Vaginal bleeding is variable. Little or absent vaginal bleeding may be a manifestation of concealed retroplacental bleeding which is an ominous sign.
         (e) Increase in size of uterus (a late sign)
      (3) **Laboratory studies**
         (a) Hct/Hb may be low.
         (b) Baseline coagulation studies may be abnormal.
   b. **Diagnosis**   In the extreme form, the diagnosis is obvious.
   c. **Treatment**
      (1) **Surgery**
         (a) If the fetus is alive, immediate cesarean section should be done, unless immediate vaginal delivery can be accomplished. Always check for possible vaginal delivery just before starting section. Expect a large amount of clots behind the placenta. If the uterus is blue and mottled, do not do a hysterectomy. The patient most probably has developed DIC and will require prompt treatment (see "Medications," below).
         (b) If the fetus is dead, more time is available for vaginal delivery if coagulation studies are satisfactory and monitored. If delivery is not expected within 2 hr, cesarean section should be done. Removal of the placenta is essential to survival.
      (2) **Medications**   Prepare for possible severe hemorrhage and coagulation defects which may require large volumes of component therapy.
   d. **Complications**
      (1) Uncontrollable hemorrhage
      (2) Renal failure

(3) Parenchymal damage possible in other organs such as pituitary and adrenal

(4) Infection

2. **Separation of the placenta, partial form** The patient may present with premature labor following abdominal trauma. The retroplacental bleeding stimulates the uterus into hypertonia and labor, which is often precipitated.

   a. **Manifestations**
      (1) **Symptoms**
         (a) Uterine pain is mild to moderate. If the pain is constant, the separation may proceed to abruption.
         (b) Vaginal bleeding
      (2) **Signs**
         (a) Uterine hypertonicity
         (b) Vaginal bleeding may be absent, moderate, or heavy.
         (c) Fetal heart rate, initially normal, may show distress patterns due to placental deprivation.
      (3) **Laboratory data** Hct and coagulation profile may be abnormal.

   b. **Diagnosis** Patient with trauma to a large pregnant uterus should be placed on fetal monitor constantly for 12–24 hr, even if asymptomatic. The heart rate pattern may be the only evidence of placental separation. Diagnosis is usually established at cesarean section for fetal distress.

   c. **Treatment** When signs are present or fetal distress is evident, proceed as for abruption of placenta. A partial separation may progress rapidly to the severe form.

Perspective

Always consider the need for tetanus prophylaxis and the possibility of subsequent development of gas gangrene in patients with uterine or vaginal trauma.

At all times, especially when the fetal welfare is considered, avoid compression of the maternal vena cava by an enlarged uterus. Use the left lateral position during procedures; during surgery when the patient has to be flat, designate someone to displace the uterus until it is empty or the patient can be moved.

Tables 1 and 2 provide guidelines for the use of drugs in the critically ill pregnant patient.

Table 1. Partial drug guide in pregnancy

Contraindicated	Use if needed	Little risk
Dicumarol	Salicylates	Demerol
Warfarin	Heparin	Morphine
Oral antidiabetics	Dilantin	Barbiturates
Isotopes of all kinds	Propylthiouracil	Aldomet
Thalidomide	Thiazides	Reserpine
Amphetamines	Benadryl	Digitoxin
Chemotherapeutic agents	Pyribenzamine	Corticoids
Tolbutamide	Chlor-Trimeton	Insulin
Marezine	Dramamine	
Antivert	Librium	
Bonine	Valium	
	Meprobamate	

Table 2. Anti-infection agents in pregnancy

Contraindicated	Use if needed	Little risk
Chloramphenicol	Lincomycin	Penicillins
Tetracyclines	Tobramycin	Ampicillin
Cloxacillin	Gentamicin	Cefazolin
Streptomycin	Kanamycin	Cephalexin
Vancomycin	Metronidazole	Cephalothin
Griseofulvin	Gantrisin*	Clindamycin
Amphotericin		Erythromycin
		Methicillin

*Short-acting sulfa drugs are preferred. Do not use sulfonamide if delivery is probable within 1 month.

12
CENTRAL NERVOUS SYSTEM INJURIES

The central nervous system is composed of the brain and spinal cord, either of which may be damaged by blunt or penetrating trauma. The morbidity that may be associated with damage to the spinal cord or brain may vary from minimal to almost total incapacitation. Functional impairment depends upon the level at which the spinal cord is injured and whether the lesion is complete or incomplete. Similarly, the sequel to brain injury depends upon which portions of the brain or brain stem are injured. The ultimate result of injury to the central nervous system depends upon the initial trauma and how well the physician minimizes subsequent metabolic and physical insult. In other words, the injured spinal cord must be immobilized and cardiopulmonary function must be stabilized to minimize insult to the damaged central nervous tissue. Any patient who has an alteration in level of consciousness associated with trauma must be considered to have intracranial pathology. Any individual who has been involved in a vertical or horizontal deceleration accident or crush injury must be suspected to have a spinal injury, until proved otherwise. A patient may have a spinal column injury without cord damage. However, if improperly handled, the patient may develop a neurologic lesion. Brain or spinal cord injury may be obvious or may be subtle at the time of admission. Since the manifestations of central nervous system injuries may be subtle, especially in the multiply injured patient, these injuries must be actively sought by the clinician until their presence has been excluded. After early stabilization and management of the patient with a brain or spinal cord injury, vigorous therapy is necessary to minimize pulmonary and urinary infections and skin problems. A great deal of functional return depends upon placement of the patient in a proper rehabilitation center to optimize mobility and interpersonal communication.

I. **Brain** The management of the acute head injury (blunt or penetrating) presents a surgical and medical challenge to the neurosurgeon and traumatologist. The diagnostic and therapeutic approach should be logical, organized, and expeditiously executed. The procedures should be flexible enough to allow sound clinical decision-making, especially if the patient has multiple trauma.

The primary goals of treatment of the head-injured patient are
—Rapid obtainment of respiratory and cardiovascular stability
—Early recognition and surgical treatment of intracranial mass lesions
—Initiation of specific measures that minimize intracranial hypertension

A. **Initial assessment** A severe head injury by definition is one that renders the patient unable to open the eyes and talk or move appropriately to painful stimulus (purposeful). A neurosurgeon is to be immediately informed at the time of, or before, the patient's arrival, if possible. Ideally, a neurosurgeon should examine the patient before sedation is administered or intubation is performed. However, if the clinical condition necessitates these interventions on an immediate basis, the admitting personnel should evaluate the **neurologic status** by answering the following questions:

—Does the patient open his eyes and to what stimulus?

—Does the patient utter recognizable words?

—Does the patient follow commands?

—Does the patient move arms and legs equally to central pain and what is the posture?

—What are the pupils' size and reactivity?

In addition, information should be obtained in regard to the time of injury, mechanism of injury, and clinical changes that occurred during the patient's transfer. This information will enable the neurosurgeon to determine the severity of the injury, the presence of any lateralizing neurologic findings compatible with an intracranial mass lesion, and the progression of the patient's condition from the time of injury.

Trauma patients may have a depressed level of consciousness due to metabolic insults. Metabolic causes of central nervous system (CNS) depression associated with trauma are

—Hypoxia/shock

—Alcohol intoxication/drugs

—Sedatives

—Hypothermia

Metabolic CNS depression is a diagnosis of exclusion after the intracranial vault has been evaluated for focal pathology. Metabolic causes of CNS depression and intracranial pathology are commonly seen in the trauma patient. An accurate temperature, arterial blood gases (ABG), and toxicology screen are mandatory.

At the initial **neurosurgical evaluation**, a neuroassessment flow sheet should be started and continued throughout the patient's hospitalization. At MIEMSS, we use a rapid but comprehensive neuroassessment sheet (Figure 1). This assessment index system is a graded neurologic scale that has two purposes:

—On admission, it is an indicator of the severity of injury and type of injury (brain stem versus hemisphere).

—Compared with subsequent scores, it is used to indicate the clinical course.

Brain death is discussed on p. 540.

B. **Stabilization** The stabilization of the patient begins and is simultaneous with the assessment. Stabilization is initiated according to the well accepted principles of assuring an adequate airway, ventilation, and circulation. A basic axiom in regard to resuscitating the injured brain is: "Perfuse the brain with well oxygenated blood and keep the intracranial pressure normal." Therefore, all patients with severe head injury are intubated and hyperventilated as soon as possible. Baseline arterial blood gases should be drawn and serial determinations made routinely. A neurologic deficit can worsen as a result of hypoxia. All patients require arterial pressure lines inserted to follow the systemic pressure. A decrease in **cerebral perfusion pressure** (CPP) leads to further cerebral damage. CPP is the balance between mean arterial pressure and intracranial pressure (ICP). If the CPP is $\leq 50\,\text{mm Hg}$, cerebral perfusion is likely to be compromised. Our experience reveals that 56% of pa-

University of Maryland
NEURO ASSESSMENT

Eye Opening:

Spontaneously	0
To speech	1
To pain	2
None	3
Untestable	U

Orientation

Time, place, person	0
2 of the 3	1
1 of the 3	2
None	3
Untestable	U

Pupil, Corneal & Caloric Reflexes and Grimace:

Normal	0
Decreased or abnormal	1
Absent	2
Untestable	U

Stimulus:

Voice	0
Shake or shout	1
Pain	2
Central pain	3

Verbal Response:

Oriented	0
Confused	1
Inappropriate	2
Incomprehensible	3
None	4
Untestable	U

Leg Motor Response:

Normal	0
Paretic	1
Abnormal or extensor	2
None	3
Untestable	U

Arm Motor Response:

Obeys - strong	0
Obeys - paretic	1
Localizes	2
Withdraws	3
Abnormal flexion	4
Extensor	5
None	6
Untestable	U

Date
Time
Initials
Sedation Meds (yes/no)
Paralytic Agents (yes/no)
Seizures
Eye Opening
Orientation
Pupils (R/L)
Corneals (R/L)
Facial grimace (R/L)
Calorics (R/L)
Stimulus
Verbal Response
Arm Motor (R/L)
Leg Motor (R/L)
Signature/Status

Figure 1. Neuroassessment chart.

tients with severe head injury have multiple injuries. In these patients, adequate perfusion to all organ systems is mandatory. We attempt to maintain the patient in a normotensive state with a systolic pressure between 100 and 170 mm Hg. Pressures higher than 170 mm Hg can cause increased cerebral blood volume leading to increased ICP, as well as aggravate the formation of vasogenic edema. Initial hyperventilation is instituted by regulating the $PaCO_2$ between 25 and 30 mm Hg. Hyperventilation causes constriction of cerebral vasculature with a resultant decrease in cerebral blood volume (not cerebral blood flow), which decreases intracranial pressure. This initial stabilization process is aimed at disrupting the vicious cycle depicted in Figure 2, thus preventing secondary brain injury.

C. **Diagnosis** After the patient has been stabilized and the severity and nature of the brain injury has been assessed, the neurodiagnostic work-up should commence and proceed rapidly. Two important facts should be remembered:
—Any unconscious head-injured patient may be harboring a spine injury (5–15% at MIEMSS, depending on the severity of head trauma).
—If a patient with a head injury is not following commands, there is about a 25% chance that the patient is harboring an intracranial lesion requiring surgery.

1. **Cervical spine x-ray** A lateral cervical spine film should be obtained immediately after stabilization of the patient to rule out a cervical spine injury which may be compounding the neurologic picture or which, if unrecognized, could result in additional neurologic deficit due to spinal cord injury.

2. **Skull x-rays** Anteroposterior and lateral skull films should be obtained immediately in those patients who have penetrating wounds of the skull and those suspected to have a depressed skull fracture. Plain skull x-rays are of value in localizing the position of foreign bodies inside the calvaria and the amount of bony depression of the skull. In severe closed-head injuries, the skull x-ray may

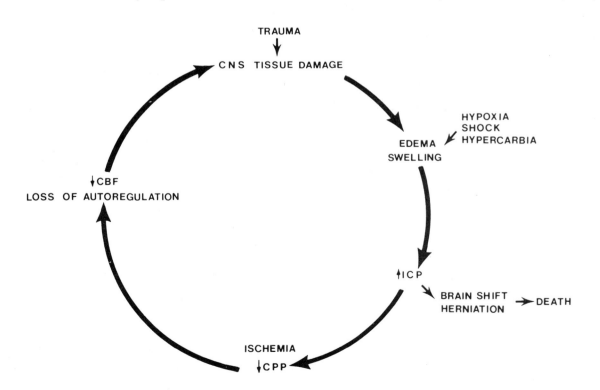

Figure 2. Vicious cycle of CNS tissue damage.

be deferred until after computed tomography of the head is performed. In these cases, the skull x-ray has generally been negative or nondiagnostic. One way in which plain skull x-rays are of help is in the identification of "high risk linear fractures." These are nondepressed linear skull fractures that cross vascular grooves of the middle meningeal artery, the dural sinuses, or extend into the foramen magnum. These fractures put the patient at risk for developing an epidural hematoma. The presence of this type of finding mandates a CAT scan regardless of the patient's neurologic condition.

3. **Computerized axial tomography**   If a patient has an intracranial mass lesion, there is the potential for sudden clinical deterioration. The burden is on the physician to diagnose or rule out these lesions as rapidly as possible. The CAT scan is the diagnostic test of choice to identify these lesions because it is rapid, noninvasive, safe to perform, and gives an actual picture of the pathology, thus avoiding some of the guesswork necessary with other diagnostic tests, and it differentiates between intraparenchymal blood and brain swelling or edema. A CAT scan can diagnose coexisting or dual pathology, e.g., the combination of a subdural hematoma and intracerebral hemorrhage or a depressed skull fracture associated with an intracerebral hemorrhage. It can be used to assess the consequences of emergency intracranial surgical procedures (burr hole, craniectomy, etc.). The patient can be taken immediately to the CAT room while remaining under anesthesia, to evaluate the effect of the surgery and to monitor evolving pathology. Sequential CAT scanning can detect the presence of delayed pathology (intracerebral hemorrhage, recurrent extracerebral hematoma, etc.), which may alter the patient's outcome or require further surgery.

The indication for CAT scan is a patient who has sustained head trauma and presents with any sign of neurologic dysfunction while in the Admitting Area. Neurologic dysfunction includes any alteration in mental status (disorientation, drowsiness, etc.), as well as localizing or lateralizing signs (hemiparesis, unilateral pupillary dilatation, etc.).

The timing of the CAT scan depends on the patient's stability in regard to other systems injuries, as well as on neurologic condition. If the patient has no other associated injuries and is comatose or has lateralizing neurologic signs consistent with a unilateral mass lesion, the patient should be scanned immediately after initial resuscitation. If the patient is hemodynamically stable, routine peritoneal lavage, x-rays, etc., may be deferred until after the CAT scan. Therefore, the patient should be studied within 30 min of admission.

If the patient has no other associated injuries and the neurologic condition is stable (i.e., patient awake but with altered mental status), there is less urgency for a CAT scan. The patient may undergo complete evaluation in the Admitting Area as long as frequent (every 15 min) neurologic checks are done. The CAT scan should be obtained within 1–1½ hr of admission. This same plan applies to patients who have other systems injuries that need attention and who are neurologically stable.

4. **Carotid angiogram**   The biggest dilemma is the patient who has both life-threatening injuries (e.g., shock and a positive peritoneal lavage) and a critical neurologic status (comatose, unilateral decerebration, a dilated or fixed

pupil(s), etc.). The ideal solution is to have the CAT scanner in the Admitting Area where stabilization of the patient can be continued while the patient is being scanned. However, few centers have this luxury. One of two things can be done: One can wait until the immediate threat of cardiovascular or pulmonary death is under control and then obtain a CAT scan, or one can perform a percutaneous, common carotid, "one shot" cerebral angiogram using portable x-ray equipment. By persisting with this latter technique, we have mastered it in a way that we can gain significant and sometimes life-saving information in this select group of patients. The angiogram assists in the identification of an intracranial surgical lesion.

5. **Laboratory data**   Included in the initial diagnostic work-up of these patients are various laboratory tests that are relevant to a patient's neurologic status. Laboratory tests of significance include: toxicology screen (both urine and blood); serum alcohol level; electrolytes; blood urea nitrogen (BUN); hemoglobin and hematocrit; glucose and serum osmolality.

D. **Treatment**

1. **Surgical**   If the diagnostic work-up reveals a surgical lesion, surgery is performed immediately. If an extracranial injury also requires immediate surgery, the procedures are performed simultaneously. The general indications for emergency intracranial surgery are:
    —Open depressed skull fracture and/or penetrating skull wound
    —Expanding intracranial hematoma (epidural or subdural) causing brain shift or clinical signs of herniation
    —Focal contusion with swelling or intracerebral hematoma acting as an expanding mass lesion

    The majority of emergency surgery for head trauma is done to decompress the brain. This is true in an operation on a depressed skull fracture, expanding hematoma, or a swollen hemorrhagic cerebral lobe. The goals are to adequately relieve the pressure and to prevent its recurrence. Additional goals are to clean, debride, and prevent infection in wounds that are contaminated.

    a. **Open depressed skull fractures**   All open depressed skull fractures require early operation (within 2–6 hr of admission). The only exception is an asymptomatic fracture overlying the sagittal sinus. The depressed bone fragments are elevated with as little disruption of the normal skull as possible. Dural tears are repaired by direct suturing or by using graft material such as temporalis fascia or pericranium. The bone fragments can be soaked and washed in aseptic and/or antibiotic solution and replaced to avoid a cranioplasty. If the wound is extremely contaminated, the bone pieces should be discarded, a cranial defect is left, and a cranioplasty is performed 6–12 months later. Meticulous attention should be paid to achieving hemostasis if the cortical surface of the lesion has been lacerated.

    b. **Gunshot wounds**   Most of the surgical principles that apply to depressed skull fractures also apply to gunshot wounds that penetrate the skull and brain. If a patient with a gunshot wound to the brain is deemed salvageable, that patient will undergo an operation. The purpose is primarily to clean and debride the entry wound and exit site, if one is present. Also, the dura is repaired. Any associated hematoma (epidural, subdural, intracerebral) is removed, as described below. Bone fragments are removed if they are easily accessible. Further cerebral damage is not risked solely to remove a bullet fragment. Antibiotics are not used routinely. If the intracranial vault has been grossly contaminated (i.e., shot through the sinuses), the patient may receive antibiotic coverage.

c. **Extracerebral hematomas**   The removal of epidural and subdural hematomas is done in a variety of ways, depending on the individual surgeon; there is no single right way. However, certain basic principles must be followed if good results are to be expected. When evacuating an extracerebral hematoma, an initial small craniectomy in the temporal region is adequate for immediate removal of a critical amount of subdural or epidural clot to achieve decompression of the brain. At this point, one should then provide wider exposure through a formal craniotomy flap. This will ensure complete removal of the clot and give access to active or potential sites of bleeding. An epidural hematoma may require extending the craniectomy to the floor of the middle fossa to control bleeding from the middle meningeal artery or to completely remove subtemporal clot. A large craniotomy is recommended for a subdural hematoma. The bone flap should expose the frontal, temporal, and parietal lobes almost to the midline. The use of a small craniotomy or burr holes as the only procedure for evacuating acute extracerebral hematomas invites postoperative complications and is to be discouraged.

d. **Emergency burr holes**   The need to perform emergency burr holes before a CAT scan or angiography is rare. There are certain times, however, when this is necessary. If a patient is admitted with a stable neurologic status and suddenly undergoes transtentorial herniation, we will do an emergency burr hole. The clinical signs of transtentorial herniation include coma, a unilateral fixed and dilated pupil, and hemiplegia or decerebrate posturing on the side of the body opposite the fixed, dilated pupil. The other occasion for emergency burr holes is a patient who experiences the same process en route to the hospital. This must be well documented by competent emergency medical personnel. In either case, a rapid temporal burr hole is **placed on the same side of the head as the abnormal pupil.** If a clot is found, the patient is taken immediately to the operating room. If no clot is found, the patient undergoes immediate CAT scanning. It should be emphasized that emergency burr holes should be reserved for those patients who are dying of brain compression "before your eyes." These patients are given intravenous mannitol (1 gm/kg) to rapidly shrink the brain and decrease intracranial pressure. We reserve the use of mannitol for patients showing clinical signs of herniation, i.e., dilation of one or both pupils in a comatose patient, unreactive pupil in a comatose patient, unilateral or bilateral decerebration, and respiratory arrest subsequent to a head injury.

2. **Medical** After evaluation and surgery, if indicated, care consists of aggressive medical therapy that is designed to minimize intracranial hypertension. The medical therapy is dictated by the ICP levels.

The general indications for **ICP monitoring** are
—A patient who is comatose and not purposeful to pain
—A multiple trauma patient who has an altered level of consciousness and must undergo prolonged anesthesia for other injuries
—Any patient who has had an intracranial hematoma evacuated

The ICP monitoring technique commonly used is ventriculostomy and placement of an intraventricular catheter for direct continuous measurement of ventricular fluid pressure. We use this method because it provides a reliable reading of ICP and it allows treatment of hypertension by draining cerebrospinal fluid (CSF), thus reducing ICP immediately. Ventriculitis may develop after the catheter has been in place for 72 hr. On the third day of monitoring, a ventricular fluid specimen is obtained by the neurosurgical staff. One cubic centimeter of fluid is obtained for culture, sensitivity, and Gram stain; protein and sugar; and cell count. If only a very small amount of ventricular fluid can be obtained, the cell count, Gram stain, and culture are first priority tests. The cell count and glucose should be obtained on a stat basis. If at any time the question of CNS infection arises—even before the 3rd day—a CSF specimen is obtained. If the CSF specimen is negative for infection, the intraventricular catheter (IVC) is left in place and each day afterwards a similar specimen is obtained. If and when the CSF specimen shows signs of infection, the IVC is removed. If continued ICP monitoring is necessary, there are two alternatives: A new IVC may be placed in the opposite side, or a subarachnoid screw may be placed on the opposite side.

If the IVC remains uninfected for 4–5 days and continued ICP monitoring is necessary, consideration is given to prophylactically removing it and inserting a new one on the opposite side.

When it is determined that ICP monitoring is no longer necessary, the IVC is removed under sterile conditions. Prior to removing the IVC, 1 cc of ventricular fluid is removed for the battery of tests described earlier. In addition, the ventricular catheter tip should be cultured. After the IVC is removed, a dry sterile dressing should be applied to the exit wound and left in place for 2–3 days.

We also use a subarachnoid bolt device which has the advantages of ease of insertion, a lower CNS infection rate than a ventricular catheter, and being used when the ventricles are compressed and cannot be punctured. The disadvantages are that the CSF cannot be drained and that this device is not quite as reliable as the catheter (Figure 3).

All patients who have sustained severe head injuries receive a standardized medical regimen specific for treating the brain injury. The variations in treatment depend on the ICP levels. Normal ICP is equal to or less than 15 mm Hg. Patients with an ICP less than or equal to 15 mm Hg are **hyperventilated** with a $PaCO_2$ of 25–30 mm Hg for 2–3 days. When hyperventilation is stopped, if the ICP rises above 15 mm Hg, hyperventilation is reinstituted. **Sedation** will often

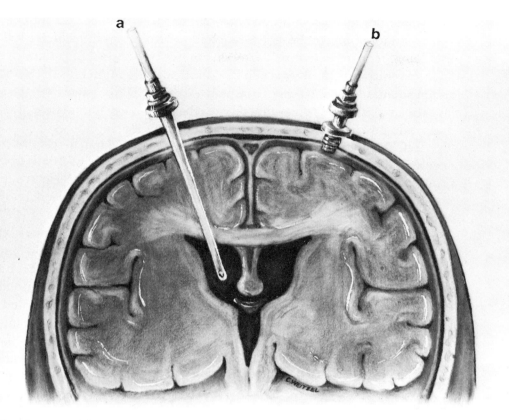

Figure 3. Intracranial pressure monitoring. *a*, intraventricular catheter; *b*, subarachnoid bolt.

reduce the intracranial pressure. Barbiturates or morphine may be used to control occasional elevation in ICP secondary to agitation. **Elevation of the head** will often lower the ICP and should be used for increases in ICP in the supine patient. **Oxygenation** is maintained by the appropriate FiO_2, level of PEEP, and chest physiotherapy. PEEP may contribute to the intracranial pressure if the brain is poorly compliant. We feel that "physiologic PEEP" (3–5 cm) is beneficial and unlikely to affect ICP. If PEEP is likely to affect ICP, usually that patient will have an ICP monitor in place and the effect of PEEP can be seen.

We feel that head-injured patients benefit from **steroids.** Steroids are begun in the initial resuscitation period with a loading dose of methylprednisolone (Medrol), 5 mg/kg i.v. The same daily dose is given in four divided doses. Dexamethasone (Decadron) in doses of 1 mg/kg may be used following the same scheme. If after 3 days there has been clinical improvement, the steroids are continued for approximately 7 days and tapered over the next 3 days. If no improvement is seen at 3 days, the steroids are stopped. Our experience at MIEMSS suggests that the efficacy of steroids may be related to individual patient factors (i.e., initial injury, hypoxia, cardiovascular instability, etc.) and the best indicator for continued use may be the patient's initial response to treatment. Antacids should be given with the steroids and the gastric pH should be monitored.

If the ICP is 16–24 mm Hg, the patient is administered the same treatment as that given to the group whose ICP is less than or equal to 15 mm Hg. In addition, **mannitol** therapy is begun with intermittent doses of 0.25 gm/kg every 4–6 hr. If more frequent doses are required, a continuous infusion is employed. If ICP still remains between 16–24 mm Hg, we will drain CSF intermittently if an intraventricular catheter is in place. Particular attention must be paid to the **serum sodium** level and **serum osmolality** during the treatment. When sodium levels reach 150 and serum osmolality reaches 320, the mannitol dose is reduced and gradually discontinued.

If ICP goes to 25 mm Hg or greater for more than 10 min at rest, the patient is entered into our high-dose **barbiturate therapy study.** The non-barbiturate group continues the same maximal therapy as the 16–24 mm Hg group. The barbiturate therapy for severe head-injured patients is based on two facts: High-dose barbiturate therapy is often able to control high levels of ICP when other therapies have failed, and barbiturates may offer some form of cerebral protective effect against the secondary insults of shock, hypoxia, and ischemia. The efficacy of this type of therapy is not known at present. Barbiturate therapy is started by the administration of a loading dose of pentobarbital (Nembutal), 10 mg/kg/hr for 4 hr. The maximum loading dose is titrated based on changes of ICP and arterial pressure. After the 4 hr of loading dose infusion, a maintenance dose of pentobarbital, 50–200 mg every 30–60 min to maintain control of ICP, is given by injection or continuous infusion. A Swan-Ganz catheter is indicated to assess cardiovascular performance, which may be affected by large doses of pentobarbital.

Barbiturate levels are drawn at least every morning. A blood level of 2.5–4.0 mg % is maintained. If the barbiturate level is > 4.0 mg %, the drug will be held. Electroencephalogram (EEG) and auditory-evoked potentials may also be used to guide barbiturate therapy.

Barbiturate therapy is stopped by tapering the dose over several days. Indications are

- —ICP ≤ 15 mm Hg for 24 hr. At this point, barbiturates are tapered off. If ICP increases again to 20 mm Hg, barbiturate treatment is reinstituted.
- —If ICP remains unstable, barbiturate therapy is continued for 4 days and then tapered off. No patient will receive barbiturates for longer than 10 days.
- —If there is no response to barbiturate therapy, it will be stopped after 24 hr.

Barbiturate therapy will be held but not necessarily discontinued if

- —Barbiturate level is ≥ 4 mg %
- —There is a deterioration of auditory-evoked potentials

A number of well controlled, randomized studies are being conducted at several centers. Since this therapy is not without risk, it is our feeling that its use should be limited to those centers that are conducting such studies and have around-the-clock critical care support.

During the first 3–5 days post-injury, when cerebral edema formation is most likely, **fluids** should be given judiciously to maintain a **serum osmolality** of around 300–310. A **urinary output** of 25–30 cc/hr is accepted unless there is multiple trauma, in which case there is a major concern for the onset of acute renal failure. No matter how many organ systems are injured, judicious fluid administration is a priority during the first 5 days after a severe head injury.

Occasionally, in the very spastic and uncontrolled patient, **Pavulon** may be administered and associated with a fall in ICP. Pavulon should be infrequently used, but if administered it should be given only if an ICP monitor is in place.

| Note | Patients with intracranial hemorrhage should have their **coagulation parameters** monitored, serially, whether they have had a craniotomy or not.

3. **Skilled observation** After the patient has been resuscitated, assessed, and initially treated (operation, ICP monitor, etc.), the task becomes one of intensive nursing care coupled with the aggressive medical treatment outlined above. Skilled observation is the ability to recognize significant clinical changes and to react appropriately.

Physical examination allows us to detect manifestations that may represent a rise in intracranial pressure. These physical findings are
—Deterioration in the level of consciousness
—Development of lateralizing signs
—Pupillary changes
—Changes in the vital signs
—Progressive depression in motor response

If one of these manifestations appear, the cause must be evaluated. The most important pathology to rule out is an expanding mass lesion. Changes in neurologic function may also be brought about by
—Over-sedation (narcotics)
—Electrolyte abnormalities (hyper- or hyponatremia)
—Sepsis
—Meningitis
—Hypoglycemia
—Hypothermia
—Hypotension
—Hypoxia/hypercarbia

Thus, evaluation of a deteriorating neurologic picture requires a work-up for structural and metabolic abnormalities.

a. **The conscious head-injured patient**
   (1) **Level of consciousness** Any deterioration of the conscious level (e.g., harder to arouse, sleeping more, responding inappropriately to questions) is an emergency. Notify the neurosurgeon and simultaneously begin evaluation by performing a neurologic examination and metabolic evaluation.
   (2) **Lateralizing signs** A lateralizing sign is the finding of a neurologic deficit on one side of the body and not the other. It implies focal brain

dysfunction and may be caused by an expanding mass lesion (i.e., epidural, subdural, or intracerebral hemorrhage or focal brain swelling). The appearance of weakness on one side of the body is the most common example. A changing speech pattern (slurring words, not following commands, and inappropriate conversation) can also be a lateralizing sign. **Call the neurosurgeon.** If these are new findings, a CAT scan is usually indicated to rule out an intracranial mass lesion.

(3) **Pupillary changes** If the pupil size changes asymmetrically, **report to the neurosurgeon.** If the reaction of a pupil becomes more sluggish, this should be watched closely and reported.

(4) **Vital signs** Many head-injured patients will be hypertensive and tachycardic during the initial phase of the injury. If intracranial pressure is increasing, this may be reflected by a rise in the blood pressure with a drop in the pulse, at which time the neurosurgeon should be alerted. ICP frequently rises without changes in the vital signs.

b. **The unconscious head-injured patient**
(1) **Level of consciousness** If the patient has been evoking a particular response (i.e., movement) to a given stimulus (e.g., pinching) and is requiring a greater degree of stimulation to obtain the same response, this constitutes deepening of coma and is an emergency. **Do not use terms like obtunded, stuporous, etc.; describe what the patient does or does not do.**

(2) **Motor response** An unconscious patient will exhibit one of the following types of movement to painful stimuli:
(a) **Appropriate** This is purposeful movement which localizes pain and attempts to remove it.
(b) **Inappropriate** This is either decorticate or decerebrate rigidity. Decorticate rigidity is flexion of the arms, wrist, and fingers with adduction in the upper extremities and extension of the legs. This is seen in large lesions of the cerebral hemisphere, internal capsule, or diencephalon (thalamus and basal ganglia), i.e., moderate to severe head injuries above the brain stem. Decerebrate rigidity is extension and hyperpronation of the arms and extension of the legs. This is seen in brain stem injuries and implies a worse neurologic condition than decorticate posturing. The flexion withdrawal response is between purposeful and decorticate, i.e., the patient will flex the upper extremities in a nonspastic manner but will not localize pain. It is sometimes referred to as "semipurposeful."
(c) **No movement** The patient is flaccid in response to central pain. This implies disruption of corticospinal fibers from higher centers. Flaccidity implies severe CNS damage and is associated with a poor prognosis.
In order of increasing severity of injury and decreasing neurologic function, the motor responses are as follows:

Condition	Movement	Injury
Good	**Purposeful**	Minor
	Flexion-withdrawal (semi-purposeful)	
Bad	**Decorticate**	
	Decerebrate	
Worse	**Flaccid**	Severe

If a patient's response moves down the scale, the patient is deteriorating; up the scale, the patient is improving in regard to motor response. When describing a patient, use these terms appropriately. If the motor response deteriorates, call the neurosurgeon and rule out superimposed metabolic complications. If the patient has an ICP monitor, evaluate its level. A deterioration in motor response may represent an expanding intracranial mass lesion.

(3) **Pupillary changes and vital signs** The same concerns and responses apply as they do in the conscious patient.

(4) **Intracranial pressure** Any elevation of ICP greater than 16 mm Hg at rest for greater than 10 min should prompt a call to the neurosurgeon.

E. **Miscellaneous problems**

1. **Basal skull fractures** The diagnosis of a basal skull fracture is usually clinical. Periorbital ecchymosis, rhinorrhea, blood behind the tympanic membrane, otorrhea, and Battle's sign (ecchymotic mastoid region) are signs of basal skull fracture. X-ray findings of fractured sinuses, air-fluid levels in the sinuses, or pneumocephalus confirm the clinical impression that a basal skull fracture is present. These patients should be watched closely for the development of meningitis, cranial nerve palsies, and CSF leaks.

2. **CSF leaks** At MIEMSS, we do not treat these patients with prophylactic antibiotics. In our experience, the incidence of meningitis following traumatic otorrhea or rhinorrhea is the same with or without antibiotics. However, if a patient is on prophylactic antibiotic coverage and develops meningitis, it is often due to a resistant strain of bacteria. Thus, the clinical course is stormy. If a patient has CSF otorrhea or rhinorrhea, packing of the ear or nose is contraindicated. The patient is nursed with the head elevated 45–90° to decrease intracranial subarachnoid pressure. The majority (75%) of CSF leaks will stop with this treatment within 5–7 days. If they do not stop or decrease significantly at 5 days, we do daily lumbar punctures to decrease the CSF leak. Sometimes an indwelling lumbar subarachnoid drain is employed for the same reason. Only 1–2% of patients will need an intracranial operation to stop a CSF leak. If at any time the patient with a CSF leak becomes febrile and/or shows signs of meningismus, we sample the CSF for evidence of meningitis.

3. **Posttraumatic seizure**   There is controversy over the efficacy of prophylactic anticonvulsants (Dilantin) to prevent posttraumatic seizures. We do not start all head-injured patients on anticonvulsant therapy. Indications for anticonvulsant treatment are
   —A CAT scan finding that is compatible with cortical disruption, i.e., large intracerebral hemorrhage involving the cortex
   —Findings at surgery that predispose to epilepsy (i.e., badly lacerated cortex)
   —Any patient put on paralytic agents (a paralyzed patient may have seizures without obvious motor activity)
   —More than two seizures in the posttraumatic period

4. **Management of the mild to moderate head injury**   Patients who present to the Admitting Area conscious are observed closely for evidence of CNS injury. The patient's treatment depends on the neurologic examination. Any trauma patient with neurologic abnormality is admitted and has a CAT scan regardless of whether or not there was loss of consciousness. If there was loss of consciousness, the patient is admitted for at least 24 hr of observation. The reason for this strict admission policy is a concern that we might miss an epidural hematoma which may be associated with a lucid interval during which the neurologic examination may appear normal before the patient deteriorates due to an expanding clot. When these patients are admitted, they are kept NPO, intravenous fluids (isotonic solution) are administered at low rates (50–75 cc/hr), and frequent neurologic assessments (every hour) are done. See p. 218 on high-risk skull fractures.

II. **Spine**   The management of spinal or spinal cord injuries begins at the scene of the accident. Unfortunately, nothing at the present time can be done to reverse the disruption of central nervous system tissue which occurs at the time of injury. Consequently, the management of these patients is aimed at preserving what spinal cord function remains by adhering to the principles of
   —Immediate immobilization and early diagnosis
   —Alignment and stabilization of the bony injury
   —Preventing the progression of the cord injury by stabilizing the patient medically
   —Early rehabilitation

The following patients should be considered to have a spine injury, until it is proved otherwise:
   —An alert patient who cannot move extremities upon command
   —An unconscious patient who fails to move an extremity (or extremities) when sternal pressure is applied
   —Any unconscious patient with a history of blunt trauma
   —A patient who has suffered penetrating trauma to the neck or torso and is unable to move an extremity (or extremities) upon command or sternal compression
   —An alert patient who complains of neck pain or back pain
   —A patient with maxillofacial trauma

A. **Immobilization** All patients suspected of having spinal injury should have that particular area of their spine immediately immobilized.

  1. **Cervical** Apply a hard collar or "sandbag" and secure the head to a spine board.

  2. **Thoracic and lumbar** Immobilize on a Stryker frame. The patient should not be moved or allowed to roll, turn, or elevate himself.

B. **Notification of consulting services** The Neurosurgical Team should be called immediately for spinal injuries if they have not been notified prior to the patient's arrival. If the patient arrives before these consultants, the Trauma Team should institute resuscitative measures that are appropriate for the patient's injuries.

C. **Initial management**

  1. **Ensure adequate oxygenation** A neurologic deficit can be created or worsened by a hypoxic insult to the injured cord. The quadriplegic has a markedly impaired vital capacity and is subject to the other causes of respiratory insufficiency following blunt trauma (see pp. 15 and 238).

  2. **Hemodynamic stability** Disruption of the descending sympathetic pathways results in loss of vasomotor tone and subsequent hypotension. The unopposed parasympathetic activity results in bradycardia; therefore, the clinical picture of hypotension with bradycardia is often seen in the quadriplegic patient. In a patient with both depressed blood pressure and cardiac rate, the impaired cardiac output may result in tissue hypoperfusion. Because of the inability to regulate vasomotor tone, caution should be exercised while replacing fluids. If the patient is hypotensive, but has a normal urinary output, the hypotension is not aggressively treated. If there is oliguria, the hypotension is treated with dopamine (Intropin) and **judicious** fluid administration (see p. 237).

  3. **An orogastric tube** should be inserted to prevent abdominal distention secondary to a paralytic ileus. If untreated, this can result in vomiting, aspiration, and respiratory embarrassment.

  4. **Urinary tract management** If the patient cannot void, immediately insert a Foley catheter. Retention of urine can develop within hours and lead to overdistention of the bladder and subsequent hypotonia. Because of sensory paralysis, there may be no discomfort. Record the patient's reaction to insertion of the catheter. If the patient is stable, ask the patient to void to assess pelvic visceral function.

D. **Physical examination** The principal symptom of fracture of the spine is **acute local pain,** which may or may not radiate into the arms, torso, or legs. If this is present, a detailed examination should be performed without moving the patient's spine. Inspection of the patient for external signs of trauma may help in localizing the spinal injury and its pathomechanism. For example, injuries to the forehead and chin may cause hyperextension of the cervical spine. A blow to the vertex of the head may cause a compression fracture of the cervical spine. Abrasion or lacerations over the posterior trunk can be a sign of thoracic and lumbar injuries. Palpation of the spine without moving the patient may reveal prominence of the spinous processes, local tenderness and pain, edema, deformity, or muscle spasm. Findings should be recorded in the admission note. There is a 5–20% incidence of spine injury associated with acute head injuries; therefore, any comatose patient may harbor a spine injury and should be treated accordingly.

E. **Neurologic examination** The traumatologist who admits the patient should perform a basic neurologic examination noting any motor and sensory deficits. The initial examination states whether or not the patient can
   —Take a deep breath (i.e., use both intercostal and diaphragmatic muscles)
   —Raise and extend arms (C_5/C_7)
   —Open and close hand (C_7/T_1)
   —Raise legs (L_2/L_4)
   —Wiggle toes (L_5/S_1)
   —Tighten anus (S_3/S_5)

A quick sensory test to pinprick should be performed beginning on the bottom of the foot—from the lateral aspect of the foot, across the dorsum of the foot, to the anterior tibial region, the anterior thigh, lateral thigh, up the torso in the midaxillary line, into the axilla, down the inside of the upper arm, to the ulnar aspect of the forearm, the ulnar aspect of hand, across the palm surface of fingertips of digits 5–1, up the radial side of the forearm, the outer (lateral) aspect of the upper arm, over the shoulder, up the lateral aspect of the neck, and to the back of the occiput. The same pattern should be followed on both sides of the body. If there is a well demonstrated point of sensory deficit, this should be marked on the body with a pen. If this pattern is followed, all the dermatomes up to C_2 are tested consecutively. Note should be made of perineal sensation and sensory response to catheterization of the bladder.

The neurosurgeon will perform a more extensive neurologic examination and record his findings on the spinal neural chart as well as in a formal admission note. The examination will assess motor, sensory and autonomic function, and reflex activity. Based on this information, the level and the type of neural involvement will then be determined.

1. The **motor examination** is done by testing individually each major muscle group in each extremity. The function of the muscle should be graded and recorded. Grading is based on whether the muscles function normally (5), weak but against resistance (4), against gravity but not resistance (3), not against gravity (2), trace movement (1), and paralysis (0). It is only through the accurate recording of this information that one can determine whether the patient is improving or deteriorating.

2. The **sensory examination** must determine any deficit of pain, temperature, and fine touch (spinothalamic function), as well as any deficit of proprioception, deep sensibility, and vibration (posterior column function). A level of sensory deficit should be determined and correlated with the motor level of deficit.

Reflex changes should be ascertained carefully. This may provide information on whether certain spinal roots were spared from injury and whether the cord injury is complete. In the evaluation of lumbosacral injuries, the reflex examination is of utmost importance, since we are dealing with nerve root injury of the cauda equina rather than the cord itself.

3. **Autonomic dysfunction** may be assessed by checking for diminished sweating, vasomotor instability, loss of bladder and rectal control, and priapism.

For the emergency room physician, one of the most important objectives of the initial clinical examination should be to determine whether the injury has resulted in a lesion that presents as a complete cord deficit or an incomplete cord deficit.

Patients will be classified as having
— Complete cord lesion (presenting)
— Incomplete cord syndrome
— Root lesion
— No neurological deficit

A complete lesion is one in which there are no clinical signs of any cord function below the level of the bony injury. Incomplete lesions have some preservation of cord function (i.e., sacral sensory sparing, minimal motor function in legs, preservation of position senses, deep tendon reflex, etc.). The importance of this differentiation lies in its prognosticating value. A lesion that presents complete on admission and remains complete over the next 24–72 hr has an extremely poor prognosis in regard to return of function. An incomplete lesion at least has the possibility of return of function. It should be noted, however, that, to date, there is no clinical way to differentiate truly between a patient who has a complete lesion and one who is in severe spinal shock. In other words, all lesions have the possibility of being incomplete and should be approached with that in mind during this early phase.

Some of the typical findings of the more commonly injured spinal levels are as follows:

C_2/C_3 **injury**
General
Complete respiratory paralysis
Motor and reflexes
Complete flaccidity and areflexia

Death will occur in a few minutes unless artificial respiration is maintained.

C_5/C_6 **injury**
General
Paralysis of intercostal respiration Diaphragmatic respiration continuing without thoracic muscle action
Motor
Quadriplegia Complete loss of motor power in hands, trunk, and lower extremities; preservation of shoulder girdle functions and some deltoid, pectoral, and biceps action

Sensory

Anesthesia beginning approximately 3 cm below the clavicles; anesthesia of at least the ulnar half of the upper extremities

Reflexes

Deep tendon reflexes, initially absent, with possible exception of biceps reflex; absent abdominal, cremasteric, and plantar reflexes

Autonomic

Bladder and bowel retention; priapism

T_{12}/L_1 injury

Motor

Paraplegia

Sensory

Anesthesia in the legs

Reflexes

Deep tendon reflexes are initially absent in the lower extremities; absent cremasteric and plantar reflexes; upper abdominal reflexes may be preserved.

Autonomic

Bladder and bowel retention

L_4/L_5 injury

Motor

Partial flaccid paraparesis, especially involving the ankle

Sensory

Numbness of lateral aspect of the feet

Reflexes

Absent ankle reflexes

Autonomic

Urinary retention and a relaxed anal sphincter

F. **Radiologic diagnosis** After the patient has been stabilized and a clinical motor and sensory level of injury has been determined, radiographic examination must be done to delineate the exact site and nature of the bony injury. This is usually done in the Admitting Area with the patient lying supine on the stretcher. Portable lateral and anterioposterior views of the suspected area of injury are generally easily obtained and demonstrate the injury. In the cervical region, an open-mouth view of the odontoid may be of considerable help in assessing fractures of C_1/C_2. Oblique films can be obtained without spine manipulation and often give valuable information in regard to the status of the posterior elements of the cervical spine. Occasionally, polytomography of the injured area is necessary to properly identify the type and extent of bony damage. The roentgenograms should be examined closely for contour and alignment of the vertebral bodies, displacement of bone fragments into the spinal canal, linear or comminuted fractures of the laminae, pedicles, or neural arches. In all cases of cervical injury, C_7 must be visualized on the lateral film. It is often necessary to pull distally on the arms to lower the shoulders. If this maneuver is unsuccessful, a swimmer's view can be attempted if the patient is alert and cooperative. A firm collar should be kept in place if these techniques fail and tomography should be employed later to rule out a low cervical fracture.

The radiologic appearance of a spine injury depends on the mechanism of injury and the force with which it occurs. In the cervical spine, flexion injuries can result in bilateral dislocation of the facet joints (jumped facets) or teardrop or anterior wedge fractures of the body (comminuted). Flexion-rotation injuries often lead to a unilateral facet dislocation. Vertical compression injuries to the cervical spine can cause bursting fractures of the vertebral bodies. Extension injuries can break spinous processes or show no fresh fracture pathology in the presence of pre-existing osteoarthritic changes and spinal canal narrowing. Finally, it should be noted that a patient may have a significant neurologic deficit with a normal-appearing cervical spine x-ray. If this occurs, careful flexion and extension views or cine-fluoroscopy should be considered, which may demonstrate instability due to a ligamentous or soft tissue injury. The other two possibilities are that a disc is herniated or there is a vascular lesion of the cord, with bone stability. Thoracic and lumbar fractures may occur by the same mechanism as those in the cervical area. In addition, a rather dramatic rotational slice fracture may occur. The most frequently injured vertebrae in this area are T_{11}/L_2 (i.e., the thoracolumbar junction), where there is often a compression injury with a kyphotic deformity.

G. **Treatment—reduction and spinal stabilization** After the patient is stable in the Admitting Area, the neurologic status assessed, and the bony injury identified by x-ray, attention is then turned to reducing the specific spine injury. The principle that applies here is rapid alignment of the spine to normal anatomic position. This restores the spinal column to its proper dimensions and thus decompresses the spinal cord. Next, stability is assessed.

1. **Cervical spine injuries**
    a. **Closed reduction** In fractures of the cervical spine, reduction is best accomplished by skeletal tongs and traction. There are numerous types of skeletal tongs, all of which are effective (i.e., Crutchfield, Gardner-Wells, halo, etc.). After the tongs are inserted, weights are applied for traction force. The only exceptions are the atlantooccipital and atlantoaxial injuries for which a firm neck brace is adequate and traction is contraindicated. The initial poundage for the other cervical injuries is around 2–3 pounds per vertebra involved (e.g., for a C_6 fracture begin with 12–18 pounds). The weight is rapidly increased with image fluoroscopy or serial roentgenograms with 5- or 10-, and occasionally 20-pound increments, depending on the age and weight of the patient. As the traction is being increased in certain injuries, the patient can be appropriately positioned, i.e., mild hyperextension or flexion, to adequately align the bones. Frequent x-rays or cinefluoroscopy must be obtained during this time to assess the consequence of each maneuver. We do not exceed 10 pounds per vertebral level involved.
    b. **Open reduction** If adequate realignment cannot be achieved by this method within several hours, open surgical reduction should follow. This is particularly true with locked dislocated facet joints.

c. **Mini-myelogram** After adequate spinal alignment has been achieved, a mini-myelogram should be performed if there is a cord deficit. The purpose of this procedure is to demonstrate possible spinal cord compression from disc material or bone fragments. Persistent compression can hinder or prevent neurologic recovery.

(1) The patient is turned prone on the Stryker frame and a repeat lateral C-spine film is obtained to recheck the alignment.

(2) A C_1/C_2 spinal puncture is performed and the head of the Stryker frame is elevated approximately 20°. Three to six cubic centimeters of Pantopaque is injected, and the head of the Stryker frame is elevated in increments to outline the entire cervical canal. Lateral C-spine films are obtained as needed to assess the presence of cord compression.

This procedure may demonstrate a complete block, an anterior or posterior filling defect, extravasation of dye from the dural tube, or no block. The first two findings are compatible with cord compression and may signal the need for surgical decompression. The third finding is compatible with disruption of the dural sac and is associated with physical separation of cord tissue in nonpenetrating spine injuries; this finding negates the need for emergency surgery.

The percentage of cervical spine injuries that warrant an emergency decompression operation is probably less than 10%. It should also be noted that the majority of these patients who undergo emergency operation will **not** improve neurologically. Nevertheless, since some patients (3%) may have significant improvement, any patient with demonstrable persistent cord compression after spinal alignment should be considered for emergency operation. Decompression does **not** necessarily mean laminectomy. If myelography reveals anterior cord compression from extruded intervertebral disc material or posteriorly displaced bone fragments, an anterior discectomy or corpectomy with fusion may be required. If spinal block or compression is due to fractured laminae, disrupted ligamentum flavum, or diffuse osteoarthritic spinal stenosis, a laminectomy may be needed. The point is that the procedure is chosen to relieve the specific compression, not just to unroof the spinal canal, which can contribute to further instability if not coupled with internal fusion. If an operation is required, it should be performed with the patient in traction. Any emergency decompressive procedure of the cervical spine should be accompanied by a stabilization procedure at the same time.

d. **Stabilization** Once the spine is aligned and no compression is demonstrated, attention must be turned toward achieving permanent stabilization of the spine. This can be accomplished either by elective surgical stabilization or by prolonged skeletal traction. The advantages of an early surgical procedure are early mobilization and rehabilitation. This helps prevent the complications associated with prolonged bed rest, especially when the patient is kept prone or supine. Mobilization allows for the early initiation of an active training program. The particular stabilization procedure should be determined by the anatomical disruption. If the fracture resulted in primarily vertebral body fracture and disrupted the anterior supporting structure of the spine, an anterior fusion should be performed. If there has been predominantly posterior ligamentous disruption and/or fracture of facet joints and lamina, a posterior wiring and fusion should be done. In a few rare cases, it may be necessary to do both an anterior and posterior fusion to stabilize the spine properly. Nonsurgical stabilization can be just as effective. The patient who is quadriplegic or has marked neurologic deficit may be maintained in skeletal traction on a frame or regular bed for approximately 6–8 weeks. After that time, the patient may be placed in a cervical brace and the process of mobilization begun. A halo vest apparatus may be used in lieu of, or as an adjunct to, surgical stabilization. The vest offers efficient immobilization and allows ambulation if the neurologic picture is appropriate. Although the most meticulous care is given, we caution against the use of halo vest traction in patients with a marked neurologic deficit because of the risk of skin breakdown in patients with anesthetic trunks. Also, the halo vest is quite cumbersome for active rehabilitation. We reserve the use of the halo vest for ambulating patients, when possible.

2. **Thoracolumbar injuries** The treatment of fractures of the thoracic and lumbar spine is based upon the same principles as that of the cervical spine injuries. If the patient has a **neurologic deficit** associated with displaced fractures and/or dislocation, urgent realignment/decompression is necessary. This usually requires open reduction. Operations should be performed as soon as life-threatening injuries have been treated. The surgical insertion of Harrington rods adequately realigns these fractures and usually decompresses the cord by restoring canal dimensions to normal.

Following maximum orthopedic reduction, the neurosurgeon should assess the adequacy of spinal cord decompression with the use of an intraoperative mini-myelogram. This can be performed by injecting Pantopaque through a C_1/C_2 or lumbar puncture site and then tilting the Stryker frame until dye passes the injured segment. If more than 12 hr has elapsed since the time of injury, cord swelling may preclude passage of the dye despite adequate decompression. If cord or cauda equina decompression is performed, an iliac bone fusion is done. If a significant myelographic defect persists, the neurosurgeon may elect to perform direct decompression. This can be accomplished in some cases by tapping an anterior fragment forward through a posterior laminotomy or by excision of the offending bone fragments through a posterolateral approach. Following decompression, any fixation appliance which has to be removed can be replaced and the adequacy of the decompression checked by additional myelographic x-rays. Patients who have thoracic or lumbar injuries with a neurologic deficit but have no demonstrable bony displacement should undergo immediate myelography to rule out traumatic herniated disc material compressing the cord or cauda equina. If a myelographic deficit is found which is compatible with the neurologic deficit, a decompression procedure should be performed immediately.

Patients who sustain a thoracolumbar spinal injury **without neurologic deficit** should be kept on a Stryker frame until full assessment of spinal stability is determined. Evaluation might require lateral tomography or computerized axial tomography. If there is widening of the space between the spinous processes, comminution of the posterior cortex of the vertebral body, or more than 50% loss of vertebral body height in a patient under age 50, clinical instability is likely to exist. Clinical instability means that the probability of progressive deformity, risk of neurologic deficit, or chronic pain is high. In these cases, consideration should be given to either hyperextension casting or internal fixation. Clinically stable injuries can be treated with Jewett bracing for lesions above L_2 or Taylor-Knight bracing for lesions below T_{12}.

3. **Open and/or penetrating injuries** In addition to the risk of neurologic damage, the patient is threatened with hemorrhage, infection of the wound, and meningitis. The soft tissue injury should be explored and debrided. A spinal operation is indicated if there is a cerebrospinal fluid leak or evidence of bone or foreign bodies in the spinal canal that are causing cord compression in a patient who has the possibility of neurologic recovery. The laminectomy should provide adequate exposure for a thorough exploration of the canal for fragments and for room to effect a watertight dural closure to prevent a spinal fluid leak. Caution should be exercised so as not to render a previously stable spine unstable. Gunshot wounds to the thoracic or lumbar spine are usually stable. If stability is present, the patient can generally be treated on a Stryker frame or with the appropriate brace.

H. **Postoperative management—spine protection and patient mobilization** Following posterior stabilization procedures for the cervical spine, most patients are adequately protected with either a Philadelphia collar for the upper cervical region or a 4-poster brace for the lower cervical region. Following anterior corpectomy and fusion procedures or in highly unstable injuries, a halo vest or halo cast might be necessary. Once the appropriate external fixation device is applied, the patient can generally be raised to a semi-sitting position and rapidly mobilized. Following the open reduction of thoracic and lumbar injuries, patients must remain on a Stryker frame for about 2 weeks. During this time, it is essential that the patient lie flat in bed and not attempt to turn, roll, or raise up. It is equally important that the patient not be directly pulled up or down in bed. Changes in bed position should be accomplished by moving the sheet so that the patient is moved without any distractive forces crossing the injured segment. After wounds are healed, a Risser cast is applied. The patient is then able rapidly to assume a sitting position and begin full mobilization.

I. **Medical treatment of cord injuries** The thrust of medical treatment of cord injuries is to optimize the conditions for the cord to recover. Adequate pulmonary and cardiovascular function should be maintained. Physical therapy beginning soon after admission should consist of frequent range of motion of all extremities and frequent turning and repositioning of the patient to prevent pulmonary emboli, pneumonia, and decubiti. Preventive medical treatment of cord-injured patients consists mainly of good nursing care to ward off the threat of infection.

1. **Steroids** Steroids are known to decrease edema formation in CNS tissue. Acutely, steroids are thought to minimize the amount of cord edema and the deleterious consequences of edema. Steroid therapy is initiated in all spinal cord injuries with neurologic deficits. Dexamethasone, 1 mg/kg, **or** methylprednisolone, 5 mg/kg, is administered upon admission. The same dose is then given each day in four divided doses. The maintenance of the drug beyond 2–3 days is dictated by whether the cord lesion is complete or incomplete. If complete, the steroids are discontinued. If incomplete, the steroids are continued for 7–10 days. An antacid should be given concomitantly to reduce the chance of gastrointestinal ulceration. The efficacy of steroid therapy in acute human cord injury has not been firmly established.

2. **Cardiovascular care** Because of the loss of sympathetic control to the heart and peripheral circulation, the quadriplegic has poor cardiovascular control and regulation. In the face of a circulating volume deficit, the quadriplegic is unable to maintain cardiac filling pressures by constriction of the venous capacitance vessels. In the presence of over-transfusion because of the lack of sympathetic induced tachycardia and contractility, the quadriplegic may develop pulmonary edema. The period of spinal shock lasts about 3 weeks, but may last as little as 3 days or as long as 6 weeks. It is characterized by bouts of hypotension, hypertension, and bradycardia. The patient is usually poikilothermic.

    a. **Bradycardia** Unless the heart rate is less than 50/min, there is usually no cause for alarm. If the heart rate is 40–50/min, but the PvO_2 and urine output are adequate and the patient is not hypo- or hypertensive, no treatment is required unless myocardial depressants are given, e.g., general anesthesia. If bradycardia is associated with hypotension and inadequate tissue perfusion, a bolus of atropine, 0.5 mg, is advisable. If this does not raise the pulse rate, it should be repeated in 0.5-mg increments, up to 2 mg (vagal blocking dose). With the reversal of bradycardia, hypotension is usually reversed. With persistent bradycardia, 40/min, an isoproterenol (Isuprel) infusion, dopamine, or a pacemaker should be considered.

    b. **Hypotension** Because of dilation of venous and arterial vessels, a fall in blood pressure is commonly seen in the early stages of quadriplegia. Dopamine is the drug of choice since it can be titrated to produce an inotropic effect and improve vascular tone if given in alpha doses (≥ 5 μg/kg/min). Before starting vasoactive drugs, ensure adequate volume replacement, but be judicious or fluid overload will result. Hypotension is not usually treated unless there is evidence of inadequate tissue perfusion such as oliguria.

    c. **Hypertension** As the effects of spinal shock resolve, hyperreflexia and hypertension may be seen, sometimes in association with bradycardia. The autonomic hyperreflexia response may occur between 3 weeks and 13 years after the injury and may be triggered by many visceral stimuli. The classic cause is rectal stimulation or compression of the bladder to ensure emptying while straight catheterization is being performed. The hyperreflexic episode may produce hypertension, bradycardia, sweating and skin vaso-dilation above the level of the lesion, or complaints of headache. If the patient is hypervolemic, the intense vasoconstriction which is precipitated by this "mass spinal reflex" may dramatically increase cardiac filling and precipitate acute pulmonary edema, a common cause of death. The treatment should involve raising the head of the patient's bed and giving morphine, 5–10 mg i.v., while an intravenous infusion of sodium nitroprusside is set up. Nitroprusside is titrated to reverse the hypertension. Nitroprusside may be hazardous since the volume status may be difficult to assess. Nitroprusside should only be given when sufficient i.v. lines are in place to allow rapid volume infusion should the blood pressure precipitously fall.

$\boxed{\text{Note}}$ A quadriplegic patient who manifests with cardiovascular instability should not be managed on a Stryker frame because the rapid change during turning may be detrimental. Cardiovascular unstable patients should be managed on the Roto-Rest bed or in a regular bed.

3. **Pulmonary care** The most common cause of death in the quadriplegic patient is related to the pulmonary system. Because of the loss of motor function below the level of the cervical lesion, innervation to the intercostal and abdominal musculature is lost. The quadriplegic usually has diaphragmatic innervation $(C_3/C_4/C_5)$ and the capacity to breathe spontaneously; however, the patient is frequently unable to cough well. Assessment of the patient's ventilatory capacity should be made. Useful guidelines which assess adequate chest mechanics are obtained by measuring the vital capacity $(>15$ ml/kg$)$, tidal volume $(>5$ ml/kg$)$, and maximum inspiratory force $(\leq -20$ cm $H_2O)$. Arterial gases should be sampled. If the patient has multisystem injury or the admission chest x-ray shows evidence of a parenchymal infiltrate, immediate tracheal intubation and ventilation should be carried out. Chest physiotherapy should be initiated in the quadriplegic patient to treat or prevent pulmonary complications. If the patient is having respiratory difficulty related to pneumonia and/or retention of secretions, access to the chest for physical therapy is mandatory. As a rule, pulmonary toiletry in the patient with atelectasis, pneumonia, or lung contusion takes precedence over external bracing or casting which constricts the thoracic cage or renders it inaccessible to physiotherapy. Daily assessment of ventilatory capacity is helpful in assessing progress and the need for pulmonary support or its withdrawal.

$\boxed{\text{Note}}$ Compounding poor chest wall mechanics, the prone position may interfere with diaphragmatic respiration in the quadriplegic patient. If a nonventilated quadriplegic patient is managed on a Stryker frame during the first 7 days after injury, while the patient is in the prone position, the nurse should

—Be at the bedside at all times to observe for respiratory insufficiency

—Make certain that the hole in the abdominal sling is large enough to allow for adequate abdominal/diaphragmatic excursion

—Build up the upper chest and pubis so that abdominal pressure is minimized

A Roto-Rest or regular bed is an alternative to the Stryker frame.

A spinal cord-injured patient is at high risk to develop a **pulmonary embolus.** Regular examinations should be performed to detect signs of phlebitis, deep vein thrombosis, etc. Changes in vital signs, respiratory function, and general well-being may signal this event. Prophylactic treatment to prevent pulmonary embolism remains controversial. At the present time, we are content to watch these patients with a high degree of suspicion and embark on a diagnostic work-up (isotope scan, pulmonary arteriogram) at the least indication of this potentially fatal complication. If clinical signs and/or tests point to this diagnosis, full anticoagulation is begun.

4. **Gastrointestinal care** The gastric pH should be controlled during the stress period whether the patient is receiving steroids or not, since **gastrointestinal ulceration** can be a fatal complication. Abdominal disease accounts for 10% of all fatalities in the cord-injured population, with perforated viscus being the most common. The sensory deficit makes the routine abdominal examination virtually useless. Persistent nausea and vomiting or tachycardia or bradycardia with a pulse that has been normal may be a sign of intra-abdominal pathology. Pain in the shoulders and clavicular regions may be referred pain from diaphragmatic irritation from gastric material. If these signs appear, one should embark upon a diagnostic work-up to rule out an impending disaster. (See p. 365.)

The aim of **bowel care** is to obtain a patient-controlled reflex evacuation. The patient is started on Colace to soften the stool. Suppositories (Dulcolax) are begun to initiate rectal stimulation. Enemas may be required from time to time. The patient should be frequently checked for fecal impaction.

5. **Skin care** Meticulous attention must be paid to the skin care of patients who have diminished sensation following spinal injury. The heels and presacral area, as well as skin under the edge of a cast or brace, must be checked and noted in the nursing notes daily.

Whether the patient undergoes a surgical procedure or is treated in prolonged skeletal or halo traction, the care of the patient from this point on should always include the following:

a. Attention to skin care should be initiated as soon as the patient arrives in the Admitting Area.

b. It is imperative to change the position of paralyzed, anesthetic body parts at least every 2 hr.

c. Specialized foam rubber mattresses or horizontally rotating frames (not vertically rotating frames) should be used.

    d. Anesthetic skin should be washed and massaged with alcohol and powdered at least once a day.

    e. Bed coverings should always be dry.

    f. Meticulous perineal and sacral skin care is obligatory.

6. **Urologic care**   The aim of bladder care is to obtain urine excretion by "automaticity." Spontaneous voiding is best accomplished by intermittent catheterization, which should be started as soon as medically possible and initiated every 4–6 hr. An attempt should be made to reduce the residual urine volumes to below 400 cc. The frequency of catheterization is decreased as the residual volumes fall. Urologic consultation should be obtained early to provide proper bladder management.

7. **Rehabilitation care**   The most important goal in the management of a spinal cord patient is to make the patient as functional and independent as the neurologic deficit will allow. This goal is the purpose of a physical and psychologic rehabilitation program. Even in the acute phase, physical therapists and nurses should begin exercise programs and patient and family instructions. Range of motion exercise to the extremities should begin immediately after admission. Upper extremity resistance exercises should begin as soon as sufficient spinal stability has been achieved. Splinting should be instituted within several days after admission; otherwise, contractures will develop and hinder ultimate function. Dorsiflexion splints should be constructed for patients who have lost active ankle dorsiflexion. Hand splints must be made for patients who are unable to maintain normal posture. External bracing should be as light as possible yet assure stability so that physical activity is facilitated.

    Psychologists and social workers should begin working with the patient and family in regard to social, sexual, occupational, and financial adjustments. After the acute phase, the patient should be transferred to an academic rehabilitation center as soon as possible.

J.   **Case responsibility**   To rule out the presence of a neurologic deficit, the initial evaluation of the spine-injured patient is performed by the neurosurgical team. If the patient has a neurologic deficit, the neurosurgical team has primary patient responsibility and will obtain consultation as they deem necessary. If the patient has no neurologic deficit, the primary patient responsibility is relegated to the orthopedic team.

    The neurosurgical and/or orthopedic team will present the treatment plan to the Surgical and Critical Care Staff. Treatment of spinal cord injuries is an urgent situation and should include alignment within a few hours, except in complex thoracic/lumbar injuries.

13
EXTREMITY INJURIES

The extremities may be injured by blunt or penetrating trauma. Any one or a combination of structural components of the extremity may be involved.

Following blunt or penetrating trauma, the following systems must be evaluated in each extremity:

—Vascular
—Neural
—Osseous
—Ligamentous
—Muscular
—Tendinous
—Skin and subcutaneous tissue

An initial survey of the extremities should be performed to detect the following:
—Absent or decreased pulse
—Pallor
—Generalized extremity edema
—Deformity
—Local swelling
—Ecchymosis
—Joint laxity
—Obvious soft tissue lacerations or defects
—Decreased motion to command or painful stimulation
—Hypesthesia or anesthesia

If these findings are noted on the initial survey, more specific diagnostic pursuit is necessary, as described in this section.

I. **Skeletal System**   Multiple trauma patients present with various combinations of fractures and joint injuries. Some are open or otherwise obvious, but many have more subtle findings. A thorough systematic approach to clinical and radiographic analysis of the limbs is necessary to discover and accurately determine the nature and severity of each lesion. This section discusses the diagnosis, prioritization, and staging of treatment of these injuries.

   A. **Diagnosis**

      1. **History**   Seek information on mechanism of injury.

      2. **Symptoms**   Focal pain is intensified by any motion of the unsplinted part.

3. **Physical findings**
   a. Visible open fracture or joint injury
   b. Deformity
   c. Crepitus
   d. Abnormal motion between or at joints
   e. Tenderness
   f. Ecchymosis
   g. Swelling
   h. Distal neural or vascular deficit

   ⎡Note⎤ Make a survey of distal neurovascular status of all four limbs and document the findings.

   The alert patient should be asked to move the hands and feet up and down at the wrists and ankles, respectively. The unconscious or confused, but responsive, patient can be stimulated in each area with a pin. In the patient with profound CNS depression, each extremity should be systematically evaluated for the previously mentioned physical findings. It is important to do this survey early and document the findings accurately in the chart because many of these patients will have general anesthesia and pancuronium bromide (Pavulon) paralysis induced early. Complete survey of the distal pulses, temperature, color, and capillary filling must also be made. Early detection of vascular injuries is important in maximizing the results of treatment. The extent of ischemia and elapsed time since injury must constantly be kept in mind. Proper coordination of subsequent diagnostic and therapeutic interventions may make the difference between survival and loss of extremities in these cases.

B. **Splinting** Obvious fractures and joint injuries diagnosed on the basis of the above criteria should be splinted as early as possible. Splinting reduces pain, bleeding, and tissue damage. Grossly displaced open fractures must be splinted as they lie, without attempt at full reduction.

   Reduction by gentle traction and manipulation can be attempted in cases where there is obvious vascular compromise due to the position of the deformity. Prefabricated splints of various materials can be used. Cotton padding, plaster strips, and elastic bandages can be used very effectively for most injuries. An important exception is femoral fractures which must be immobilized by continuous traction applied with a Hare or Thomas splint.

   Whenever possible, the injured part, once splinted, should be elevated to decrease edema formation. Splinting should be done prior to radiographic studies.

C. **Radiographic studies** A true AP and lateral view of all obvious or suspected injuries should be obtained. This will often require repositioning the limb to eliminate rotation. It is essential that the joint at either end of a long bone fracture be visualized. Special views, stress studies, arthrography, angiography, or tomography may be necessary subsequently to more clearly delineate some injuries.

D. **Notification of orthopedic trauma team**   The orthopedic trauma team member on first call should be notified by beeper and/or home telephone by the Team Leader as soon as a significant orthopedic injury is diagnosed. In some cases, injuries will be obvious from their physical findings at first sight and, in others, suspicions will need confirmation by x-ray. It is preferable to err on the side of premature notification of the orthopedic team, although there will often be delays before the definitive intraoperative orthopedic therapy can begin. The orthopedic team member can help in splinting the injured extremities or spine and in obtaining and evaluating x-rays.

Plastic surgery consultation should be obtained for the evaluation of open fractures of the lower extremity where soft tissue loss is going to necessitate reconstruction.

E. **Priorities of management**
   1. **Emergencies**
      a. **Open fractures**
         (1) **Grading** indicates extent of injury:
            (a) **Grade 1**   Puncture wound, usually caused by sharp bone end from inside
            (b) **Grade 2**   Wound not greater than 6–8 cm without sign of contamination or muscle damage
            (c) **Grade 3**   Larger open wounds with associated muscle damage, contamination, or bone or soft tissue loss
         (2) Cover wounds immediately with Betadine-soaked dressings.
         (3) Formal intraoperative debridement and jet lavage irrigation are performed within 6–8 hr of injury, whenever possible, to best decrease the risk of wound infection and osteomyelitis. If significant delay is expected due to the need for further diagnostic studies, other more pressing surgery, or lack of access to an operating room, the wounds should be thoroughly irrigated in the Admitting Area with the jet lavage irrigator.
         (4) After debridement and irrigation, the fracture or joint is stabilized. Hoffman external fixation is used when there is a significant soft tissue wound, bone loss, comminution, or after fasciotomy. Limited internal fixation with lag screws and K-wires is employed for articular realignment, but plating and rodding are avoided. Traction and Robert Jones splinting is used for injuries not requiring external fixation.
         (5) Primary wound closure is avoided since it increases ischemia of already edematous tissue, prevents drainage, and increases the risk of gas gangrene. Wound cavities are loosely packed with 1% neomycin-soaked roll gauze.

   Loose 000 wire retention sutures are placed in the wound edges. These can subsequently be drawn up and twisted down serially at the bedside to effect a safe progressive delayed primary closure. In cases where this is not possible, serial debridement and open wound care are continued. When a granulated wound is attained or wound biopsy shows fewer than 10^5 colonies/gm, secondary wound closure can be undertaken by split skin graft, flap coverage, or suture (see p. 248).

(6) Prophylactic antibiotics (cephalosporin or nafcillin) are administered for 3–5 days.

b. **Dislocated hip** A dislocated hip requires early recognition and prompt treatment. The posterior dislocation is most frequently seen and presents with a flexed, shortened, and internally rotated hip that cannot be extended. Because of the abnormal tension on the blood supply to the femoral head and the increasing incidence of avascular necrosis with prolonged dislocation, early reduction of the hip is important. An x-ray should be taken to document an associated acetabular rim fracture. Reduction usually requires general anesthesia. Closed reduction is usually successful. After reduction, the hip is moved through its range of motion and its stability, i.e., resistance to dislocation, is noted. Open reduction may be necessary for irreducible hips and those with bone fragments in the joint or unstable acetabular rim fractures. Skeletal traction is employed for 3–6 weeks following reduction.

c. **Displaced fractures of the femoral neck** Displaced fractures of the femoral neck result in traction on the blood supply to the femoral head and are associated with avascular necrosis. For this reason, they are best treated by early internal fixation.

d. **Fracture or dislocation associated with vascular injuries** Keep elapsed ischemic time constantly in mind. Formal skeletal stabilization need not precede vascular repair. Limited external fixation can be applied provisionally. After vascular repair and fasciotomy, fixation is augmented by adding more pins and frame components (see p. 252).

e. **Open joint injuries**
   (1) **Diagnosis**
      (a) When communication of a wound with a joint is not obvious, it can be delineated by injecting saline into the joint at a site distant from the wound. If the injected saline pours out of the wound, communication with the joint is confirmed. This technique is most useful for wounds around the knee.
      (b) Stress testing should be done to discover associated ligamentous injury.
      (c) X-ray should be obtained to detect associated fractures.
   (2) **Treatment**
      (a) All open joint injuries must be taken to the operating room for exploration, debridement, and thorough irrigation.
      (b) Grossly contaminated or macerated wounds should be left completely open. In other cases, the synovium and capsule may be closed over Hemovac drains and the skin left open.
      (c) Prophylactic cephalosporin is administered for 3–5 days.

(d) Immobilize the joint for 5 days to minimize inflammation; then begin motion as early as permitted by associated ligamentous and bony injuries.

2. **Special requirements**
   a. **Femoral shaft fractures** The multiple trauma patient needs frequent turning and chest percussion/postural drainage of all pulmonary segments. If these procedures are not performed, atelectasis and subsequent pneumonia or shunting will develop. Traditional balanced skeletal traction prevents these goals.

   The method chosen for treatment must allow significant patient mobility as well as fracture stabilization.
   (1) **Immediate open reduction and internal fixation** achieves rigid fracture stabilization but risks significant additional blood loss and a higher incidence of infection and nonunion.
   (2) **Immediate closed intramedullary rodding** is an excellent method but requires an image intensifier and surgical expertise.
   (3) **The Neufeld single rope, roller-traction cast system** is an excellent method if closed nailing is not available or precluded by excessive comminution of the fracture, open wound, or poor patient condition. In this method, a skeletal pin is inserted distal to the fracture. A long leg cast is then applied in two sections. The thigh portion is applied first and molded with a sling. The cast is then completed by incorporating the skeletal pin. Three sets of wire loops fashioned from coat hangers are then attached to the anterior, medial, and lateral aspects of the cast at the knee. The single rope for suspension and traction from the roller on the traction frame can now be attached to the cast at variable points with an "S" hook. This allows complete turning in bed and mobilization out of bed to a chair while traction is maintained. This system can be used to maintain the fracture prior to delayed internal fixation or as the definitive method of therapy. At 14 days, the solid cast is converted to a cast-brace. Ambulation is possible in those patients with intact upper and contralateral lower extremities. In this procedure, the patient is brought to physical therapy, the traction is unhooked, and the patient stands and walks with the injured leg dependent, but nonweight-bearing. At the end of the session, the patient returns to bed and traction is resumed.

   Traction is discontinued when sufficient callus has formed to prevent shortening and translation of the fracture (usually 6 weeks). The patient is then treated as an outpatient for 3–4 months with some type of external cast support. Distal fractures are treated with cast braces, while those in the proximal one-half of the shaft require hinged spica cast braces.

   Complications include vascular compromise, pressure sores from the cast, and nonunion and malunion. The incidence of each of these complications is very low when patients are carefully managed and closely followed.

(4) **Hoffman external fixation** is used to treat complex open fractures.

(5) **Bilateral femur fractures** cannot be managed with single rope roller traction-cast on a regular bed. There is so much distal traction that this restricts turning and results in a Trendelenburg position, which has an adverse effect on tracheobronchial toiletry. Treatment alternatives include internal or external fixation of at least one femoral fracture or use of the Roto-Rest bed with bilateral traction.

b. **Central acetabular fractures** in which the femoral head is displaced into the pelvis represent a problem. Treatment with traction requires combined lateral and distal pull with skeletal pins in the trochanter and distal femur. This severely limits the turning of the patient in bed and leads to inadequate tracheobronchial toiletry. Treatment alternatives are open reduction and internal fixation or triangulation through Hoffman external fixation with pin groups in both iliac crests and the intertrochanteric region of the affected hip.

c. **Intra-articular fractures**

(1) Anatomic realignment of the joint surfaces must be achieved.

(2) Articular fragments must be rigidly fixed under compression.

(3) Early joint motion is essential.

(4) The best results are achieved through early operation.

d. **Major ligamentous injuries**

(1) Diagnose by stress-testing joints and confirm with stress x-rays, if necessary.

(2) Complete disruptions are best treated by early repair prior to ligament retraction.

e. **Compartment syndrome**   The forearm and leg by virtue of their dense fascial covering, the presence of two bones, and an interosseous membrane are compartmentalized. Excessive pressure within these compartments will damage the muscles and nerves within that space and lead to ischemic contracture. Increased pressure can be caused by

—Swelling of bluntly traumatized muscle

—Postischemic edema

—Intracompartmental arterial bleeding

—Venous injuries

See p. 253.

(1) **Symptoms**   Unusual pain out of proportion to the injury

(2) **Signs**

(a) Palpable firmness of fascial compartment

(b) Exquisite tenderness on passive stretch of muscles in the compartment

(c) Pulse diminution ±

(d) Pallor

(e) Hypesthesia

(f) Motor weakness

Clinical assessment is not 100% reliable and is impossible in patients who are unresponsive as a result of head injury or anesthesia.

Physical examination should be supplemented with direct measurement of intracompartmental pressure.

(3) **Techniques**

    (a) **CVP manometer, IV tubing, and sterile needle**

       i. Fill the manometer, tubing, and needle with saline.

       ii. Insert the needle into the compartment to be tested.

       iii. Slowly elevate the manometer above the limb until the saline just begins to run in, then steady the manometer.

       iv. The number of centimeters from the needle (extremity) to the top of the fluid column equals the pressure in the compartment in centimeters of H_2O (mm Hg = cm $H_2O \div 1.36$).

    (b) **Wick catheter** is a more sophisticated system for continuous direct intracompartmental pressure monitoring.

       i. Fill the catheter, needle, and strain-gauge manometer with saline.

       ii. Insert the needle into the compartment.

       iii. Advance the wick.

       iv. Balance the system.

       v. Record intracompartmental pressure in millimeters of Hg.

(4) **Treatment** Generally, a compartment pressure that is 50 mm Hg does not need a therapeutic fasciotomy. If the compartment pressure is 60 mm Hg, a therapeutic fasciotomy is usually required. The 50–60 mm Hg pressure range is a gray zone. If the patient is in the gray zone and is alert, the decision to perform a therapeutic fasciotomy is based on clinical examination. If the patient is not alert and is in the gray zone, a fasciotomy is strongly considered. These objective guidelines should complement the physician's clinical judgment.

    (a) Decompression requires fasciotomy of each involved compartment.

    (b) Fasciotomy wounds should not be closed primarily. Closure is best effected by progressive delayed primary closure with progressive delayed primary wire suture technique or split thickness skin grafts.

Perspective

Since it is not possible in a work this size to discuss the diagnosis and treatment of fractures and dislocations of each anatomic area, we have focused on problem areas that are relevant to multiple trauma. The discussion has covered the general approach to diagnosis and prioritization of treatment of skeletal lesions in the multiple trauma patient. Injuries requiring early surgical care have been stressed. Injuries with special treatment requirements have also been discussed. For a comprehensive and detailed discussion of specific fractures, the reader is referred to a standard fracture textbook.

F. **Soft tissue coverage in open fractures of the lower extremity**   Management of open wounds of the lower extremities associated with underlying fractures requires a joint effort between the orthopedic and plastic surgeons. Adequate bony stabilization is of paramount importance, since instability will impair soft tissue healing. Despite adequate fixation, inadequate soft tissue coverage can lead to delayed healing and prolonged morbidity. This is especially true in situations where the remaining soft tissue has been damaged.

The use of the Hoffman external fixation device allows direct access to the wound for management and observation while maintaining bony fixation. The use of local muscle and musculocutaneous flaps, as well as distant flaps through either microvascular or cross-leg techniques, supplies the needed soft tissue to enhance wound healing and fracture union.

The initial management of the open wound involves the principles that have been outlined on p. 261. Once a surgically clean wound is established and the bone has been stabilized, the proper timing and technique of wound closure are considered. If delayed primary closure can be accomplished without tension, this is the optimal method.

1. **Local muscle flaps**   The gastrocnemius muscle or gastrocnemius musculocutaneous flap and the soleus muscle flap are the flaps of choice for use in lower extremity reconstruction.
    a. **Gastrocnemius**   Either the medial or the lateral head of the gastrocnemius muscle may be used in the development of the gastrocnemius muscle or musculocutaneous flap. The muscle is supplied by paired arteries, the sural arteries, which are direct branches of the popliteal artery. By maintaining its proximal blood supply, the muscle is detached distally from the Achilles tendon and rotated to cover defects of the proximal third of the tibia. Its location is deep to the gastrocnemius muscle; therefore, it should both muscles be sacrificed since this will weaken the Achilles tendon significantly. The muscle can be used as a pedicled muscle or musculocutaneous flap or as an island musculocutaneous flap for more proximal coverage.
    b. **Soleus**   The soleus muscle flap has a segmental blood supply but has a dominant proximal blood supply which allows its detachment from the Achilles tendon and rotation for coverage of defects of the middle third of the tibia. Its location is deep to the gastrocnemius muscle; therefore, it can only be used as a muscle flap. This requires subsequent skin grafting of the muscle after its transfer for complete closure of the defect.

2. **Cross-leg flaps**   A cross-leg gastrocnemius musculocutaneous flap may be used to cover lower extremity defects. The primary disadvantage of the cross-leg flap is the necessity for immobilization of the patient in a cross-leg position for approximately 3 weeks before the flap can be divided. This precludes its use in older patients where joint stiffness would be a major problem following prolonged immobilization.

3. **Microvascular free flaps**   For extensive defects where inadequate local soft tissue is present or in defects involving the lower third of the tibia or ankle

where no uniformly successful flaps are available, the use of free transfer of distant tissue becomes necessary. The most commonly used free flaps are the latissimus dorsi musculocutaneous or muscle flap, and the groin flap (skin and subcutaneous tissue).

Perspective
It must be emphasized that the management of soft tissue defects associated with lower extremity injuries mandates cooperation between the orthopedic surgeon and the plastic surgeon. Many other flaps and techniques can be used, but require expertise (see p. 267).

II. **Peripheral Vasculature** The management of peripheral vascular trauma has been largely influenced by military and civilian experiences with penetrating injuries. Blunt and penetrating trauma are seen at MIEMSS, with the former predominating. Similarities and differences in the diagnosis and management of these two types of vascular injury are discussed. Circulation may be impaired by

   —Arterial injury
   —Venous injury
   —Compartment syndrome and/or
   —Microcirculatory damage secondary to the contusive effect of blunt or missile trauma

Damage to the artery may result in
   —Occlusion (intimal injury/thrombosis)
   —Laceration
   —Transection

The presence of a peripheral arterial injury should be suspected in any patient sustaining an extremity injury. Certain types of trauma should raise suspicion regarding the likelihood of such an injury:
   —A knee or elbow dislocation, as suggested by history or physical findings
   —Any long bone fracture, particularly if there is supracondylar humeral or femoral fracture
   —Crush injury to an extremity, as evidenced or as suggested by history
   —A wound produced by a knife (or similar object), a low velocity bullet wound, or shotgun blast that could **conceivably** have encountered a vessel
   —A high velocity missile which may produce a vascular injury remote to the entrance and exit wounds

A. **Manifestations of arterial injury**

   1. External **hemorrhage**

   2. A **pulse deficit** This sign can be evaluated both qualitatively and quantitatively. The qualitative method consists of comparing distal pulses of the injured extremity with those of the noninjured side. Quality of the pulse is

graded + to 4+. To detect a pulse deficit more accurately in a quantitative fashion, comparative Doppler pressures are obtained. It is important to note that the presence of a distal pulse does not negate the possibility of a major arterial injury.

3. **Acute ischemic changes** include extremity pallor or cyanosis, coolness, hypesthesia, and partial or complete paralysis.

4. **Bruit**

5. **Thrill**

6. **Hematoma**

> **Note** Pulse deficit and/or ischemic changes should not be attributed to arterial spasm.

An unreduced fracture or dislocation may make the diagnosis of an arterial injury difficult. A nonreduced dislocation or a fracture not "pulled out to length" may compress the artery and give the impression that an arterial injury is present. On the other hand, an ischemic extremity secondary to an arterial injury may be fallaciously credited to the bone injury. If the injury is reduced and/or the fracture is "pulled out to length" and vascular abnormality is still present, an arterial injury must be excluded.

Perspective
Penetrating arterial arteries are **usually** singular and easily recognized. Blunt arterial injury may go undetected while attention is directed to more obvious and/or life-threatening injuries. In blunt trauma, the extremities must be examined specifically for the presence of an arterial injury when stabilization has been obtained. Initial and serial neurologic examination of the extremity should be performed.

B. **Arteriography** In general, when there is clinical evidence of an extremity arterial injury associated with a penetrating wound, particularly if there is a rapidly expanding hematoma or profuse hemorrhage, a preoperative angiogram is not required. Angiography for penetrating wounds is suggested for multiple penetrating wounds, a missile that appears to have traveled parallel to the artery of concern, or a shotgun blast to an extremity.

Blunt arterial injury usually requires angiography to diagnose and identify the site(s) of injury. Dislocation of the knee is so frequently associated with a popliteal artery injury that an arteriogram should be routinely performed. In the multiple trauma patient, single exposure, hand injection angiography performed in the resuscitation area or operating room is preferable to moving the patient to the radiology department. The presence of a proximal limb injury in the axillary or groin area requires transportation to the radiology department for central angiography. (For a description of angiography, see p. 32.)

C. **Treatment** The timing and treatment of a peripheral vascular injury in the trauma patient are dictated by the presence and severity of associated injuries. Life-threatening extravascular injuries, commonly seen with blunt trauma, must be treated before the peripheral arterial injury is addressed. Isolated peripheral arterial injuries are treated as soon as stabilization is obtained.

External hemorrhage is a life-threatening condition which must be addressed immediately. Bleeding can usually be controlled by direct pressure, preferably with sterile gloves and gauze. Blind clamping into the area of bleeding is not recommended because of the risk of damaging neurovascular structures. Tourniquets may aggravate an existing injury by causing further ischemia. Tourniquets may be used when immediate amputation is to be performed. An **ischemic extremity** requires immediate revascularization to maintain neuromuscular function. An extremity with an **arterial injury and the absence of ischemia** requires less emergent attention. In other words, if there is no ischemia associated with an arterial injury and the patient has multiple injuries, the repair is deferred until the patient is stable. If there is a delay in vascular repair, the extremity must be followed closely for evidence of ischemia. Doppler pressures provide an objective tool for following nonischemic arterial injuries.

The basic principles of vascular surgery are applicable to peripheral arterial trauma. The operative field must allow access for proximal vascular control. An uninjured extremity should be prepared to allow for the harvest of a venous graft, usually the thigh to obtain a saphenous vein. Harvesting of veins from the injured extremity may enhance posttraumatic edema and failure of a repaired arterial injury.

The following classification of arterial injuries provides a useful management plan.

1. **Type I** These injuries consist of simple arterial laceration or transections and are associated with minimal soft tissue injury. The injuries are produced by sharp objects such as a knife or ice pick.

   Type I injuries can generally be repaired by simple suture closure. Associated venous injuries are usually repairable. Sharply severed nerves can often be approximated by standard techniques. Postoperative problems are few and results are generally good.

2. **Type II** These injuries involve segmental arterial damage and local soft tissue trauma with or without associated fractures. Such injuries are produced by gunshot wounds, localized blunt trauma, and/or fracture.

   a. **Vascular structures** Type II injuries usually require debridement or resection of a portion of the vessel. Primary anastomosis must be accomplished without tension. About 4 cm of a vessel must be mobilized for each centimeter of resected vessel to prevent tension. Generally, patent collaterals should not be sacrificed to gain sufficient mobilization; therefore, interposition vein grafts should be used. An arteriotomy is performed over the injured area to rule out an intimal injury. Thrombotic lesions without intimal damage can be successfully treated with thrombectomy.

Repair of venous injuries, if possible, is preferable to ligation, to minimize posttraumatic edema and improve the likelihood of a successful arterial repair.

b. **Soft tissue** Nonviable soft tissue should be debrided and the wound copiously irrigated. Delayed closure is preferable if the tissue is of questionable viability or if the wound might be closed under tension. Neurovascular structures must be covered with viable tissue; this may involve mobilization of adjacent muscle pedicles. Damaged nerves should not be repaired initially because the limits of neural damage are ill defined. Always suspect gas gangrene in a crushed and ischemic extremity injury when confronted with fever, toxemia, skin color changes, crepitus, or odor.

c. **Fractures** Fractures are stabilized by using external skeletal fixators (Hoffman device). Casts are not used because they preclude the ability to observe the extremity and may impede venous return. Revascularization takes priority over orthopedic procedures when limb ischemia is present. When the fracture is unstable, one side of a Hoffman device is rapidly applied and the vessel is repaired. If a Hoffman device cannot be rapidly applied, an arterial shunt may be inserted to reconstitute circulation until stabilization can be applied. Failure to stabilize a fracture prior to vascular repair has the disadvantage of subjecting the vascular reconstruction to orthopedic manipulation.

3. **Type III** Type III injuries involve segmental arterial injury and massive soft tissue damage. Shotgun and high velocity missile wounds, crushing trauma, and explosions produce these injuries.

Guidelines for the treatment of type II injuries are applicable. Revascularization of the limb is essential for healing of the extravascular tissues. More than one arterial site and/or arteries may be damaged and should be repaired, if possible, beginning with the most proximal injury. If the soft tissue damage and contamination are severe, an extra-anatomical bypass should be attempted if there is ischemia. Coverage of neurovascular structures may be accomplished with porcine grafts early and muscle flaps and/or skin grafts later. Early use of muscle flaps usually results in necrosis of the flap due to compromise of its vascularity. Open wounds must be inspected daily and debrided, if necessary, until skin grafts are applied.

When there is massive soft tissue damage or signs of ischemia and revascularization cannot be accomplished, **early amputation** is recommended. When a successful repair has been accomplished, one must watch for signs of muscle necrosis secondary to soft tissue trauma (crush). The patient's life should not be placed in jeopardy to save a necrotic/septic limb. Should muscle necrosis develop, amputation should be performed despite the presence of a funitioning anastomosis and a distal pulse. Nerve injuries that are not amenable to treatment frequently accompany type III injuries. Since recovery is not predictable, a neurologic deficit alone is not an indication for early amputation (see p. 277).

D. **Adjuvant therapy**

1. **Anticoagulation** Systemic anticoagulation is not necessary in peripheral arterial trauma and may be dangerous in the patient with multiple injuries. Local heparinization of clamped arteries and veins helps prevent thrombus formation. **Dextran 40 or aspirin** may be useful to prevent thrombosis when long interposition grafts are used or small caliber arteries are repaired. Dextran therapy may minimize the microcirculatory disturbances associated with massive soft tissue damage seen in type III injuries.

2. **Antibiotics** Antibiotic coverage is not necessary for all vascular injuries. A 5-day course of antibiotics (Keflin) to cover Gram-positive organisms is routinely administered when open fractures are present. When a prosthetic graft is inserted, coverage should be continued until all vascular lines or other sources of bacteremia are removed.

3. **Fasciotomy** Compartment syndrome is the development of impairment of microcirculation secondary to a rise in soft tissue pressure. The compartment syndrome usually develops secondary to prolonged ischemia, muscle contusion, and/or impairment of venous outflow. Signs of compartment syndrome include
   a. Hypesthesia
   b. Loss of motor function
   c. Pain with passive stretch
   d. Palpable compartment tension

The first three signs may be due to neurologic and/or ischemic-producing vascular injuries without elevated compartment pressures. When there is prolonged ischemia or muscle contusion, palpable compartment tension, and a high compartment pressure, the diagnosis of a compartment syndrome is confirmed.

Decompression is advised as soon as muscle ischemia develops or if it is likely to develop. Considerations for compartment decompression are
   —Prolonged ischemia
   —Palpable tension in a muscle compartment
   —Concomitant arterial and venous injury
   —Major venous injury which requires ligation and is associated with major soft tissue injury

Compartment decompression is performed by fasciotomy.

Compartmental pressures are helpful in determining the need to perform a fasciotomy. An 18-gauge needle is connected to a water manometer and the needle is inserted into each compartment. A therapeutic fasciotomy should be considered according to the criteria described on p. 247. All compartments should be decompressed. An open fracture is less likely to develop a compartment syndrome than a closed fracture, but an open fracture does not guarantee compartment decompression.

4. **Hypothermia** An ischemic extremity should be cooled with ice as soon as possible to decrease the ischemic insult.

E. **Venous injuries** Signs of extremity edema and venous engorgement warrant venography and/or operative exploration. Acute extremity edema may be secondary to venous thrombosis, venous transection, or an arterial-venous fistula. Hemorrhage secondary to a venous laceration is usually apparent. An injured major vein should be repaired, if possible, especially when there is an associated arterial injury. Adequate venous drainage is necessary to minimize tissue congestion, which may compromise arterial inflow and/or the ability of injured soft tissues to survive. Small isolated venous injuries are not critical and may be ligated. Major venous interruption may result in chronic edema. Anti-platelet drugs are suggested for use if a major vein is repaired or ligated.

Perspective

The management of peripheral vascular injuries requires a consideration of the patient's total injuries. After control of hemorrhage from peripheral vascular injuries, the timing of the surgical management is dictated by the presence or absence of associated life-threatening injuries. The degree of local extravascular injury must be assessed. Neurologic injury and compartment injury must be suspected, particularly if there is a long period of ischemia and/or the presence of type II or type III injuries. When indicated, fasciotomy should be performed early. If possible, major venous injuries should be repaired. Systemic sepsis from soft tissue injury, despite the presence of a competent vascular anastomosis and a distal pulse, requires aggressive debridement, often amputation.

III. **Peripheral nerves** The management of peripheral nerve injuries is an extremely controversial area of surgery. Proper treatment of these injuries includes early diagnosis, proper evaluation, follow-up, and sound decision-making in regard to timing of diagnostic tests and possible surgery. When a peripheral nerve injury is suspected, an examination should be performed at the first opportunity that the patient's condition allows.

A. **Clinical anatomy and examination**

1. **Upper extremity** The **brachial plexus** originates from the roots of C_5 to T_1. Basically, the C_5 root gives rise to deltoid function; the C_6 root to bicep func-

tion; the C_7 root to tricep function; the C_8 root to deep flexors of the forearm; and the T_1 root to the intrinsic muscles of the hand and fingers.

The upper two roots (C_5 and C_6) and the lower two roots (C_8 and T_1) join to make upper and lower trunks. The C_7 root progresses to form the middle trunk (Figure 1). Therefore, the upper trunk is responsible for deltoid and bicep function; the middle trunk for tricep function; and the lower trunk for hand function. Each trunk subsequently divides into anterior and posterior divisions. The three posterior divisions unite and form the posterior cord, which in turn gives rise to the **axillary and radial nerves.** Therefore, the posterior cord supplies deltoid and tricep function, as well as extension of the wrist. The anterior divisions from the upper and middle trunk unite to form the lateral cord. The lateral cord gives rise to the **musculocutaneous nerve** to the bicep muscle and a branch that forms part of the median nerve, which accounts for the distal sensory distribution of that nerve. The anterior division of the lower trunk becomes the medial cord. The medial cord divides to form the **ulnar nerve** and part of the **median nerve.** Therefore, the medial cord provides intrinsic hand movement and wrist flexion and grip.

There are other cutaneous sensory nerves to the arm, as well as nerves that come off higher in the plexus to innervate muscles in and about the shoulder. Clinical examination of peripheral nerve function will help determine the location of the injury site in the plexus or a specific peripheral nerve. For injuries involving the shoulder, careful evaluation of the associated structures in this area (bones, joints, and muscle) is imperative. After the initial evaluation, a more detailed evaluation of neural function is performed.

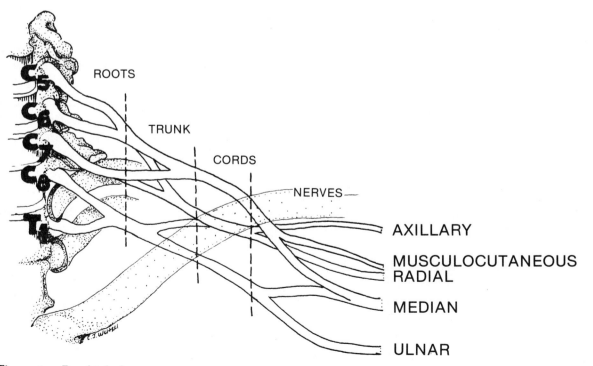

Figure 1. Brachial plexus.

In **shoulder injuries,** the first clinical test of peripheral nerve function should be abduction of the shoulder. Injury to the brachial plexus will become apparent if the patient is unable to raise the arm from the side to a position over the head or the patient is unable to extend the elbow against resistance.

For **injuries in the axilla,** all five major nerves to the upper extremity may be affected. The axillary nerve to the deltoid muscle is usually spared. The musculocutaneous nerve is evaluated by testing for bicep function and hypesthesia on the lateral (radial) aspect of the forearm. Radial nerve injuries in the axilla often spare tricep function; however, wrist extension is usually impaired. There is no reliable sensory deficit from injury to the radial nerve. Deep flexors of the fingers and opponens of the thumb are tested for median nerve function. Sensation on the volar surface of the index finger is supplied only by the median nerve. Motor function of the ulnar nerve is evaluated by having the patient abduct and adduct the extended fingers to test the interosseous muscles. The distal volar surface of the little finger is tested for sensory ulnar function.

There may be direct injury to the bicep and tricep muscles associated with injuries of the arm. Uncommonly, there is direct injury to the nerves that innervate these muscles; however, the radial nerve may be injured (especially with fractures of the humerus) and result in a wrist drop. If the injury involves the medial aspect of the arm, the median and ulnar nerves are suspectible, and the appropriate muscle tests should be performed.

Injuries to the forearm, wrist, and hand most commonly involve the median and ulnar nerves; however, movements of the fingers may be good if the tendons of more proximal flexors are intact. The extensor tendons from the extensor muscles along the forearm will readily open the hand. The deep flexors that are supplied by the median nerve proximal to the injury will allow the fingers to close. Distal median nerve function is tested by asking the patient to bring the extended thumb across the palm and touch the little finger. For sensory testing, the volar surface of the index finger should be checked since this is autonomously innervated by the median nerve. To evaluate ulnar function, the patient should be asked to abduct and adduct the extended fingers. In most cases, the patient cannot fully extend the fourth or fifth digit. These digits remain flexed to give the classic deformity called the "ulnar claw" or the "Benedictine" hand.

Injuries to the hand may cause damage to branches of both the median and ulnar nerves. Finger injuries most often involve digital nerve damage and result in sensory deficit of the finger involved (see p. 273).

2. **Lower extremity**   Peripheral nerves of the lower extremity come from the lumbosacral plexus via the anterior rami of spinal nerves L_4, L_5, S_1, S_2, and S_3. Plexus injuries in this area are not as common a problem as those of the brachial plexus. The intrapelvic portion of this complex may be involved in cases of severe fractures of the pelvis, particularly those involving the sacrum. Root avulsion frequently occurs in this type of injury and, in such cases, surgical repair is impossible.

The **sciatic nerve** is essentially a continuation of the plexus. It makes its exit from the pelvis through the greater sciatic foramen. As the nerve leaves the pelvis, it descends through a tunnel between the ischial tuberosity and the greater trochanter. Although the sciatic nerve is well protected from external trauma by the gluteal musculature and its adipose padding at this point, it is easily threatened by dislocations and fractures of the hip joint.

Inferior to the gluteus maximus, the sciatic nerve is quite superficial, almost subcutaneous, before passing under the lateral head of the biceps femoris. Externally, the gluteal fold marks this site of vulnerability. Lacerations and even deep burns in this area may injure the nerve.

The sciatic nerve trunk bifurcates into two divisions which form the **tibial and peroneal nerves.** The common peroneal nerve crosses the popliteal fossa and then winds around the neck of the fibula before reaching its destination in the anterior compartment of the lower leg. In its course around the neck of the fibula, external protection is minimal. Such vulnerability renders it susceptible to lacerations and contusions.

The tibial nerve descends through the popliteal fossa and is susceptible to trauma. On reaching the inferior aspect of the fossa, the nerve dips between the two heads of the gastrocnemius to pursue a relatively deep and safe course through the posterior compartment. Its main hazard at this point lies in its susceptibility to fractures or the compartment syndrome. The nerve becomes a subcutaneous structure medial to the Achilles tendon. Further descent along the posterior aspect of the tibia brings it around the internal malleolus with subsequent division to form the medial and lateral plantar nerves.

The **femoral nerve** arises from the lumbar plexus with root supply from L_2 through L_4. It enters the thigh along the lateral border of the psoas muscle, behind the inguinal ligament and just lateral to the femoral artery. The nerve supplies the quadricep, sartorius, and pectineus muscles, as well as the skin of the anterior thigh. Injury to this nerve can result from penetrating wounds or blunt trauma to the anterior thigh.

The quadricep muscles are solely innervated by the femoral nerve; thus, knee extension provides a motor index of its integrity. Hypalgesia over the anterior thigh from the inguinal ligament to the knee implies femoral nerve injury.

Sciatic nerve evaluation is accomplished by testing the common peroneal and tibial nerves. Injuries to the thigh may inflict complete sciatic disruption or may be partial, affecting only one division. The common peroneal nerve innervates dorsiflexors of the foot and toes and evertors of the foot; the tibial nerve innervates plantar flexors of the foot and toes and invertors of the foot. A foot drop occurs with a peroneal nerve injury; inability to tiptoe follows tibial nerve damage.

It is frequently difficult to evaluate strength in a painfully traumatized limb. In such circumstances, plantar flexion and dorsiflexion of the great toe will suffice for initial assessment. Sensory disturbances from common peroneal injury may be ascertained by testing the skin (web) between the great and second toe. Tibial nerve injury causes sensory changes over the heel and plantar surface of the foot. Injuries to the branches of the common peroneal and tibial nerves may occur individually and cause selective dysfunction.

B.   **Principles of peripheral nerve repair**   The mechanism by which the peripheral nerve and its associated extremity are injured is of utmost importance when planning the repair of an injured nerve. Even the strongest proponents of primary nerve repair have made exceptions for gunshot wounds and war injuries. With a high-velocity injury, the associated tissue damage is often considerable. Secondary infections readily occur. Accurate assessment of the extent of nerve injury is often not possible until 15–20 days have elapsed. In a gunshot wound, the extent of disruption of a peripheral nerve is often greater than one would anticipate on the basis of the "obvious" nerve damage; accurate early repair is simply not possible. Repair of a peripheral nerve injury should be delayed whenever extensive injury to soft tissues and bones has occurred. This type of injury invariably contains considerable devitalized tissue and, frequently, there is communication with the external environment, which predisposes to infection. Many of these injuries require delayed or secondary closure. As soon as all evidence of infection has subsided and devitalized tissue has been eliminated by granulation and debridement, surgical repair of the injured nerve can be planned.

Primary nerve repair is considered in clean lacerations, especially for the digital nerves of the hand and certain very clean lacerations of the wrist. The digital nerves heal quickly and should be repaired primarily. Injuries to the median and ulnar nerves at the wrist lie in the gray zone between primary and secondary repair. Results are much the same whether the nerve is repaired primarily or secondarily. In all other clean lacerations of peripheral nerves, including the brachial plexus, primary repair should be considered if it is apparent that only a single operation will be required to repair both the nerve and the associated soft tissues. If the nerve stumps are not retracted, they can be located easily and anastomosed without extensive mobilization. Ideally, the wound is not more than 3 hr old, the approach to the problem is deliberate, and the surgeon has substantial experience in repairing peripheral nerves. If exploration reveals the stumps to be contused or irregular, repair should be delayed for 4–6 weeks. The divided ends of the nerve are tacked down into separate areas of soft tissue to maintain proper stump length for the eventual repair.

In traction (stretch) injuries, the nerve remains in continuity and is usually partially functional. The decision of whether or not to operate depends upon which nerve trunks are damaged. In the pelvis, operations on the lumbosacral plexus are generally useless. For sciatic nerve injuries at the hip, exploration is rarely indicated because the length of axonal regeneration precludes repair. For the shoulder, a delayed procedure may be considered. Traction injury in the shoulder can be explored if the lesion is not a root avulsion. An extradural lesion can be documented by the presence of normal paraspinalis muscles on electromyogram (EMG), by sensory conduction (which is slow but present), and by a normal myelogram. Decompression, external neurolysis, and nerve grafts can be considered, but less than 15% of shoulder traction injuries benefit from surgery. If the brachial plexus is explored for an associated vascular injury or to debride a penetrating wound, the degree of injury to the plexus can be assessed to some degree. If the brachial plexus is disrupted and is repaired, a functional hand is not likely. By the time the intrinsic muscles of the hand are reinnervated, they are usually significantly atrophic and the joints are contracted. This point must be remembered if the patient has multiple injuries and is unstable, since a prolonged operative procedure which may gain minimal limb function may jeopardize the patient's life.

When an upper extremity fracture is associated with a peripheral nerve injury, exploration is not usually indicated initially. Three out of four patients recover spontaneously, especially if the injury is in the radial nerve. However, if evidence of peripheral nerve regeneration is overdue or if surface neurography indicates lack of nerve regeneration, surgical exploration is indicated. Fractures of the humerus often cause radial nerve damage; however, if the fracture is in the upper two-thirds of that bone, the radial nerve usually recovers spontaneously (axonotmesis). If the fracture in the arm is oblique and involves the lower third of the humerus, the radial nerve is often damaged extensively and cannot be repaired at the time of exploration. When a great length of the radial nerve has been damaged, an autograft may be attempted, but failure is common. Fractures of the elbow may involve the median nerve. If recovery is slow, exploration should be carried out. The nerve is often disrupted and/or trapped in the bony callus. The ulnar nerve can also be affected by fractures of the elbow, especially if the medial epicondyle of the humerus or the olecranon and/or ulna are involved.

If a fracture of the femur damages the sciatic nerve, exploration 3 or 4 weeks after injury is usually helpful. Even if anastomosis is not required, the external neurolysis is often dramatically beneficial immediately after the operation. In fractures and dislocations of the knee, the tibial nerve usually recovers spontaneously if injured. Knee injuries involving the common peroneal nerve may be treated surgically, but results are usually poor. More distal leg fractures rarely require surgical nerve repair.

Timing of the repair of lesions in continuity is a debatable topic. A delay of 8 to 10 weeks is generally acceptable for repair. During that time, the patient should be followed with clinical examination, as well as electrophysiologic tests. Periodic electromyography (EMG), nerve action potentials, etc., should be done to evaluate the progression or deterioration of nerve function. Intraoperative stimulation should be employed to aid in the decision to resect the injured portion of the nerve or simply perform a neurolysis.

C. **Flow chart for peripheral nerve repair**

1. **Clinical finding** Sensory/motor deficit is identified after extremity trauma.

2. Following admission:
   a. If the neural deficit is associated with a clean laceration, the nerve is repaired at this time.
   b. If the soft tissue needs debridement (gunshot wound, open fracture, or shotgun wound), the nerve is tagged, if it can be identified.

c. If the soft tissue does not need debridement (closed blunt trauma), the patient is observed.

3. If nerve endings were not found at the initial exploration or the patient suffered closed trauma, an EMG is performed at 3 weeks to confirm the presence or absence of neural function.

4. Exploration of the nerve is indicated for neurolysis or repair if
    a. The nerve was found to be transected and not repaired at the time of admission
    b. EMG 7 weeks after injury reveals poor or absent nerve conduction
        (1) Nerve entrapment
        (2) Nerve transection
        (3) Failure of initial repair

IV. **Soft Tissues**   The results of improper management of soft tissue injuries may be disastrous. A prompt evaluation of the extent of the injury, appropriate initial management, and a definitive plan of surgical debridement, wound care, and subsequent wound closure are essential. Injuries to underlying structures, i.e., nerve, tendon, bone, muscle, or vessels, must be considered in any soft tissue injury and their repair incorporated into the treatment plan. Vascular injury with distal ischemia requires emergent surgical intervention to salvage the extremity. Reconstruction of the other structures may be delayed until more favorable wound conditions can be achieved. Soft tissue wounds of major magnitude are frequently associated with other life-threatening injuries. This will often postpone definitive management of the wound. Because of this unavoidable delay, it is mandatory that a thorough initial cleansing of the wound with removal of any foreign material and debridement of all obviously nonviable tissue be carried out early. Wounds are then protected with a sterile dressing until further therapy can be undertaken. Primary closure of soft tissue wounds is preferable; however, the age of the wound, the degree of contamination and the extent of shearing, avulsing, and crushing forces will dictate the timing and method of wound closure.

The main objectives are maximum return of function and restoration of as normal an appearance as is possible. It is impossible to obtain optimal function if an infection develops or if there is a large degree of scar tissue formation. If infection is present, it must be eradicated prior to wound closure. Early wound closure, when safe, and good technique are the key to minimizing scar tissue formation.

A. **Classification**   An attempt to organize a rational program for treating wounds must start with a classification that is both comprehensive and simple. Wounds can be placed into the following classification based on their etiology, the degree of contamination, the presence of associated injuries to underlying structures, and the likelihood that primary wound healing will occur.

1. **Tidy wounds**   The wound is clean. The wound edge and surrounding tissue have minimal damage. There is minimal or no loss of tissue and the wound is unlikely to become infected.

2. **Untidy wounds** These wounds have a significant amount of soft tissue damage or destruction by crushing or avulsing forces. There may be loss of superficial or deep tissue. Tissues are likely to be devitalized. Traumatized fat or subcutaneous tissue is especially subject to subsequent necrosis. There may be contamination of deep structures that cannot be debrided and an extensive soft tissue hematoma.

3. **Wounds with soft tissue loss** These are most commonly burn wounds or avulsive injuries. Chronic ulcerations with extensive skin loss and necrotizing wounds that have been aggressively debrided fall into this category.

4. **Infected wounds** These are wounds in which infection is firmly established or wounds in which the degree of contamination is so great that infection is certain. This latter category consists of human bites or wounds that contain foreign material, e.g., abrasive and blast injuries. This group includes wounds that have been open for a prolonged period prior to initial management. The so-called "golden period" in wound closure relates to the time it takes for the initial inoculum of bacteria in the wound to reach a level where invasive infection is present. This length of time is variable and is based upon the initial inoculum and the degree of devitalized tissue in the wound. Generally, the period is 3–6 hr from the time of injury.

B. **Wound management**

1. **Tidy wounds** Following initial examination to rule out injury to underlying structures, these wounds should be prepared by application of an antiseptic solution to the skin surrounding the injury. Thorough irrigation of the wound with normal saline and minimal debridement of any tissue fragments along the wound edge is performed. Following this preparation, these wounds can be closed primarily by approximation of deep tissues with absorbable suture material, such as cat gut or Dexon to obliterate the dead space. The skin is closed with simple skin sutures and the application of a dressing.

2. **Untidy wounds** Following initial examination, preparation of the skin, thorough irrigation, and surgical debridement, a decision is made whether to close the wound or leave it open. If there is injury to underlying structures, a repair can be performed primarily, if primary coverage or closure is planned, or may be delayed. The decision to close the wound primarily or to perform a delayed closure will be based upon the surgeon's judgment as to the viability of the surrounding tissues following the initial debridement and his estimation of the degree of the contamination of the wound. If primary closure is accomplished, these wounds should be drained with suction drainage catheters and dressed. If there is a question regarding the safety of primary closure, it is safest to do a delayed primary closure 3–5 days later, if the wound is clean. While the wound is open, moist dressings (saline) should be applied as often as necessary to prevent desiccation.

3. **Wounds with soft tissue loss** Initial management consits of thorough examination, preparation of the skin, irrigation of the wound, and removal of all

foreign bodies. Debridement is performed to obtain a surgically clean wound. If there is extensive soft tissue loss and vital structures are exposed, a biologic dressing should be used to protect these structures prior to wound closure. Secondary closure of the wound is then performed with skin grafts or flaps (see p. 267).

4. **Infected wounds**   The best management is aggressive surgical debridement of devitalized tissue and treatment of the wound in an open fashion. Application of moist heat, elevation if it is an extremity, immobilization, and systemic antibiotics, if there is systemic stress, are recommended. Frequent dressing changes are utilized using moist dressings to protect underlying structures and to prevent desiccation and further tissue loss. Once the wound is clean and the bacterial contamination has been controlled, wound closure can be accomplished. This can be done as a delayed closure, if possible, or may require skin grafts or skin flaps for reconstruction.

C. **Wound healing**   Wound healing involves repair of deep connective tissue by formation of collagen and resurfacing of the wound by epithelialization. This process occurs normally in all wounds whether they are closed primarily or allowed to heal secondarily. Primary repair is the term used to describe a sharply made wound that is accurately reapproximated within hours of its creation and heals with minimal space between its edges. Delayed primary closure is wound closure that occurs within 7 days after injury. Healing of a dead space or open wound by secondary intention involves filling the tissue defect with large quantities of connective tissue, which will become covered with epithelium. Primary or delayed primary wound closure is preferred, when possible, to minimize subsequent scar tissue formation.

The reparative process begins instantly at the time of injury with the influx of leukocytes, platelets, red blood cells, and other serum proteins into the wound. Collagen synthesis begins within 2–3 days following the initial injury. This fibroblastic phase lasts from the 3rd to the 5th day. During this time, the strength of the wound increases rapidly and epithelial cells begin to proliferate to cover the narrow gap between the edges of the reapproximated wound. Usually by the end of a week, a wound has reached significant tensile strength to allow suture removal without wound disruption. Following this period, the phase of wound maturation or wound contracture follows and lasts for several months. At this time, the new blood vessels become obliterated, the young fibroblasts mature and the scar begins to contract. The scar is red, raised, indurated, and firm to palpation. After resolution of this phase, the scar becomes soft, pliable, and begins to fade in color. The absolute amount of fibrous tissue in a wound that heals by primary intention is rather small and is represented by a thin sheet of scar tissue inferfacing between the surrounding normal tissue.

In wounds that heal by secondary intention, the duration of healing depends upon the dimensions of the wound, the presence or absence of infection, the mobility of surrounding structures, and the general condition of the patient. While the depths of the wound are being filled in with granulation tissue, epithelialization occurs on the surface, peripherally. At the same time, obliteration of the blood vessels and deposition of collagen in the granulation tissue takes place. Wound contraction and migration of epithelial cells from the periphery of the wound occur simultaneously. This contracture of the wound is to be distinguished from later scar contracture. Eventually, a new epithelium covers the entire granulated surface of the open wound. There is much more scar tissue in this type of wound and additional scar contracture can be expected to a much greater degree than in wounds that have healed by primary intention. The epithelium overlying the granulation tissue is not skin and in no way mimics or replaces normal skin. This epithelium is easily traumatized and ulcerations may occur causing the cycle of healing by secondary intention to be repeated with the formation of even more scar tissue.

D. **Factors affecting wound healing**

1. **Anesthesia** Use of local or topical anesthetics should only be initiated following an adequate sensory and motor examination to rule out a peripheral nerve injury. The use of local anesthesia not only comforts the patient, but aids the physician in management of the wound. Adequate cleansing of the wound to remove bacteria, soil, and other debris, necessary surgical debridement, and examination for injury to underlying structures cannot be properly carried out without adequate anesthesia. Lidocaine hydrochloride (Xylocaine) is the most commonly used local anesthetic. The loss of sensation occurs almost instantaneously and is usually complete by 5 min. The period of anesthesia lasts from 1½–2 hr in almost all circumstances. Lidocaine does not damage local tissue defenses. In selected cases, epinephrine is useful as a hemostatic agent; however, the vasoconstrictive effect damages local tissue and decreases local tissue defenses through its ischemic effect. The infection-potentiating effect of epinephrine is proportional to its concentration. **In heavily contaminated wounds, and distal structures such as digits, the use of epinephrine is to be condemned.** Surgical judgment should prevail in choosing the proper anesthetic agent with or without a local vasoconstrictor.

2. **Hair removal** The use of a razor to remove hair adjacent to a wound increases the incidence of wound infection. In planning hair removal at the time of traumatic wound closure, careful consideration should be given as to how much the removal of the hair will facilitate wound management. Consideration should be given to clipping the hair with scissors or shaving the hair with a razor that has a recessed blade, so that damage to the skin will not occur.

3. **Antisepsis** The most commonly used skin preparation compounds are the iodophors (e.g., Betadine). They are fast-acting and have a broad spectrum of antimicrobial activity. There is some absorption of Betadine and other complexed iodophor solutions; therefore, it is prudent to limit their use to intact skin. The iodophors may impair local tissue resistance to infection. Cleansing of the open wound is accomplished with more physiologic solutions, such as saline.

4. **Surgical debridement** The process of debridement is the most important single factor in the management of a contaminated wound. Debridement

removes tissue that has been heavily contaminated by particulate matter from soil or road surface or a heavy inoculum of bacteria. Debridement also removes devitalized tissue that would impair the wound's ability to resist infection and heal normally. The identification of the exact limits of debridement is a challenging problem and requires surgical judgment and careful, repeated examination of the wound.

5. **Mechanical cleansing**   The two most commonly employed forms of mechanical cleansing in the management of open wounds are hydraulic force (wound irrigation) and direct contact. In an open wound, bacteria and other particulate matter are retained on the wound surface by adhesive forces. The mechanical force must exceed the adhesive force of the contaminants, but not damage the tissue, thus decreasing resistance to invasive infection.

   a. **Hydraulic force**   A high velocity irrigating stream is desirable since it cleans the wound better than a low velocity jet. The pressure exerted by fluid delivered through a 19-gauge needle using a 35-cc syringe is a high-pressure system, while irrigation with a bulb syringe is a low-pressure system. High-pressure irrigation systems successfully clean the wound of small particulate matter, including bacteria. Conversely, low-pressure irrigation systems, even with large volumes of solution, have almost no effect on removing small particles. There is little measurable therapeutic effect except in wounds that contain only large particulate matter.

   If a period of 4–6 hr transpires prior to initial debridement and cleansing, bacteria in the wound become lodged even if there was minimal contamination initially. A fibrin coagulum protects the bacteria from the action of antibiotics and increases the resistance to removal by low pressure irrigation. Once lodgement has occurred, bacteria can proliferate to potentially infective levels (10^5/gm of tissue) and invade the soft tissues. This lodged material can only be effectively removed by sharp debridement or pressure irrigation.

   b. **Direct contact**   The other commonly used mechanical force to cleanse a wound is direct contact, usually by means of a sponge or scrub brush. This is a very effective means of removing bacteria and small particulate matter from wounds; however, this method is traumatic to the soft tissue and may impair the wound's ability to resist infection. Injudicious cleansing by scrubbing the wound, especially if vital structures are exposed, should be avoided.

6. **Antibiotics**   The timing of antibiotic administration greatly influences the success of therapy. The length of time the wound has been open and exposed is inversely related to the effectiveness of systemic or topical antibiotics. As the fibrin coat forms in the wound, bacteria are protected from antibiotics. Cooling or desiccation of the wound surface further reduces antibiotic effectiveness. The degree of contamination within the wound can affect the outcome of the antibiotic treatment. When a wound is contaminated by exceedingly large numbers of organisms (greater than 10^9), infection is usually unavoidable, despite antibiotic therapy. These large numbers of organisms

are encountered in circumstances where frank pus or fecal material contaminates the wound.

The indication for the use of antibiotics in a traumatic wound depends upon multiple factors including the mechanism of injury, the amount of inflammatory response present at the wound edge and on the wound surface, and the total bacterial count. In **crush or avulsive injuries** there is a significant degree of tissue ischemia and antibiotics are indicated in almost all instances. The impaired local tissue defenses make these wounds susceptible to invasion by a relatively small inoculum of bacteria. If the mechanism of injury is a sharp shearing force such as a knife or piece of glass, the resistance to infection is much greater. A bacterial count of 1,000,000/gm of tissue or greater is needed to establish an infection. This high level of contamination is present in only a few such wounds. If there is a question regarding contamination, a **rapid slide technique** is performed to determine bacterial counts within the wound. The technique employs the excision of a 2×1-cm sample of tissue, which weighs approximately 0.5 gm. The biopsy is taken to the laboratory where it is weighed and then homogenized in a measured amount of normal saline. The specimen is then processed by routine quantitative culture and direct microscopic examination by wet prep. Bacteria will be seen when the specimen contains greater than 2.5×10^5 organisms/gm of tissue. If smaller numbers of bacteria are present, bacteria are not detectable on microscopic examination. If bacteria are not seen, the quantity of organisms that may be present is of little clinical significance. The rapid slide technique can be performed and the information delivered to the surgeon within 20 min. Microscopic examination does not replace quantitative serial dilution and plating techniques. These should also be performed to classify the bacteria and obtain antibiotic sensitivities.

7. **Dead space**   The obliteration of dead space is an accepted principle in managing wounds. There are two principal types of wounds in which dead space or potential dead space is created. In the first, there is an elevation of skin and subcutaneous tissue from underlying structures forming a flap. After this injury is sutured, there may be an accumulation of blood or serum beneath the flap. In the second type of wound, there is loss of underlying tissue, secondary either to the original injury or to surgical debridement. There is a true dead space that will be filled by transudation and exudation of fluids and blood into the wound. The presence of clot will delay wound healing because of the time necessary for the obliteration of the hematoma with fibrous tissue. This increases the amount of scarring that may impair the functional or aesthetic result. The presence of blood or serum is an ideal culture medium for producing wound sepsis. Sutures may be used to obliterate dead space; however, the use of foreign material such as sutures to close dead space in contaminated wounds should be avoided since this is a nidus for infection. Sutures cause local tissue ischemia, which can impair local tissue resistance. Another method for obliterating or closing dead space is the use of suction drainage catheters. Suction drainage is rapidly performed and does not introduce a permanent foreign body into the wound. In most instances, cer-

tainly in potentially contaminated wounds, the use of suction catheters is more appropriate than the use of buried suture material for obliteration of dead space. If drainage is used as a prophylactic measure, its potentially harmful effects become important. Drains may act as a retrograde conduit for skin contaminants to gain entrance into the wound. If a sump drain is used, the air vent is a potential route for wound contamination. The presence of a drain impairs the resistance of tissue to infection. Therefore, in wounds without dead space and without known fluid collections or a significant potential for fluid collection, drainage is unnecessary and may be detrimental. In situations where significant dead space exists, the use of a drain for **at least** several hours in the postoperative period is a helpful adjunct in wound management. The drainage should be a closed system.

E. **Wound closure** When considering wound closure, timing and the degree of tissue loss are important factors. A significant degree of tissue loss prohibits simple approximation of the wound edges. In wounds in which there has been major tissue loss, the use of skin **grafts** or **flaps,** either local or distant, will be required to close the defect. If a wound has minimal tissue loss, **primary** or **delayed primary closure** can usually be accomplished. If a wound has major tissue loss, primary closure is generally not advised. Primary closure of contaminated wounds will frequently result in the development of wound sepsis and dehiscence. The fresh wound, when left open, will gain resistance to infection with time and permit safe closure. The development of host resistance to infection is concomitant with the development of young granulation tissue. Delayed primary closure should be used in all contaminated wounds or in wounds with a significant degree of tissue damage and decreased host resistance. Delayed primary closure is usually performed in 5–7 days after injury if an infection has not developed. If there is any question regarding primary wound closure, delayed closure is advisable.

When a wound is being considered for delayed closure, a **quantitative tissue culture** should be obtained if there is a question about the safety of closure. The wound can be closed if there are fewer than 10^5 organisms/gm of tissue. The type of materials used for wound approximation is a matter of surgical choice. The four available methods for reapproximating wound edges are tissue adhesives, clips or staples, sutures, and tapes or steri-strips.

Although there have been some encouraging reports on the use of **tissue adhesives,** primarily cyanoacrylate, for repair of visceral injuries or as hemostatic agents in large wounds, they should **not** be used for closure of skin or subcutaneous tissue injuries. The polymer forms a barrier between the wound edges which prevents wound apposition and delays healing. Also, the incidence of infection is significantly higher than when other methods of closure are used.

Metal clips markedly decrease the time required for approximation of wound edges. There are recent studies that indicate there may be decreased elasticity and less ability of the wound to absorb energy without disrupting when closed with clips as compared to monofilament nylon suture. In animal studies, stapled skin edges have been shown to be considerably more susceptible to infection than taped wound edges.

Sutures are the most common means employed for wound closure. Sutures may or may not undergo degradation and absorption within the wound. Some of the so-called nonabsorbable sutures (silk and nylon) lose their tensile strength rapidly after the second month and add little to reinforcement of the wound. The absorbable sutures are either gut or synthetic, e.g., polyglycolic acid. Gut sutures can be treated with chromium salts to increase their tensile strength and resistance to absorption. The nonabsorbable sutures are made from organic naturally occurring materials such as silk, cotton, or linen; synthetic materials such as nylon, dacron, and polypropylene; or stainless steel. Nonabsorbable sutures are either monofilament or multifilament.

There are several mechanisms by which suture material may enhance infection. The surgeon's technique in placement of the suture should be as atraumatic as possible to avoid additional tissue damage. Care should be taken not to tie sutures too tightly—"approximate, don't strangulate."

All suture materials elicit an inflammatory response. The magnitude of the local injury to the host defenses is related to both the quantity of suture within the wound and to the chemical composition of the suture material. The incidence of infection in contaminated wounds is lower when monofilament sutures such as nylon or prolene are used when compared to other nonabsorbable sutures. Among the absorbable sutures, polyglycolic acid appears to elicit the least inflammatory response.

The incidence of wound infection is much lower in **taped** wounds when compared to other methods of closure. This is related to the minimal tissue injury caused by tape as compared to other methods of closure. The use of tape in potentially contaminated wounds is a useful clinical tool and is limited by the site of injury. In areas where there is a great deal of mobility, e.g., joints, or areas where there is a large amount of secretion, e.g., the axilla, tape is impractical. In abraded wounds where the skin surface is wet, no amount of preparation will allow the tape to adhere.

Closing a wound without undue tension is necessary to obtain primary healing. The impairment of circulation at the wound edge caused by excessive tension can lead to delayed healing, secondary infection, and subsequent wound breakdown. This is especially true in tissue that has been contused by recent trauma. Unless the wound can be closed without tension, consideration should be given to another means of wound closure, such as a skin graft or flap.

A **skin graft** can be used to cover any wound that has enough inherent vascularity to support granulation tissue. This does not imply that granulation tissue must be present prior to grafting. The choice of a full thickness versus a split thickness skin graft is determined by several factors. The availability of full thickness skin grafts is limited in that the donor site must be closed primarily or with a split thickness graft; therefore, only relatively small defects can be closed with full thickness skin grafts. Because of its greater thickness, the revascularization of a full thickness graft requires more ideal conditions as compared to a split thickness skin graft. Because of their greater thickness, a more stable cover and better protection for the underlying structures is provided by a full thickness graft. Since a much larger number of skin appendages are transferred with a full thickness skin graft, the texture and color of the skin is more normal compared to a split graft. When large open areas need covering, a split thickness skin graft is more feasible, but less cosmetic. The split thickness skin graft can be meshed to facilitate drainage through the graft, which enhances the "take," as well as to enable the graft to drape into the contours of an irregular surface.

When avascular areas need coverage (e.g., exposed bone without periosteum, exposed tendon without peritenon), or when vital structures are exposed, a skin graft may not provide adequate protection. In this case, a **flap** is necessary for wound closure. Flaps may be either simple or complex (composite) and either local or distant.

Most skin flaps have a random blood supply and are called **random flaps.** This means that the blood supply to the skin and subcutaneous tissue in the flap is derived only through the subdermal plexus of vessels and no specific named artery or vein is responsible for delivering blood to the area of the flap. Because of their random blood supply, it is necessary to maintain a base of the flap that is equal to the length to assure that all of the flap will survive. If this length to width ratio of 1:1 is exceeded, the risk of flap necrosis is increased. The 1:1 ratio can be broken in areas where the blood supply to the skin is very generous, such as on the scalp or the face. On the trunk and the extremities, it is necessary to plan flaps so that the 1:1 ratio is maintained.

The second type of skin flap is the **axial pattern** or **arterialized flap.** These flaps have a central vascular bundle that supplies blood flow to the skin in the flap. Anatomically, there are relatively few axial pattern skin flaps. Some of the more commonly used axial pattern flaps are the groin flap which is supplied by the superficial circumflex iliac artery and vein, the deltopectoral flap which is supplied by perforating branches from the internal mammary artery, and the forehead flap which is supplied by the superficial temporal vessels.

Other flaps, such as **composite flaps** of multiple types of tissue, are used. The most common composite flap used is the **musculocutaneous flap** which is composed of a muscle and its overlying skin. These units are well vascularized axial pattern flaps in that the muscle unit has a specific arterial blood supply and the skin overlying the muscle is supplied by direct musculocutaneous perforators which enter the subdermal plexus. These units can be transferred in continuity with good success. In many circumstances, the muscle alone is transferred to provide coverage of vital or devascularized structures, and a split thickness skin graft is then placed over the muscle to obtain wound closure.

Axial pattern flaps can be transposed or transferred to another area in three ways. First, the flap can be transferred as a pedicled flap, which includes the vascular bundle, the overlying skin, subcutaneous tissue, and muscle (musculocutaneous flap). This type of pedicled flap (indicating that the flap is left patched by an intact pedicle to its donor area) is called a **peninsular flap** because a broad peninsula of tissue is left attached at the donor area. Second, an **island pedicled flap** may be formed by skeletonizing the vasculature so that the pedicle supplying the flap is the only tissue left attached to the donor area. Third, the tissue can be transferred by completely separating it from the donor area after dissecting the vascular pedicle. The vascular pedicle is anastomosed at the recipient site to available vessels.

The use of this **microvascular free flap** has greatly expanded the reconstructiv capabilities of the plastic surgeon who deals with large soft tissue injuries.

Local flaps are used when tissue adjacent to or very near a wound is used for coverage. There are four means of local flap transfer. First, a simple **advancement flap** may be performed by undermining an edge of the wound and incising the tissue for a distance along the lines of greatest tension and advancing the tissue to cover the defect. Second, a **rotation flap** is designed so that a long sweeping arc is incised adjacent to the wound, and the skin that is contained within this arc is undermined and rotated into the defect. The third manner of transfer is a **transposition flap.** In this flap, the tissue adjacent to the defect is used for coverage. The edge of the wound makes up one side of the flap. The other two sides of the flap are created by incising a rectangular-shaped flap of adjacent skin and undermining the flap completely and then transposing it into the adjacent defect. The transposition flap usually requires a skin graft for coverage of the donor site. The final method of transfer is an **interpolation flap,** which uses local tissue that is not directly adjacent to the wound. Thus, the pedicle has to cross over normal tissue to reach the defect leaving a bridge of tissue interposed between the donor site and the recipient site.

Distant flaps involve the transposition of new tissue from a distance. The most common example is the application of a groin flap to the dorsum of the hand for coverage. Distant flaps can be pedicled such that the flap is left attached to the donor area or can be transferred as a free flap.

In general, wounds that will require a flap are not clean enough to perform the flap at the time of admission. A distant flap may be used as a delayed primary closure. Delayed primary closure is usually safe after the wound has been debrided two or three times. Local flaps cannot be used before 10–14 days since the local tissue is usually so contused that a successful take is unlikely.

The choice of the proper method of wound closure requires a great deal of surgical judgment and experience in dealing with traumatic wounds. The foregoing discussion is not meant to be an oversimplification of this complex problem, but merely an introduction to the various types of wound closure that are available to the reconstructive surgeon. The timing of wound closure is just as important as the method chosen. Adequate debridement and meticulous wound cleansing are necessary for successful wound closure. Quantitative cultures are suggested to assist the surgeon in selecting the best time for wound closure.

F. **Biologic dressings**   As an adjunct to wound management prior to the definitive wound closure, the use of biologic dressings may play an important role in the overall care of the traumatized patient.

Types of biologic dressings include allografts or homografts usually from cadaver donors, human amnion with or without the attached chorion, and heterografts or xenografts, the most common being porcine or pigskin. The porcine grafts may be further divided by the manner in which they are prepared, i.e., fresh, fresh-frozen, irradiated, or lyophilized.

Biologic dressings are a complex and, at best, poorly understood subject, and many opinions regarding their use can be found in the literature. Our preference is the use of allograft or homograft human skin from cadaver donors; however, the availability of homografts limits their use. When biologic dressings are indicated, we use a porcine xenograft. The fresh-frozen preparation is preferable because it can be stored for long periods and thawed immediately prior to use. We do not feel that biologic dressings are indicated for wound debridement or as a primary dressing for partial thickness skin losses. There is no evidence that biologic dressings increase the rate of epithelialization or the formation of granulation tissue. They are useful for the reduction of pain in open wounds and for protection of exposed vital structures, both from further contamination and from dessication. They markedly reduce water, protein, and erythrocyte loss from the wound. We find them useful in determining whether or not a particular recipient wound is ready for ultimate skin graft closure. If the porcine xenograft adheres to the wound, the bed is conducive for successful skin grafting. If, on the other hand, the porcine slides around without adhering, additional debridement and wound care should be carried out prior to skin grafting.

G. **Dressing** The major purpose of a dressing is to prevent contamination of the wound. A primarily closed wound rapidly gains resistance to infection and does not need a dressing after the first 24–48 hr because the fibrin seal resists bacterial invasion. The dressing should be multilayered. The inner layer should be non-adhering and porous to allow egress of fluid from the wound. The second layer should be an absorbent layer to collect fluid which may egress from the wound. A third support layer is necessary to protect the wound.

In facial lacerations, there is more concern about the development of blood clots between the edges of the wound than about potential contamination. These clots will be replaced by scar tissue. Swabbing of the wound with half-strength peroxide hemolyzes and removes the clot. Swabbing the wound should be performed every 6 hr until there is no clot present. Coagulum (scab), which may form on abraded skin, makes suture removal painful. Antibacterial ointments are useful in limiting coagulum formation on abraded skin. (See p. 85.)

H. **Immobilization** Immobilization of an injured part is of value for patient comfort and wound healing. When the site of the wound is immobilized, lymphatic flow is reduced, thereby minimizing the spread of microflora. Immobilized tissue demonstrates superior resistance to the growth of bacteria compared to mobile tissue. Whenever possible, the site of injury should be elevated above the patient's heart. Elevation limits the accumulation of fluid within the interstitial spaces of the wounded tissue. Nonedematous wounds are more readily rehabilitated than wounds that have been allowed to swell.

I. **Tetanus immunization** Tetanus immunization must be considered in all traumatic wounds (see p. 429).

J. **Degloving injuries** A degloving injury is characterized by avulsion of skin with or without deeper soft tissue from the underlying skeletal or musculoskeletal framework. These injuries usually involve the entire circumference of an extremity. If the skin is attached, it is usually attached distally. A classic example of this type of injury is the ring avulsion injury which occurs when a ring worn on the finger is caught on a fixed object and strips the soft tissue from the underlying phalanges. The same type of injury results when a shearing force is applied to an extremity, thus elevating the skin from the underlying soft tissue circumferentially. Such trauma markedly compromises the circulation to the skin by direct damage to the skin and subcutaneous tissue, as well as by disrupting the perforators that enter the skin from the underlying muscle. The extent of vascular compromise will depend upon the regional nature of the arterial blood supply to the skin and the overall size of the avulsed segment.

As soon as the patient is resuscitated and stabilized, the following sequence should be carried out for **management** of the wound.

—The degloved extremity should be initially wrapped in a sterile towel or sheet pending initial management.
—While wearing sterile gloves, mechanically remove large foreign materials.
—Any bleeding should be controlled by direct pressure. The temptation to clamp vessels without proper exposure should be avoided.
—The wound should be irrigated with copious amounts of sterile saline and pulsatile pressure irrigation.
—Appropriate antibiotic therapy is instituted intravenously, and the patient is covered for tetanus prophylaxis.
—Peripheral pulses and capillary filling should be observed and recorded and, where practical, 2-point discrimination of sensation should also be recorded as baseline values.
—While awaiting definitive surgical debridement, the wound should be covered with a sterile, soft bulky dressing and elevated. If the wound is grossly contaminated, a dilute Betadine-soaked dressing is used.
—The initial operative debridement should include only obviously nonviable tissue, or tissue that is badly crushed or cannot be cleansed of imbedded materials. Repeated, copious pressure irrigation is performed at the time of initial surgical debridement.
—If there is an associated fracture, this should be stabilized at the time of the initial operative procedure. Thorough exploration of the wound and evaluation of damage to underlying vital structures, such as nerves, should be done.
—The skin should be simply replaced over the wound and not sutured under any tension. This may require leaving large portions of the wound open temporarily.
—The wound should be dressed with xeroform gauze and another soft bulky dressing and elevated in the postoperative period.
—A second-look operation should be carried out 24 hr following the initial debridement. Debridement of all nonvital tissue is carried out at this time.
—Eventual closure of the wound is performed as a delayed primary closure, secondary closure, or by the use of skin grafts or skin flaps. Skin grafts ranging from .010–.014 inch in thickness are usually the preferred method of wound closure. Meshing of the graft will provide for egress of fluid from

beneath the graft and allow the graft to fit into convoluted surfaces of the wound. Flaps are used when indicated, i.e., to cover exposed bone devoid of periosteum or exposed tendons, arteries, or nerves. Other indications include the need for additional padding over vital structures or to fill in a contour deformity.

V. Hand The functional prognosis for the injured hand depends primarily on the treatment given in the Admitting Area and the early definitive surgery.

This protocol is designed to minimize wound contamination, prevent further damage, and initiate measures that will make definitive surgery possible.

Since impaired hand function is associated with major disability, hand injuries demand immediate, expert care. All hand problems beyond superficial injuries require consultation by a specially trained surgeon.

A. Admitting Area

    1. First priorities

        a. Emergency assessment of injury (At this stage, do not attempt to carry out a detailed examination.)

        b. Control hemorrhage by moderate compression dressing. (Do not clamp blindly in the wound; obtain hemostasis by direct pressure.)

        c. If the patient has been admitted with a tourniquet in place, release it as soon as possible and control bleeding with adequate pressure dressing. (Clamping is **rarely** necessary.)

        d. Remove visible foreign bodies.

        e. Irrigate the wound with 1–2 liters of lactated Ringer's solution or normal saline solution.

        f. Cover the wound with sterile dressing and apply a thin board splint. Cover with a stockinette and elevate from an i.v. pole.

    2. Second priorities The patient's general state should be stable, thus allowing a more detailed assessment.

        a. Review available history. (Is wound clean or contaminated?)

        b. Remove dressing; **examine entire hand carefully, not just the wound.**

        c. Examine and **record** the specific injury by categories.

            (1) Soft tissue The soft tissue defect and injury is usually obvious to inspection; however, debridement will further delineate the extent of injury.

            (2) Tendon A wound located on the hand or wrist should raise the likelihood that there may be an associated tendon injury. Flexion, extension, abduction, and adduction should be checked in each digit and at the wrist. If the middle phalanx is immobilized and the patient is unable to flex the distal phalanx, injury to the flexor digitorum profundus is likely. Injury to the flexor digitorum superficialis is suspected if all but the suspected digit are held in extension and the tested digit is unable to be flexed. A laceration involving the dorsum of the hand and the inability to extend fully a digit(s) is likely to be associated with the division of a common extensor tendon, extensor indicis (index finger), or extensor digiti quinti proprius (fifth digit). A laceration that involves the dorsal aspect of the thumb or first metacarpal and is associated with an inability to extend fully the distal phalanx of the thumb represents a laceration of the extensor pollicis longus tendon. A laceration over the thumb, first metacarpal, or radial aspect of the wrist associated with an inability to extend and abduct the thumb represents injury to the short extensor and long abductor tendons; the long extensor may be divided.

(3) **Nerve** Anesthesia distal to an injury suggests a neural lesion.

  (a) **Ulnar nerve** Injury at or distal to the wrist results in an inability to abduct or adduct the index finger; sensation of the fifth finger may or may not be intact.

  (b) **Median nerve** Injury may cause the inability to oppose the thumb to the base of the fifth finger or abduct the thumb at a right angle to the palm of the hand; there is usually hypesthesia to the volar aspect of the index finger.

  (c) **Radial nerve** A proximal injury will result in impairment of wrist and finger extension. A distal injury will result in hypesthesia in the area of the anatomical snuff box and the radial, dorsal hand.

(4) **Vascular** Major vascular embarrassment will result in a cold, pale, pulseless, and painful hand. Evaluate the color of the fingertips. Note the rate of capillary refill after pressing on the fingertips. Check the radial and ulnar pulses.

(5) **Bone** Examination usually reveals deformity, excessive tenderness, and/or excessive motion.

(6) **Joint** A ligamentous injury, subluxation, or dislocation will result in local swelling, excessive tenderness, or excessive motion.

d. Position partially amputated parts in an approximately normal anatomical relationship.

e. Cover wound with sterile 4 × 4 gauze and apply voluminous light dressing. Use moderate compression to control bleeding.

f. Apply light wooden splint, holding wrist slightly dorsiflexed, digits in the position of grasp with fingertips exposed where possible.

g. Obtain x-rays of extremity (AP, lateral, and oblique) at the end of x-ray protocol, i.e., C-spine, chest, etc.

h. Start appropriate intravenous antibiotic and obtain tetanus immunization history.

i. Team Leader plans definitive treatment and discusses treatment with Hand Consultant when indicated.

B. Operating Room

1. **Cleansing** Protect the wound with sterile gauze, thoroughly wash the surrounding area with Betadine soap, and rinse copiously with sterile normal

saline solution or lactated Ringer's solution. Cover the hand and arm with Betadine solution and drape.

Note The pneumatic tourniquet may need to be elevated during the prep to prevent bleeding.

2. **Debridement** This involves meticulous and atraumatic removal of all devitalized tissue and hematoma, and irrigation with lactated Ringer's solution.

3. **Inspection** Careful assessment of injury and development of plan of treatment.

4. **Definitive treatment**
   a. **Vascular** Reestablish circulation; an isolated radial or ulnar artery should be repaired, if possible.
   b. **Bones and joints** Position and mold into alignment. Use Kirschner wire fixation when indicated.
   c. **Nerve** Meticulous repair is needed for maximal recovery, but this may not be possible at the initial operation. A delayed primary repair or a secondary repair may be the procedure of choice if
      (1) The wound is grossly contaminated
      (2) An element of crush trauma prevents a determination of the limits of injury
      (3) Other injuries mandate termination of surgery
      Major nerve endings, when seen in the wound, may be tagged together with a single suture for later repair.
   d. **Tendon** In the severely injured patient and/or in the patient with severe wound contamination, delayed primary repair or secondary repair may be the procedure of choice; otherwise, primary repair is performed.
   e. **Soft tissue** See p. 260.

   Note In the severely contaminated wound, open wound treatment followed by secondary debridement and wound closure is the procedure of choice. Primary repair is indicated if contamination is minimal, the patient's condition is good, and the surgeon's experience with hand injuries is adequate.

VI. **Replantation and Revascularization** It is possible with microvascular techniques to anastomose 1-mm vessels; thus, replantation of digits is possible. Thumb, multiple finger, wrist, transmetacarpal, forearm, arm, and some lower limb amputations should be replanted. Amputated single digits should be replanted only under unusual circumstances, i.e., for occupational or aesthetic reasons. Useful function with recovery of sensibility can be achieved.

The protocol is designed to minimize warm ischemia time and minimize physical damage to the exposed donor and recipient vessel and nerve ends.

A. **Admitting Area**

1. **First priorities**
   a. **The patient**   Control hemorrhage by either direct pressure, hand elevation, or, if necessary, with blood pressure cuff on the upper arm. Do not clamp blindly in the wound.
   b. **The amputated part**   Handle with sterile technique. Irrigate with lactated Ringer's solution to remove foreign debris (sawdust, grass). Wrap the part in sterile gauze, place it into a sterile plastic cup or bag, and place the container on top of ice in a larger container. Label the container with the patient's name and content and put this into a safe place until needed in surgery.
   c. Evaluate the rest of the injured extremity for additional injuries.
   d. Complete immediate care to the amputation site.
      (1) Remove visible foreign bodies.
      (2) Irrigate with 2 liters of lactated Ringer's solution.
      (3) Cover with sterile gauze. **Do not put on Betadine dressings.**
      (4) Support the extremity on a board and elevate.
   e. **The partially amputated part**   Irrigate with 2 liters of lactated Ringer's solution; then, wearing sterile gloves, reposition (untwist or straighten out) the part into an anatomical position, cover with sterile gauze, and support on an arm board.
   f. For the partially amputated part that requires revascularization, include a coolant in the dressing, e.g., ice bags, volarly and dorsally.

2. **Second priorities**   When there is a completely amputated part or when a partially amputated part is avascular, the Team Leader will discuss transfer with the Hand Trauma Center as soon as the patient's condition will permit. If the patient's condition does not permit transfer, the Team Leader will arrange for the Hand Trauma Center replantation team to come to MIEMSS for the surgery.

   At this time, a decision should be made whether to attempt replantation. Ideally, two teams of microsurgeons should be notified: one to work on the patient and one to prepare the part, thereby reducing operating time. A detailed discussion of risks and expected results (both of successful replantation and future function) should begin. The prognosis is best with local crush or guillotine-type amputations and worst with avulsed or severely crushed amputations.
   a. After an evaluation by the replantation team, the partially amputated part which will be revascularized should have a coolant incorporated into the dressing.
   b. Tetanus prophylaxis should be considered.
   c. Systemic broad-spectrum, penicillinase-effective antibiotic should be administered. Systemic penicillin should be added if the accident occurred on a farm.
   d. X-ray (PA, lateral, and oblique) the hand, wrist, and any amputated parts. For suspected proximal injuries, include elbow views. For unusual

fractures or wrist dislocation, include contralateral views for comparison.

    e. If upper arm or elbow injuries are present, consider the possibility of a more proximal (second) vascular injury and the need for an arteriogram.

B. Operating room

1. Under the operating microscope, using sterile technique, the amputated part is examined first to identify a usable artery and at least one vein. Nerves and tendons are also identified. The wound is surgically cleansed of foreign bodies, but skin is not debrided at this time.

2. Bone stabilization is achieved after identifying the appropriate vessel, nerve, and tendon structures proximally.

3. Depending on the degree of bone shortening, nature of injury, and gap in vessels, a decision as to whether to use vein grafts is made. The volar forearm is a good source for these donor veins.

4. Ideally, primary tendon repairs are carried out.

5. Ideally, two veins are repaired for each artery repaired in the replant. In the revascularization, a skin bridge may count as one repaired vein.

6. Ideally, primary nerve repairs are carried out.

7. Appropriate pharmacologic agents may be used:
       a. Heparinized saline, 10 units/ml
       b. Buffered Xylocaine, 2%
       c. Tissusol
       d. Thrombolytic agents (urokinase, streptokinase)
       e. Antiplatelet agents (dextran 40, aspirin)

8. Skin closure must be loose.

9. Dressing must not be constrictive and must allow easy inspection of tips of the fingers.

10. Postoperative monitoring of circulation
       a. Visual
       b. Temperature probe
       c. Doppler monitor

C. Transfer procedure

1. Contact SYSCOM with reference to transfer to the Hand Trauma Center.

2. The amputated part, wrapped in gauze, is placed in a plastic bag which, in turn, is placed in a styrofoam container that holds ice in a separate plastic bag.

3. The partially amputated part which requires revascularization should have a coolant incorporated into the dressing, e.g., ice bags volarly and dorsally.

VII. Amputation Limb salvage in the multiply injured patient is one of the most challenging problems facing the trauma surgeon. Every effort should be made to conserve usable structures, especially in the upper extremity. The overall condition and clinical course of the patient following his injury will dictate to some degree what reconstructive and salvage steps should be taken. By no means should a life be placed in jeopardy to salvage a limb. The expected capability of functional return is based upon evaluation of the entire extremity including soft tissue coverage, the skeletal framework, musculotendinous units, motor and sensory nerve supply, and its vascularity. Parts should not be salvaged that can neither be restored as useful members nor contribute tissues for overall reconstruction of an extremity. **Crush injuries may cause myoglobinuria** (see p. 351).

Although each case must be individualized and surgical judgment used, there are certain guidelines that remain fairly standard.

A. Absolute contraindications to attempted limb salvage

1. **Vascular damage** An absolute indication for amputation is the absence of blood supply to an injured extremity in which there is no possibility of restoring vascularity. This is not to say that all extremities with the capability of being revascularized should be salvaged.

2. **Significant associated injuries** Multiply traumatized patients are not best served by a prolonged operative time necessary for replantation, revascularization, and reconstruction of an extremity that is a poor risk for salvage. These patients may not be able to undergo the numerous trips to the operating room, which are frequently necessary if limb salvage is to be accomplished. If the necessary procedures for limb salvage will compromise the patient's chances for survival, an amputation should be seriously considered.

3. **Extensive injury to the affected limb** Successful repairs are uncommon when injuries involve multiple levels or when extensive degloving and crush injuries involve a large portion of the distal extremity.

4. **Chronic illness** Underlying disease, such as cardiovascular disease or renal disease, which is sufficient to make prolonged surgery hazardous, may represent a contraindication to attempted limb salvage or replantation.

5. **Neural damage** If the nerve injury is so severe that it is unlikely that the extremity will have sensory function, the most prudent course is amputation.

Perspective
If vascularity and sensory function are intact, although skeletal deformity or ankylosis is likely, a "sensate prosthesis" is often functional. An insensate extremity is essentially worthless.

B. **Relative contraindications**

1. **Patients over 50 years of age** The amount of degenerative changes in the vasculature is variable, but if degeneration is advanced, the survival rate following revascularization or replantation will be markedly reduced. More importantly, recovery of function is not nearly as complete in the older patient as it is in the younger patient following either replantation or revascularization.

2. **Avulsion injuries** In comparison to sharply amputated or sharply traumatized extremities, those with avulsion or shearing-type injuries are much more difficult to reconstruct or salvage. This is because the damage, which may seem localized at initial evaluation, is not limited to the site of the tissue defect but extends for some distance both proximally and distally. This widespread damage results in either microvascular failure (thrombosis) or, if the vascularization is successful, in poor regeneration of nerve function.

3. **Lengthy warm ischemia time** Muscles undergo some irreversible changes after about 6 hr at room temperature. Connective tissues, nerves, tendons, skin, and bone remain viable for varying periods in excess of 12 hr. With immediate cooling of the distal extremity, the tolerable ischemia time can be markedly prolonged to as long as 24 hr or longer.

4. **Extreme contamination** This rarely prevents replantation; however, oil or grease that has been driven into the tissues may make debridement impossible and lead to late infection and loss of the extremity.

5. **Previous injury or surgery** An extremity that has already been compromised by previous injury has less chance of suitable recovery following revascularization or replantation.

Perspective

It is not uncommon that an extremity of questionable salvageability will eventually require amputation. There are many extremities that are obviously salvageable but many that are obviously not. However, some extremities are in a gray zone regarding salvageability; these require evaluation on a day-by-day basis to determine if they are a detriment to the patient's life. If there is soft tissue necrosis and/or sepsis, multiple systems deterioration is a common sequel. Frequently, it is difficult to ascertain the precise limits of nonviable soft tissue. Soft tissue defects associated with blunt extremity trauma are often much smaller than the underlying soft tissue damage. Often, the surgeon is satisfied with the tissue that is exposed.

The standard criteria for evaluating "exposed" muscle for viability at the time of surgical debridement are color, bleeding, and contractility. On the other hand, the surgeon frequently terminates muscle exposure when healthy tissue is identified within the wound. Multiple systems function is important in detecting "unseen" areas of tissue necrosis and/or sepsis (see p. 369).

If the patient becomes septic and/or develops manifestations of multiple systems stress or dysfunction, especially if other sources cannot be identified, we recommend extension of the limited wounds to allow for more thorough examination of the extremity. Frequently, the most expeditious modality to save the patient's life is extremity amputation.

There is often a fine line between amputating too early, in order to save the life, and amputating too late in an attempt to save the limb but risk losing the patient.

It must be emphasized that each case is based upon its individual merits. What is a suitable function for one patient may not represent a suitable function for another. What would be considered a reasonable period of hospitalization and rehabilitation for one patient may be absolutely devastating to another who needs to return rapidly to work and to the support of the family. Many considerations toward the rehabilitation and ultimate return to society of the patient have to be taken into account. The patient's occupation, emotional status, age, and overall medical condition must form the background against which the injured extremity is viewed. With all things being equal, it is usually safer to attempt salvage of extremities, provided that amputation can be performed at any time.

Principles of Managing Major Extremity Trauma

—Decide whether the extremity is salvageable.
—Rapidly stabilize fractures with a Hoffman device.
—Repair major arterial injuries.
—Repair major venous injuries, if possible; otherwise, ligate the vessel.
—If there is inadequate soft tissue coverage, an arterial repair should be extra-anatomical or covered with porcine grafts until delayed primary closure can be obtained (transposition or free muscle flap).
—All soft tissue must be adequately debrided.
—The wound should not be closed, because the tension will create capillary congestion and thrombosis.
—Tag severed nerve ends.
—Consider fasciotomy **early** if there has been prolonged ischemia or concomitant arterial and venous injury.
—Perform vascular contrast studies before and after surgery, when indicated.

Section IV
SPECIAL CONSIDERATIONS

14
BURNS

A broad range of burn patients confront the trauma surgeon. At one end of the spectrum is the large surface area injury, which in its early stages requires no operative intervention, but taxes the surgeon's medical skills. At the other end are the small, seemingly insignificant burns in the multiply injured patient. However, these small wounds complicate the management of the patient by providing an ever present avenue for sepsis, and frequently are responsible for prolonged hospital stay after more serious injuries have been dealt with.

Designated burn centers, which provide specialized care by a team of physicians, nurses, therapists, and social workers who deal with acute burn resuscitation and rehabilitation on a day-to-day basis, are the preferred site for the management of most major thermal injuries. This discussion addresses the critical judgments that must be made in the initial evaluation and stabilization of the patient with a burn wound in the setting of multiple system trauma.

I. **Initial Patient Stabilization**

   A. **Emergency cardiopulmonary resuscitation**   Potential airway problems are the same as for any multiple trauma patient. Significant laryngeal edema usually does not become manifest for several hours after injury. The earliest ventilatory problem seen is frequently respiratory depression due to cerebral hypoxia. Cyanosis may not be a reliable index in patients with carbon monoxide poisoning, in which case the arterial PO_2 may also be normal. Patients with clinical hypoventilation or whose blood gases on admission reveal carbon dioxide retention require intubation. Because of the possibility of carbon monoxide toxicity, all patients are placed on 100% oxygen (see p. 509).

   In conjunction with the assessment of the ventilatory status, venous access is established with multiple large bore lines and infusion of Ringer's lactate is begun. Preferred i.v. sites on the arms, chest, neck, or groin may be burned. When necessary, it is acceptable to place i.v. lines through the eschar, since these are usually sterile, and these sites may no longer be available once the wound becomes colonized. Lines should be sutured in place to prevent dislodgment. Tachycardia and hypotension present on admission are treated with rapid infusion of Ringer's lactate until further investigation proves volume replacement to be adequate.

   B. **Nonemergent adjunctive measures**

      1. **Foley catheter**   In patients with greater than 10–15% body surface area burns, this is the most dependable way of following urinary output.

2. **Nasogastric tube**   Patients with 20% or more body surface area burns commonly develop an ileus with gastric retention lasting 2–3 days. Following the return of bowel sounds, this tube or a pediatric feeding tube replacement may be used to aliment the patient enterally. Burn patients have an increased susceptibility to gastric ulceration and therefore should receive 30 cc of antacid by tube every 2 hr until tube feeding is begun. Cimetidine (Tagamet, 300 mg i.v. every 6 hr) and vitamin A (50,000 units i.v. every 6 hr) may be added to offer protection against ulceration.

3. **Admission laboratory studies** include electrolytes, glucose, blood urea nitrogen (BUN), complete blood count (CBC), and urinalysis. In addition, consider carboxyhemoglobin, serum myoglobin, hemoglobin, additional chemistries dictated by prior cardiac, renal, or hepatic history, and serum and urine toxicology for alcohol or other drugs which may explain an altered state of consciousness.

4. **Chest x-ray**   The chest x-ray is necessary as a baseline for comparison should cardiac or pulmonary problems develop, and as a check for intravenous and endotracheal tube position. Even with severe ventilatory injury, the admission chest x-ray is typically normal.

5. **Electrocardiogram**   The EKG may demonstrate evidence of previous ischemic heart disease or recent injury precipitated by acute stress. Rhythm disturbance must be sought with electrical burns.

6. **Pain medication**   Demerol (0.2 mg/kg) or morphine (0.05 mg/kg) i.v. q1–2h is appropriate.

7. **Streptococcal prophylaxis**   Aqueous penicillin (50,000 units/kg/day) is given i.v. q6h for 72 hr. Erythromycin is substituted for patients who are allergic to penicillin.

8. **Tetanus prophylaxis**   See p. 429.

II. **History and Physical Examination**   The history and physical examination are appropriate for any patient. The following points should be considered.

A. **History**

1. **Mechanism of injury**   A more precise estimate of burn depth is possible if the mechanism of injury can be defined. Because the ultimate tissue damage from thermal injuries is proportional to temperature and duration of exposure, a flash fire will produce a less severe injury than direct flame contact. Tar, because of its higher specific heat and adherence, causes a deeper burn than scalding water. Without a careful probing of observers, the patient's significant deep tissue necrosis from a high voltage electrical injury may not be appreciated because of the superimposed flame injury from ignition of clothing at the time of the accident. Determination of the agent in-

284   Special Considerations

volved in a chemical burn will influence both immediate therapy and prognosis.

2. **Location of injury** This factor is of major importance in determining the severity of pulmonary injury. The size of the space in which the patient was trapped determines the density of smoke and carbon monoxide. Of particular importance are the products of combustion of synthetic materials used in the upholstery of automobiles and home furnishings. These superimpose a severe lower airway chemical injury on that produced by inhalation of smoke.

3. **Preexisting medical illnesses** Those medications that can be monitored with serum levels should be carefully followed and doses adjusted as appropriate. Burn patients hypermetabolize a variety of medicines, particularly cardiac glycosides, hydantoin, and aminoglycoside antibiotics. Doses may need to be increased as much as 50% to maintain therapeutic levels.

B. **Physical examination** All clothing must be removed and all body surface areas examined at the time of admission to reveal occult injury, particularly of the back and lower extremities. Quite helpful in calculating the percentage of surface of burn area and as a ready reference throughout the patient's course is a drawing showing anterior and posterior projections with partial thickness areas which may be shown in one color and full thickness burns which may be shown in a contrasting color. This sheet should be the first page in the patient's chart. The computation of the fluid resuscitation is also shown on this sheet. Also included on the burn diagram and of considerable importance in guiding therapy is an accurate determination of the patient's weight on admission.

III. **Determination of Burn Depth and Size**

A. **Depth of injury** Wounds are traditionally classified in three degrees of depth. The first is the most superficial and the third is the deepest. Imprecision, particularly with regard to second degree injury, has led to the adoption of a nomenclature based on depth involvement. The division of partial thickness wounds into superficial and deep groups has definite prognostic and therapeutic implications. Figure 1 shows diagrammatically the level of epidermal and dermal injury. A precise characterization of all parts of the wound as to depth is impossible and, furthermore, ignores the fact that the depth changes with time. However, the process of classification forces a careful examination and the result is a satisfactory approximation for guiding initial therapy.

1. **Erythematous nonblistering wounds (first degree)** Damage is limited to the epidermis. The magnitude of the physiologic derangement from edema formation and alteration of the evaporative barrier is minor. The major disability is pain.

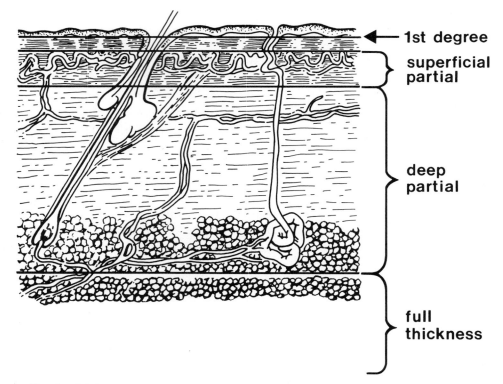

1st degree

superficial partial

deep partial

full thickness

Figure 1. Depth of injury.

2. **Superficial partial thickness wounds (second degree)** Damage is limited to the outer layers of the dermis with sparing of a majority of dermal appendages (hair follicles, sebaceous glands, and sweat glands). These wounds blister, are erythematous, and blanch on pressure. They are painful and hairs do not yield to gentle pull. The margin of the wound is raised with respect to adjacent unburned skin due to edema within the wound and is slippery to the touch due to the presence of proteinaceous exudate.

3. **Deep partial thickness wounds (second degree)** Only the deepest dermal appendages are spared. The wounds are generally more white than pink, although on occasion a nonblanching cherry red is seen. The skin is blistered and edematous but of a more woody character than the superficial partial thickness burn. The wounds are typically painless and hairs yield to gentle pull.

4. **Full thickness wounds (third degree)** All epithelial elements are destroyed. The wound is depressed relative to unburned skin or to adjacent partial thickness burn due to the lack of circulation which prevents edema. It is leathery to the touch, anesthetic, and may vary in color from white to brown to black.

B. **Size** Burn size is expressed as a percentage of the total body surface area and is of particular importance in determining fluid requirements for resuscitation.

In the adult, two rules of thumb provide a quick and reasonably accurate estimation of the extent of injury. The first, the "Rule of Nines," divides the body into eleven units of equal area (Figure 2). The second method of particular benefit for small, scattered patches is the "palm rule" which states that the surface area of the patient's palm is equal to 1% of the total body surface area.

These general guidelines cannot be applied to patients less than 10 years of age because of the disproportionately large size of the head and small size of the lower limbs of young children compared with adults. The Lund and Browder chart adjusts for these variations (Figure 3). For the purpose of inpatient burn management, nonblistering wounds (first degree) are disregarded. For ready reference, the Lund and Browder chart is included on the initial evaluation form.

IV. **Fluid Resuscitation** One of the earliest physiologic derangements apparent in burned skin is a massive capillary leak which allows intravascular fluid to escape into the extracellular space. With large surface area burns, this same phenomenon also occurs in skin and visceral organs remote from the burn site, adding further to the resultant hypovolemia and shock. A variety of formulae have been proposed to serve as guidelines to the restoration of intravascular volume. The Parkland Hospital Formula is

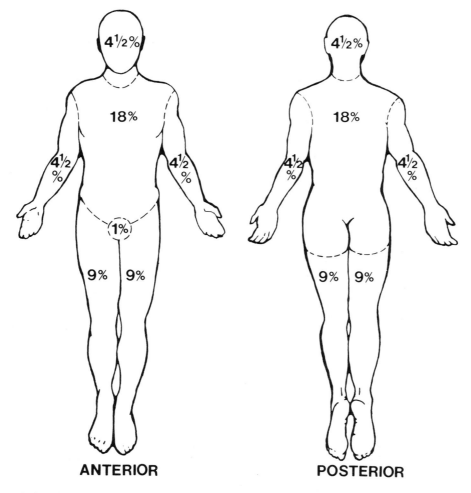

Figure 2. "Rule of Nines."

LUND AND BROWDER CHART

AREA	AGE — YEARS					% 2°	% 3°	% TOTAL
	0–1	1–4	5–9	10–15	ADULT			
Head	19	17	13	10	7			
Neck	2	2	2	2	2			
Ant. Trunk	13	17	13	13	13			
Post. Trunk	13	13	13	13	13			
R. Buttock	2½	2½	2½	2½	2½			
L. Buttock	2½	2½	2½	2½	2½			
Genitalia	1	1	1	1	1			
R. U. Arm	4	4	4	4	4			
L. U. Arm	4	4	4	4	4			
R. L. Arm	3	3	3	3	3			
L. L. Arm	3	3	3	3	3			
R. Hand	2½	2½	2½	2½	2½			
L. Hand	2½	2½	2½	2½	2½			
R. Thigh	5½	6½	8½	8½	9½			
L. Thigh	5½	6½	8½	8½	9½			
R. Leg	5	5	5½	6	7			
L. Leg	5	5	5½	6	7			
R. Foot	3½	3½	3½	3½	3½			
L. Foot	3½	3½	3½	3½	3½			
					TOTAL			

Figure 3.   Lund and Browder Chart.

presented as a reference for fluid administration; other formulae may work just as well for other surgeons. All formulae are intended as guidelines, since no one formula can be applied to every case.

A. **Parkland Hospital Formula**   The fluid replacement given during the first 24 hr is estimated to be 4 cc of Ringer's lactate/percentage of total body surface area (TBSA) burned/kg of pre-injury body weight. No additional maintenance fluid is given. One-half of this amount is administered in the first 8 hr. The remainder is given in the subsequent 16 hr. The timing of fluid replacement begins from the time of injury. Because of the rapid loss of intravascular colloid if administered during the first 24 hr following injury, plasma replacement is withheld until the second 24 hr. The second day's fluid replacement begins with sufficient plasma to restore intravascular volume, one indication of this being the restoration of the hematocrit to the normal range. Typically, 0.5 cc of 5% albumen solution (plasmanate)/kg/percentage of TBSA burn is sufficient. Additional balanced salt solution is given to maintain a normal serum sodium concentration. Fluids beyond this point are dictated by clinical and laboratory parameters. Burn patients with normal renal function tend to retain sodium and waste potassium, requiring adjustment or replacement of these ions. The insensible loss through the burn wound area per day is estimated to be 20 cc/m² (body surface area)/percentage of burn.

B. **Monitoring adequacy of resuscitation**

1. **Sensorium** Simple clinical signs are frequently overlooked, but are quite helpful. Confusion in a previously oriented patient frequently indicates hypovolemia or hypoxia.

2. **Pulse and blood pressure** A diastolic blood pressure above 60 mm Hg and pulse below 120/min are desirable.

3. **Urine output** This is the most easily accessible and reliable indicator of the adequacy of resuscitation. Output should be maintained at or just above 0.5 cc/kg/hr. Additional fluid to push the urine output over this level leads to increased wound and pulmonary edema. Diuretics are seldom indicated during the early phase of resuscitation, except in the case of myoglobin- or hemoglobinuria when a forced diuresis is indicated to protect the renal tubules.

4. **Central venous and pulmonary artery wedge pressure** Central venous and pulmonary artery pressure measurements are indicated when the patient is not responding to usual resuscitation measures. This will be particularly true in older patients with underlying cardiopulmonary disease. Perhaps the most beneficial use of the Swan-Ganz catheter is to obtain the cardiac index, which should be maintained at 3 liters/min/m² or greater.

5. **Serum chemistry** Metabolic acidosis on blood gas determination or examination of electrolytes usually indicates hypoperfusion from hypovolemia. Bicarbonate concentration should be above 18 mEq/liter. Hypernatremia implies inadequate volume administration.

V. **Pulmonary Injury and Management** True thermal burns of the lower respiratory tract are extremely rare due to the cooling capacity of the upper airway. The most common cause of injury is the inhalation of smoke and noxious gases, which excite a chemical inflammatory reaction. A restrictive type of respiratory embarrassment may also develop from circumferential eschar of the chest. See p. 379.

VI. **Wound Management** On admission, the wound is cleansed with normal saline or saline and povidone-iodine (Betadine) to remove surface debris. Blisters are ruptured and debrided. The wound is then dressed with a topical antimicrobial. Wounds are cleaned daily with saline.

A. **Topical antimicrobials** No single agent is universally applicable. However, the following are listed in order of popularity.

1. **Silver sulfadiazine (Silvadene)** Apply as a 15% cream every 12 hr and cover with gauze bandage. Antibacterial spectrum is broad and side effects

are few. Sulfa allergy is a contraindication and leukopenia is a side effect which is reversible on withdrawal.

2. **Mafenide (Sulfamylon)** Apply as a 10% cream every 8 hr and leave the wound open. Mafenide has better eschar penetration and a broader spectrum than silver sulfadiazine. However, it has the significant side effects of metabolic acidosis due to carbonic anhydrase inhibition, particularly when applied to surface areas greater than 10%, and severe pain on application. Sulfa allergy prohibits its use.

3. **Silver nitrate solution** Apply as a warmed 0.5% solution to saturate the dressings every 4 hr. The antibacterial spectrum is unsurpassed, but eschar penetration is poor, heat loss must be controlled, and electrolyte depletion is relatively common. The solution stains the skin and objects black.

4. **Iodophor (Efodine)** Apply as a 1% cream twice a day and dress with gauze. Used as a second alternative for small surface areas and when resistance develops to other agents. Renal toxicity has been reported.

5. **Antibiotic ointments** such as Bacitracin have little antibacterial effect, but serve well in exposed areas, such as the face, to prevent crusting of superficial burns.

B. **Wound monitoring** Surface cultures are of little benefit in identifying predominant wound flora and the likelihood of invasive sepsis. Whenever possible, quantitative cultures performed on biopsy material should be used to monitor the wound and sensitivities should be obtained for topical agents. Colony counts of less than 10^5 organisms/gm of tissue are not associated with wound problems. Levels of 10^6 to 10^8 may respond to a switch to a more effective topical agent. Levels of 10^9 and above are associated with invasive and generalized sepsis requiring systemic antibiotics.

C. **Extremity burns**

1. **Assessment of circulation** Circumferential full thickness burns may compromise distal circulation and require escharotomy. The presence of distal pulses is a notoriously unreliable indicator of adequate circulation. A better indication is deterioration of neurologic function. Sensibility and intrinsic function should be documented on admission and followed; if deteriorating, escharotomy should be performed. Compartmental pressures are easily measured. Pressures within 20 mm of the diastolic pressure require release (see p. 246).

2. **Technique of escharotomy** The full thickness burn requiring escharotomy is anesthetic, allowing the release to be done in bed without anesthesia. Incisions are in the midlateral line of the arms, hand, and fingers to a level where edematous deep tissues bulge freely. If incisions are confined to full thickness areas, bleeding is minimal. Better positioning of the fingers can be achieved if a transverse incision is placed dorsally across the metacarpalphalangeal joints.

3. **Splinting** Considerable secondary deformity is prevented by adequate positioning of the joints from the time of injury. Splints of waterproof, thermoplastic material are serviceable and may be easily modified as necessary as edema resolves. Preferred positions for various joints are as follows:
   a. Hips and knees: full extension
   b. Elbows: extension and supination
   c. Shoulders: 90° abduction, neutral flexion and extension
   d. Wrist: 30° extension
   e. MP joints: 80° flexion
   f. PIP and DIP joints: full extension
   g. Thumbs: abduction and opposition
   h. Ankles: neutral dorsiflexion

4. **Therapy** Occupational and physical therapy with active and passive range of motion is begun with the first dressing change and encouraged, in and out of dressings 4–6 times/day.

D. **Natural history**

1. Wound healing in first degree burns is complete in a matter of days, and no scarring results.

2. Superficial partial thickness burns heal by re-epithelialization from intact dermal appendages in 7–14 days with minimal scarring.

3. In deep partial thickness burns, healing is slow with uneven progression of epithelialization. The quality of the healed wound may be unacceptable, particularly over joints where pliability is necessary. Poor resistance to repeated trauma may result.

4. Full thickness burns heal by a combination of epithelialization and contraction. Spontaneous healing, which can take months to complete, not infrequently results in functional impairment from contractures. For this reason, these wounds are usually skin-grafted to achieve early closure. The therapeutic objective in third degree burns is to remove all dead skin and to cover the defects with autografts. Multiple operations may be required. Xenograft or homograft is an acceptable temporary substitute if there is insufficient skin for autografting.

   The depth of the burn wound is not fixed. Partial thickness wounds may convert to full thickness wounds due to any one or a combination of the following factors: local infection, peripheral hypoperfusion due to hypovolemia, septic or cardiogenic shock, or hypoxia or local capillary stasis due to pressure. Of perhaps as great a significance as these factors is the apparently usual occurrence of widespread small vessel thrombosis within the burn wound 3–4 days following injury. This change occurs in severely damaged tissue at the margin between areas of deep partial thickness and full thickness injury. This interface is called the "zone of stasis" and may by various manipulations, including early skin grafting, be prevented from undergoing thrombosis and necrosis. The existence of this zone may explain the common observation that partial thickness damage may fail to heal and ultimately require skin grafting.

E. **Early excision and grafting** A very attractive alternative to allowing spontaneous eschar separation from areas of full thickness injury before grafting is early excision (within 3–4 days) of the eschar with immediate grafting. The wound is generally not colonized at the time of excision, thus improving graft take. Early grafting may prevent extension of the wound via the "zone of stasis." This procedure has a practical limit of 15% body surface area burn. This technique is particularly attractive for areas of functional importance, such as the hands, for which delay in grafting frequently results in increased edema, fibrosis, and stiffness. A short hospital course is an added advantage. Early excision is best done in a tangential fashion using a free hand knife or mechanical dermatome. Capillary bleeding is used to determine adequate excision. Grafting is done immediately with thin split grafts. A high percentage of take is achieved with meshed, unexpanded grafts.

VII. **Electrical burns** Electrical injuries possess unique problems, which occur at the time of injury and immediately following.

A. **Mechanism of injury** Any one or all three mechanisms may contribute to the injury in a given patient.

1. **Electrical arc** The completion of a circuit at household voltage (110) generates temperatures in excess of 2000°F. This is the mechanism at work in electrical cord injuries of the commissure of the lips in young children. There is apparently no conduction of current through the tissues; however, a high-temperature arc is generated by saliva shorting across the contacts of an extension cord plug.

2. **Secondary flame burn** The high temperatures mentioned above may secondarily ignite clothing.

3. **Generation of heat within tissues due to conduction of electrical current** Voltages in excess of 500 are necessary to damage tissue. The current follows the path of least resistance, seeking, in order, nerves, blood vessels, muscle, skin, tendon, fat, and bone. In terms of destructive potential, the quantity of current (amperage) is of much greater significance than the voltage.

B. **Wound characteristics and points of contact ("entrance" and "exit")** Wounds experience the greatest concentration of current and thus the greatest damage. The deep tissue destruction is much greater than with a similar surface area thermal injury; this is frequently underestimated. Hemoglobinuria and myoglobinuria are common and must be looked for and treated to prevent secondary renal damage. Wound necrosis is frequently progressive. Sulfamylon is the topical agent of choice because of its penetrating ability.

C. **Distant effects**

1. **Peripheral neuropathy**   This is a direct effect of current conduction. Recovery is rare.

2. **Cardiac arrhythmia**   This is due to disturbance of the myocardial conduction system. Patients should be monitored for 24 hr or until the rhythm normalizes.

3. **Fractures**   Tetanic muscle contractions at the time of injury may produce spinal or long bone fractures.

4. **Cataracts**   These may appear any time up to months following injury.

5. **Seizures**   These reflect cortical damage and scar.

VIII. **Chemical Burns**   These wounds differ from those that are thermally produced in that the injury progresses as long as active chemical is in contact with the tissue. The severity of injury can be modified by copious irrigation begun as soon after the accident as possible. This treatment is generally more beneficial for alkali burns than for those due to acids or other chemicals, since alkalis produce a liquid eschar which retains penetration ability and ionic strength. Acid burns, in contrast, produce a barrier of coagulated protein which limits penetration. As a rule, all burns are lavaged, either by immersion, continuous saline drip, or by showering for 12 hr, followed by implementation of the usual treatment modalities appropriate for other burns. Very few specific antidotes exist, with the following exceptions:

—**Hydrofluoric acid**   Calcium carbonate solution (10%) may be injected directly into the wound, or benzalkonium chloride (Zephiran) or magnesium oxide may be applied, topically, with questionable success.

—**Phenol**   Systemic absorption and toxicity can be reduced by topical application of polyethyl alcohol to the wounds.

—**Phosphorus**   The fragments of retained metal may be more easily seen (stained black) and removed if copper sulfate solution is added.

Neutralization of acid or alkali burns is specifically contraindicated because of the risk of superimposition of a thermal injury from the heat of neutralization. Systemic toxicity from skin absorption varies with the individual chemical involved, the concentration, the surface area, and the length of exposure. No general rules can be formulated except for the maintenance of an appropriate level of suspicion when unusual and unfamiliar agents are involved.

15

GUNSHOT WOUNDS

AND

BALLISTICS OF WOUNDING

Today, there is little to differentiate between gunshot wounds of war and peace. Weapons that produce wounds equivalent to war wounds may also be found in the hands of civilians. A cursory examination of gun/ammunition sales catalogs shows that cartridges are available with bullet weights and muzzle velocities ranging from about 15–500 grains (7,000 grains = 1 pound) and 700–5,000 feet/sec, respectively. The bullet types are manifold. We list, but we do not describe or explain, some of the types.

H.P., hollow point

O.P.E., open point expanding

S.P., soft point

P.S.P., pointed soft point

F.P., full patch

S.T., silver point

M.C.B.T., metal case boattail

Mush., mushroom

Br.P., care-lokt

M.C., metal-cased

T.H., tapered heel

M.C.L., mushroom care-lokt

Ptd., pointed

P.P. Exp., protected point expanding

Sp.P., spire point

R.N., round nose

Because of the potpourri of combinations of types, weights, and velocities, much research remains to be carried out before generalized models are developed for describing in sufficient medical detail resultant wound tracks. The problem is further magnified when one considers that a bullet can impact randomly on a person in different postures from many different directions and, consequently, thousands of different wound tracks can be produced. Moreover, anatomical components (particularly internal organs) are not fixed with respect to position and are subject to gross displacements, depending on whether or not the victim is standing, crouching, prone, supine, or moving at the time of wounding.

In spite of the complexity of the problem, many excellent military studies have been (and are still being) carried out in the field of wound ballistics for the purpose of forecasting wound tracks, associated physiologic dysfunctions, and the development of improved surgical procedures. This Institute is aware of some of these studies and is extracting from them information pertinent to the treatment of victims of gunshot wounds.

I. **Factors Governing Wound Configuration**   Wound tract shapes and dimensions depend strongly on the following five bullet parameters: weight (m); striking velocity (v); frontal area (a); type; and stability factor (associated with the rapidity with which a bullet starts to tumble along the wound track). A bullet of high sectional density (defined as m/a) can penetrate quite deeply.

Of interest is Figure 1, which shows a generic sketch of some of the resultant temporary wound cavities caused by different bullets. During the course of penetration, tissue is displaced laterally, depending on bullet characteristics. We depict maximum temporary cavities associated with four different bullets.

—Stable bullet
—Less stable bullet
—Very unstable bullet
—Soft-nose bullet

II. **Myths Related to Wounding**   Some myths on wounding should be dispelled. It is "reported" that critical impact velocities exist, above which wounds are massive; this is not so because careful experimentation and analysis show that wound tracks increase smoothly with an increase in velocity. Another myth alludes to the "stopping power" of specific bullets; however, the "stopping power" or "shocking power" is a strong function of the part of the anatomy struck. Another myth refers to the ability of the bullet to propel the victim backwards. For example, consider a person weighing 150 pounds hit by a 150-grain bullet at a velocity of 3,000 feet/sec. Invoking the physical principle of the conservation of momentum, the maximum rearward velocity of the person is less than ½ foot/sec.

III. **Effects of Bullet Wounding**   Some of the physiologic/biologic effects of bullet wounds are local tissue necrosis, regional and local circulatory metabolic changes, cell injury at significant distances from the wound tract, effects on the central nervous system, and centers regulating circulation and/or respiration, etc. In general, surgical treatment, including debridement, should start early, i.e., within 1 hr.

A total systems approach must be used for multiply injured victims of gunshot wounds, just as for victims of automobile accidents. To reduce patient morbidity/mortality, it is mandatory to reduce the total time from the event to effective emergency medical response. Of interest is a MIEMSS study showing a reduction in deaths of patients treated for gunshot wounds of the chest at hospitals after they converted to trauma centers.

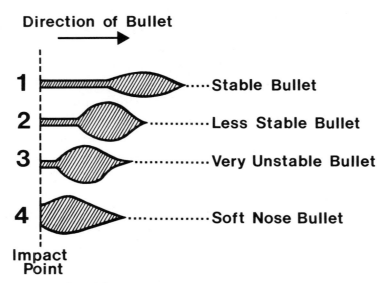

Figure 1.   Temporary wound cavities.

16
SOFT TISSUE INFECTIONS

There are numerous varieties of soft tissue infections; they may be localized or widespread and may be secondary to one organism or multiple organisms. Since MIEMSS has a hyperbaric chamber, patients with soft tissue infections are frequently referred to this center to treat "gas gangrene." The patient usually has a soft tissue infectious process which has been present for a variable period of time. Soft tissue gas is usually identified by palpation or it is seen on a plain radiograph. The majority of these patients have a synergistic soft tissue infection and only rarely is isolated *Clostridium perfringens* the cause of the septic process. The Gram stain is very helpful in making the differential diagnosis between gas gangrene and a synergistic infection. Generally, gas gangrene is associated with a more toxic patient and a more **rapidly** spreading soft tissue sepsis as compared to synergistic infection. We feel that surgical and hyperbaric therapy are complementary in managing these devastating diseases.

I. **Gas Gangrene** Clostridial gas gangrene must be differentiated from tissue gas production by other organisms. The lethality of the clostridial form relates directly to the effect of the many liberated exotoxins. Over 20 exotoxins have been identified from the major six clostridial bacteria (*Clostridia perfringens, novyi, septicum, histolyticum, bifermentans,* and *fallax*) capable of producing gas gangrene in humans. Of these toxins produced, alpha toxin, a lecithinase C_1, is the only lethal one; working synergistically with nonlethal toxins (hyaluronidases, hemolysins, and elastases) it results in a rapid-spreading liquefaction necrosis. Theta toxin is highly cardiotoxic and causes severe hemolysis and necrosis. Kappa toxin lyses protein, mu toxin alters DNA, neuraminidase destroys immunologic receptors on erythrocytes, and hemagglutinin inactivates group A factor on erythrocytes.

The progressive nature of gas gangrene depends on the continuous production of alpha toxin which is fixed in tissues and detoxified within 2 hr of its elaboration. There is very little host reaction to clostridial invasion, with minimal inflammatory response and no purulent discharge. On Gram stain, there are only a few white cells in the face of many Gram-positive rods. The disease is thus best described as an intoxication and not an infection.

A. **Manifestations**
1. **Clostridial myonecrosis with toxicity** is associated with a rapid diffuse spread from the initial site. An incubation period of 4 hr to 2–3 days is followed by rapid advancement. The initial symptom is pain that is out of proportion to the appearance of the wound. The area around the wound may be blanched, edematous, and bronze-like in color. The skin darkens as tissue dies and is associated with the formation of blebs and bullae. Unless there is secondary in-

vasion with a mixed infection, the patient has a fever of only 100–101°F, but the pulse is usually disproportionately elevated, frequently over 140/min. Blood pressure normally is maintained until late in the disease; once shock develops, the prognosis is grave. The patient usually remains oriented but has a flattening of the affect ("la belle indifference"). Serosanguineous drainage occurs with a mousey sweetish odor, unless mixed infection exists. Hemorrhagic bullae usually contain **few** polymorphonuclear leukocytes and many Gram-positive rods. Gas bubbles may be seen or felt as crepitus in soft tissues or demonstrated radiographically. Nonclostridial organisms may be associated with gas production. Patients with true gas gangrene may succumb within hours.

2. **Localized clostridial myonecrosis** This is a localized consequence from the injection of nonsterile drugs. Few, if any, toxic symptoms are present. Local incision, drainage, and antibiotics are appropriate therapy.

3. **Clostridial cellulitis without toxicity** These patients present initially with a cellulitis that becomes rapidly spreading and then develop toxic symptoms. If untreated, the prognosis is as grave as that associated with myonecrosis.

B. **Clinical management** The clinical management of the advanced toxic gangrene patient is a major clinical challenge. These patients require intensive fluid resuscitation for circulating volume expansion; blood and blood component replacement for hemolysis and coagulopathies; tetanus prophylaxis; antibiotic therapy which should include penicillin, an aminoglycoside, and clindamycin for coverage of associated anaerobic organisms; and intensive invasive monitoring with central venous, direct arterial, and Swan-Ganz pulmonary artery monitoring. Surgical intervention is undertaken early with extensive fasciotomies to decompress all compartments involved in the extremities. In the early phase, extensive tissue debridement is not necessary because following hyperbaric oxygen therapy much of what looks necrotic is, in fact, viable.

Alpha toxin production is inhibited by exposure of the clostridial organism to 3 atmosphere absolute (ATA). Hyperbaric oxygen overcomes the effects of catalase, which is present in necrotizing tissue.

On notification of an expected gas gangrene admission, the chamber operator and chamber nurse on call are notified. The usual admission protocol is followed with these additions:

1. The wound is inspected and the boundaries or line of demarcation are clearly marked with a pen.

2. All sutures in the wound and area of the wound are removed.

3. A direct Gram stain is obtained.

4. A swab for aerobic and anaerobic culture is taken.

5. The involved area is x-rayed.

6. Volume resuscitation is undertaken; if Hct and Hb are low (below 33 and 11, respectively), blood should be transfused as soon as possible in order that optimal benefit may be received from hyperbaric therapy.

Once the decision is made to submit the patient to hyperbaric oxygen therapy, the appropriate routine for patient preparation must be followed. The diving schedule consists of seven dives at 3 ATA for 90 min with 100% oxygen, if intubated; if on mask, intermittent 5-min air breaks are given every 30 min. The first three dives are at 6-hr intervals and the remaining four dives are at 12-hr intervals. This schedule should be strictly adhered to for maximum inhibition of alpha toxin production. The only exception is the nonresponding critical patient. The second dive can be 2 hr after the first, at the discretion of the physician in charge of hyperbaric medicine, after which the routine schedule is followed.

Fasciotomy should be performed before the first dive to allow for maximum circulation of hyperbaric oxygen to the area. Debridement of necrotic tissue should be performed after the first dive. Definitive surgery should be delayed until the patient is nontoxic, with a well demarcated area for excision or amputation, unless frank necrosis is present and/or a superimposed nonclostridial component is present.

Toxic and critical cases must have a physician and nurse in attendance during the dive. Between dives, the critical patient is kept adequately sedated, intubated, and on mechanical ventilation.

The spontaneously breathing patient is treated by breathing 100% oxygen by mask while in the chamber. When breathing O_2 by mask, the patient receives a 5-min air break every 30 min.

II. **Synergistic Soft Tissue Infections** Massive soft tissue wound infections develop from a number of different causes:

—Severe crushing, avulsing, or high velocity missile trauma with gross disruption of the capillary circulation

—Post-intra- or extraperitoneal surgery with contamination and secondary infection

—Devascularized (e.g., diabetes or atherosclerosis) areas with secondary infection following minor trauma

Associated factors frequently found include obesity, malnutrition, diabetes, chronic alcoholism or drug addiction, age, and/or compromised vascular supply.

In this setting, the host's defenses to minor infections and normal commensals of the bowel and epithelium are disrupted. These organisms become frank invaders of the host tissues. The infections are mixed with aerobic and anaerobic organisms. The predominant anaerobic organisms are *Peptostreptococcus*, bacteroides, and *Fusobacterium*; the predominant aerobic organisms are the coliforms. The infectious process primarily involves the skin, subcutaneous tissue, and the fascia; muscle is usually spared.

Classical manifestations of these infections are

Absence of the classical signs of local tissue inflammation

Gas production and putrid discharge

A tendency to burrow through soft tissue and fascial planes

A. **Manifestations** An elderly or debilitated patient usually presents with crepitus of soft tissues, cutaneous erythema, and/or blister formation. The patient is often toxic, with fever, leukocytosis, and hemodynamic instability. There is usually extensive dissection and necrosis of superficial fascia and undermining of adjacent tissue. Gram stain from the blisters and necrotic tissue usually reveals Gram-positive and Gram-negative cocci and rods.

The course of the disease, despite surgery and antibiotics, is often one of progressive multiple organ failure with death in 7–14 days. The unanswered question is whether this is the result of ongoing inadequate control of wound sepsis or an overwhelming septic process in a compromised host which has initiated the "domino effect" of multiple organ failure prior to medical intervention.

B. **Management**

1. The **initial management** consists of correction of fluid, electrolyte and erythrocyte mass deficiencies. Appropriate **aerobic and anaerobic wound cultures** and a **Gram stain** of the wound exudate are obtained. **Intravenous antibiotics** are begun immediately after cultures have been obtained and should include activity against aerobic and anaerobic, Gram-positive and Gram-negative rods and cocci. Our present parenteral antibiotic regimen includes penicillin, clindamycin, and gentamicin. Aminoglycoside levels should be frequently monitored, since these patients frequently have multisystem instability. Antibiotics should be changed in accordance with culture results and patient response. **Pulmonary instability** may require intubation and ventilation with the addition of positive end-expiratory pressure (PEEP). **Cardiovascular instability** may require Swan-Ganz catheterization and close monitoring of the hemodynamic parameters. Prior to surgery there should be optimization of cardiac and pulmonary function and judicious administration of volume and/or cardiotonic agents.

2. **Surgical debridement**   The primary therapy in necrotizing fasciitis or cellulitis is **radical surgical debridement** of all affected tissue. Once hemodynamic and pulmonary stability is gained, the patient should be taken to the operating room for adequate debridement. The usual objective is to debride soft tissue until it bleeds. This policy is probably the best clinical indicator of adequate debridement; however, with the eventual poor outcome of these patients, we must ask if our macroscopic evaluation is adequate. We suggest that quantitative tissue cultures be taken from the wound margins after debridement.

When a patient with a mixed soft tissue infection is admitted to MIEMSS, the Plastic Surgery Service is consulted and a coordinated effort is initiated in the management of this difficult problem. The Team Leader, Plastic Surgeon, and Traumatology Attending Surgeon then take the patient to the operating room for debridement. The cutaneous margins of the debridement are defined by cutaneous abnormalities such as erythema and blister formation and are extended to a point at which the skin bleeds. If there is difficulty in determining the cutaneous extent of the debridement, intravenous fluorescein may be administered; this will define the point at which nutrient cutaneous flow ceases. Adequate debridement of the subcutaneous tissues is achieved when fat is resected until bleeding, bright yellow tissue is seen. Muscle should be debrided to the point of bleeding and where contractility occurs secondary to a mechanical stimulus. Obviously, in checking for muscular contractility, the patient must not be under the influence of a paralytic agent. It is difficult to define the limit of adequate fascial debridement. Grossly infected fascia is usually shredded and dull gray, while healthy fascia is usually a glistening white structure. It is difficult to tell at which point between these extremes there is viable fascia. Immediately superficial to the fascia is a capillary bed that supplies nutrition to the fascia. If this capillary complex fails to bleed upon incision, the fascia should be excised.

Arterial or capillary thrombosis frequently propagates; therefore, the tissue immediately adjacent to an incision following debridement may be nonviable in the subsequent 24–36 hr. For this reason and the fact that the septic process may rapidly advance, the patient should be initially taken to the operating room on a daily basis. The general philosophy should be taken that the patient should go to the operating room every 24 hr until it is obvious, microscopically and macroscopically, that the wound is viable in all of its perimeters. Hypotensive episodes propagate capillary thrombosis along the edge of the surgical wound; therefore, hypotension should be aggressively treated.

There is a tendency toward conservatism regarding the extent of debridement. Frequently, the patients have a coagulopathy and are prone to significant blood loss from the wound. The larger the wound the more protein and water that is lost; therefore, the greater the propensity for a hypermetabolic insult. Despite this fact, the wound must be aggressively controlled to terminate the septic insult.

At the end of the debridement, quantitative tissue cultures should be obtained to assess the adequacy or inadequacy of wound debridement. Quantitative tissue cultures are arranged with the infectious disease department. There is a 24-hr delay in obtaining the results from the quantitative tissue cultures. The Gram stain slide test can be performed within 30–45 min to give immediate feedback regarding adequacy of tissue debridement. (See p. 265.)

The initial infection and subsequent phases of wound management should be followed with photography. Photography is important to provide information to subsequent consultants who may not have seen the original wound, for future use in lectures and papers, and for medico-legal purposes in which a question may arise regarding the validity of radical debridement.

3. **Post-debridement wound care** It is important that the wound not be allowed to dry, since dessication will impair local tissue resistance and thus propagate wound sepsis. Soaked gauze sponges or Kling is used as the transport agent for moistening the wound. Caution must be exercised in choosing the medium that is used to moisten the wound. There is a tendency to use caustic agents in a wound to kill bacteria. Since a medium that kills bacteria also insults tissue host resistance, the agent must not be too caustic. The suggested medium is hydrogen peroxide which is diluted with an equal portion of saline. The sponges should be wet and gently wrung out. To maintain moisture of the wound, the dressing should be changed every 4 hr.

4. **Hyperbaric oxygenation**   The exact role of hyperbaric oxygenation in these infections is not well defined. The purpose of hyperbaric oxygenation is two-fold, i.e., to stimulate formation of granulation tissue, thus preparing the wound for subsequent closure, and to provide oxygen to the tissue to enhance local resistance. Since the CCRU and hyperbaric chamber are some distance apart, there is some inherent risk in transporting patients with cardiovascular and/or pulmonary instability. If the patient has cardiovascular and pulmonary stability, the surgical debridement is complemented with hyperbaric oxygenation. If the patient has pulmonary and/or hemodynamic instability and the wound sepsis is controlled, the hyperbaric oxygenation will be interrupted until hemodynamic and/or pulmonary stability are gained. If the patient has cardiovascular and/or pulmonary instability, yet the wound is grossly infected and rapidly deteriorating, the patient should be taken to the hyperbaric chamber despite instability. Inability to control wound sepsis will usually be obvious within 48 hr after admission, but may become apparent at any time during the patient's course.

5. **Whirlpool**   When the patient is stable from the cardiovascular and pulmonary standpoint, surgical debridement may be complemented with whirlpool therapy. The primary benefit from whirlpool therapy is mechanical debridement. Since significant water and electrolyte imbalance may develop, caution must be exercised in using whirlpool therapy.

6. **Diverting colostomy**   The role of a diverting colostomy in patients with perineal lesions is debatable. The diversion of the fecal stream from the wound helps reduce wound reinfection and contamination. The colostomy is placed such that the stoma will not contaminate the wound. The distal bowel must be thoroughly irrigated and the perineal wound protected from contamination by a barrier antibiotic/antiseptic cream which can be washed off once the washout is completed. The colostomy, if needed, should be done early in the course of the disease.

Section V
SYSTEMS FAILURE

INTRODUCTION

Systems failure or dysfunction may develop in any organ or physiologic system following trauma. Multiple systems may be affected at a given time. The patient may have a single system failure which improves or is followed by sequential systems dysfunction. Systems failure is not well understood, but there are several pathologic conditions that are associated with it. Hypoxia, shock, and/or the injury itself are frequent factors that are identified in patients with systems dysfunction. Physical destruction of an organ, e.g., pulmonary contusion or liver fracture, commonly leads to failure in that organ. Environmental hypoxic insults such as hypothermia, smoke inhalation, and near drowning commonly cause multiple systems deterioration. All of these insults generally occur at the time of injury; however, sepsis, drug-induced problems, and other iatrogenic sequelae may be acquired during the hospital course as a cause of post-injury systems dysfunction. The impact upon the homeostasis of the patient is variable. A patient with only a single system injury and dysfunction, such as a severe brain injury with herniation, may die within minutes of injury. On the other hand, a patient may have multiple systems involved, yet rapidly recover. In general, the greater the number of systems that are affected and the greater the degree of dysfunction, the worse the prognosis. If the insult is not too severe and the physiologic systems are aggressively supported, recovery of each system is likely and the patient will survive. However, if the patient in shock acquires additional insults, e.g., renal failure, during the hospital course, the patient is less likely to survive than if additional insults had not occurred. Systems dysfunction, e.g., oliguric renal failure, may be obvious soon after injury, or may not become obvious until subtle manifestations become overt. For example, a patient who is tachypneic at the time of admission and is immediately placed on ventilatory support may not develop fulminant respiratory failure until the ensuing 2–3 days. Physiologic parameters of the trauma patient should be closely followed, because any dysfunction that is treated early is more likely to be reversed than if not treated until the impairment is blatant.

The critically ill patient may have a multitude of problems. It is frequently difficult for the uninitiated to know where to begin in evaluating such a patient. Each problem must be addressed or the patient's outlook may be significantly affected. Frequently, the physician will focus on the patient's major problems; however, problems that are currently minor may become major problems, if not addressed.

The following outline is a format for the systematic appraisal of the complex patient. The evaluation begins with a brief history which entails injuries incurred at the time of trauma and major complications which have developed during the hospitalization. The second major area provides a list of items which review the major physiologic systems. Each item should be carefully assessed so that subtle manifestations of pathology are not overlooked. The third section lists problems that are a result of admission injuries and the ensuing hospital course. The last facet of the evaluation states the plan to evaluate and/or treat the patient's problems.

Patient_____ Age_____ Admitted _____

I. **Brief history**

II. **Systems review**

    A. **Cardiovascular**

Heart rate	CVP	$P\bar{v}O_2$
BP	SVR	$A-V\ O_2$
CO	PVR	Cardiovascular medications
PA/wedge	EKG	

    B. **Respiratory**

Spontaneous rate	MIF	
IMV rate	Compliance	
CMV rate	Chest tube	MS
$FIO_2/PEEP/PaO_2$	1. Air leak	Pavulon
$Q\dot{s}/Q\dot{t}$	2. Drainage	Valium
$PaCO_2$	3. Functional	Phys exam
pH	4. When inserted	CXR
Vital capacity		

    C. **Neurologic**

1. Level of consciousness
    a. Oriented
    b. Agitated
    c. Follows command
2. Motor function
    a. Purposeful
    b. Semi-purposeful
    c. Decorticate
    d. Decerebrate
    e. Spastic
    f. Flaccid
3. Brain stem
4. ICP
5. Mannitol
6. Cord function
7. Steroid dose
8. Misc medications
    a. Dilantin
    b. Phenobarb.
    c. MS
    d. Pavulon
9. CAT scan

    D. **Gastrointestinal**

PO	Diarrhea
NPO	BM
Gastric drainage	Drains
Abdominal exam (soft, distended, bowel sound ($\pm$), wound)	Bilirubin
Flatus	Gastric pH
Gastrointestinal bleeding	Amylase

    E. **Renal**

UOP	BUN	Ur Na^+	FWC
Ur creat	Ur osm	Ur K^+	
Ser creat	Ser osm	Cr Cl	

F. **Metabolic-electrolyte**

Na   K   HCO$^-_3$ Ca   Mag   Phos

Input
1. IVS (cc)
2. Enteric feedings (cc)

Output
1. Foley catheter
2. Gastrointestinal drains
3. etc.

I/O
Calories
Protein
Cal/N$_2$

G. **Hematologic**

H/H   Fibrinogen
Blood received   Platelets
PT   Platelets received
PTT   Clinical bleeding
FFP received

H. **Extremities**

Sensation   Soft tissue
Motor   Skeletal
Vascular

I. **Septic profile**

Temp max
Blood cultures
WBC
Sputum Gram stain
U/A—Urine C&S (pyelo, cystitis, prost, epid)
Wounds/drains
IV sites (new & old)
Length of time IVs present
Arterial line site

Organ dysfunction (CV, pulmonary, renal, hematologic, biliary, gut, CNS)
CSF—meningismus ($\pm$)
Serum glucose
Platelet count
Sinuses
Gallbladder
Heart murmur
Antibiotics

III. **Problem list**

IV. **Medication**

V. **Plan** (for each problem)

This outline may serve as a patient presentation format. It is not necessary, nor is it desirable, to mention each item during the presentation. It is valuable for the audience, at least, to be informed that a given system is felt to be clinically intact. If there is a major problem, it should be substantiated with objective information. It is helpful to give current data and compare it to previous information, e.g., "the serum creatinine is 4.8 and was 3.9 yesterday."

In summary, the patient's outcome depends upon the severity of the initial insult, control of the shock process, adequate metabolic support, appropriate surgical management, and acquisition of nosocomial complications.

17
CEREBRAL DYSFUNCTION

Cerebral dysfunction may present as an alteration in level of consciousness and/or as a focal neurologic deficit. An alteration in level of consciousness such as a depressed awareness of the environment, a decreased level of arousal, agitation, or confusion, may be a manifestation of primary or secondary CNS derangement. A focal neurologic deficit that presents at the time of admission (e.g., hemiparesis, decortication, aphasia) usually implies primary CNS pathology. Cerebral dysfunction may occur in the trauma patient as an isolated entity or as a component of multiple systems dysfunction.

The investigation of cerebral dysfunction includes consideration of the following entities.

I. **Primary Brain Insult**

   A. **Trauma**

      1. Concussion

      2. Contusion

      3. Reactive cerebral edema

      4. Intracranial hemorrhage
         a. Epidural
         b. Subdural
         c. Intracerebral

      5. Delayed traumatic hydrocephalus

   B. **Infection**

      1. Meningitis

      2. Brain abscess

   C. **Cerebral vascular accident**

II. **Systemic Diseases**

   A. **Hypoxic encephalopathy**

      1. Near drowning

      2. Pulmonary contusion

3. Aspiration

4. Traumatic asphyxia

5. Hypotension (shock)

6. Carbon monoxide intoxication

B. Systemic sepsis

C. Toxicities

1. Carbon monoxide or cyanide intoxication

2. Drugs (narcotics, barbiturates, benzodiazepines)

3. Alcohol (excess or withdrawal)

D. Environmental insults

1. Hypothermia

2. Hyperthermia

E. Metabolic derangements

1. Hypoglycemia

2. Diabetic ketoacidosis

3. Hyperglycemic nonketotic hyperosmolar state

4. Uremia

5. Hepatic encephalopathy

6. Hyponatremia

7. Wernicke's encephalopathy

8. Hyperalimentation disorders
   a. Hyperammonemia
   b. Hypophosphatemia

9. Dehydration

F. Fat emboli syndrome

Investigation of cerebral dysfunction includes a history, physical examination, routine laboratory investigation, toxicology screen, and special evaluation procedures. The history of an accident and cerebral dysfunction suggests that primary central nervous system injury is present. Metabolic derangements, such as ethanol intoxication, hypothermia, etc., are common causes of cerebral dysfunction in the trauma patient. Metabolic derangement as a cause of cerebral dysfunction in the trauma patient is always a diagnosis of exclusion until intracranial pathology has been ruled out.

The physical examination is often important in providing a clue to the etiology of the cerebral dysfunction. A meticulous general and neurologic evaluation should be performed. Examination should be aimed at finding manifestations of focal or generalized neurologic alteration and evidence of systemic disease.

Routine investigation consists of the following: CBC, urinalysis, electrolytes, BUN, creatinine, glucose, calcium, phosphate, liver function tests, osmolality, EKG, chest x-ray, and an arterial blood gas. If there is alteration in the level of consciousness at the time of admission, special examinations that may be appropriate include a carboxyhemoglobin level, toxicology screen, and cervical spine and skull x-rays. The most important investigation is usually the CAT scan.

Each etiologic entity must be considered until the clinician is satisfied that the specific origin of the cerebral dysfunction is identified. More than one etiology is often present, e.g., an intracerebral contusion and superimposed systemic sepsis.

Progressive cerebral dysfunction may be due to an expanding intracranial mass lesion or may be secondary to the development of a systemic complication. If the patient develops progressive cerebral dysfunction following admission, repeat performance of previous studies is usually indicated. A normal CAT scan or a scan that reveals minimal pathology on admission does not exclude the possibility of an intracranial lesion developing into a space-occupying mass. Therefore, a repeat CAT scan may be indicated in the presence of progressive cerebral dysfunction. Studies that may provide useful information include: blood cultures, electroencephalogram, serum ammonia level, cerebral spinal fluid sampling, and evoked potentials.

Treatment is directed at removing the etiologic insult, if possible, and instituting general support.

—Brain   (see p. 215).
—Systemic disorders   (see appropriate sections).
—General care

Provide cardiovascular support (see p. 335).
Administer respiratory support (see p. 313).
Provide nutritional support (see p. 454).
Administer antacids during the stress period (see p. 366).
Provide bowel stimulation to prevent constipation.
Prevent pressure sores by turning the patient at least every 2 hr.
Prevent corneal abrasions (see p. 77).
Use an external urethral catheter in the male patient to prevent perineal maceration.
Provide perineal care.
Perform passive exercises of the extremities.

18

PULMONARY INSUFFICIENCY
AND COMPLICATIONS

I. **Insufficiency** Conceptually, acute respiratory insufficiency is an impairment of CO_2 excretion and/or an absolute or relative hypoxemia. The PaO_2 may be "normal," but may be low relative to the FIO_2. For example, a PaO_2 of 90 is "normal," but on 45% oxygen it represents approximately a 20% shunt.

A. **Impairment of CO_2 excretion**

  1. **Causes**

    a. **Decreased minute ventilation volume**
      (1) Excessive administration of narcotics or sedatives
      (2) Paralytic drugs
      (3) Obstruction of natural or artificial airway
      (4) Airway leaks (on ventilator)
        (a) Dislodged translaryngeal tube
        (b) Dislodged transtracheal tube
        (c) Tracheal cuff leak
        (d) Bronchopleural fistula
      (5) Ventilator leaks
      (6) Decreased pulmonary compliance (high airway pressure)
        (a) Compression of tidal volume (TV) within ventilator tubing
        (b) Ventilator "pop-off"
      (7) Quadriplegia
      (8) Compensatory for a metabolic alkalosis
      (9) Ventilator asynchrony ("out of phase")
      (10) Inadequate ventilation volume setting on the respirator
      (11) CO_2 absorber dysfunction

    b. **Increased dead space** (increased $\dot{V}/\dot{Q}$)
      (1) Hypoperfusion
      (2) Alveolar overdistention
      (3) Pulmonary embolus
      (4) Sepsis

    c. **Increased CO_2 production**
      (1) Fever
      (2) Shivering
      (3) Excess carbohydrate administration

2. **Clinical manifestations**
   a. Decreased chest wall motion and/or retractions
   b. Out of phase on the ventilator
   c. Tracheal cuff leak
   d. Bronchopleural air leak
   e. Dislodged tracheal tube
      (1) Increased peak airway pressure
      (2) Inability to pass suction catheter
      (3) Air leak into pharynx or tracheostomy stoma
   f. Ventilator leak may be reflected in a decreased expired volume or low airway pressure
   g. Poor compliance may lead to increased airway pressure, which results in wasting ventilation into the ambience by ventilator pop-off or by volume compression into the ventilator tubing.

3. **Objective manifestations**
   a. CO_2 greater than 45 (patient without chronic obstructive pulmonary disease)
   b. Respiratory acidosis
   c. Increased dead space with variable $PaCO_2$

$$V_D/V_T = \frac{PaCO_2 - P\bar{E}CO_2}{PaCO_2} \; (normal = 0.3)$$

$$P\bar{E}CO_2 = mixed\ expired\ CO_2$$

   d. Usually the patient has a low PaO_2, unless he is receiving supplemental oxygen.
   e. $PaCO_2$ greater than 35 with a minute ventilation volume greater than 100 cc/kg/min, i.e., increased dead space

4. **Treatment**
   a. Patients with the following problems are treated on a ventilator by providing an adequate minute ventilation volume.
      (1) Narcotic or sedative excess
      (2) Anesthetization
      (3) Residual paralytic drugs
      (4) Quadriplegia
      (5) Inadequate minute ventilation volume setting
      (6) Ventilator leak
   b. Airway leak
      (1) Cuff leak
         (a) Inflate the cuff
         (b) If the cuff is ruptured, change the tube.
      (2) If there is bronchopleural fistula, lower the airway pressure.
      (3) Reinsert transtracheal or translaryngeal tube, if dislodged.
   c. Decreased compliance   Manipulate the respiratory rate and tidal volume to decrease the airway pressure and minimize wasted tidal volume.

d. Correct metabolic alkalosis with chloride administration.

e. Ventilator asynchrony   Identify the specific cause and normalize PaO_2 and $PaCO_2$.

   (1) Head-injured patient may need light sedation.

   (2) Sepsis must be eradicated.

   (3) Pneumothorax must be evacuated.

   (4) Mucous plug and endobronchial secretions must be suctioned.

   (5) Ventilator malfunction—New ventilator system must be obtained.

f. Airway obstruction (see p. 17)

g. Hypoperfusion   Improve cardiac output.

h. Alveolar overdistension   Decrease PEEP and/or tidal volume to improve the compliance.

i. Pulmonary embolus   Heparinize or consider vena caval interruption.

j. Control fever.

k. Control shivering (Thorazine).

l. Reduce carbohydrate infusion, if excessive.

B. Hypoxia   In acute respiratory failure, hypoxia which does not respond to supplemental oxygen is usually secondary to a decreased ventilation/perfusion ratio (shunt). Hypoxia may be secondary to CO_2 retention, since CO_2 displaces oxygen from the alveoli. If the patient has retained CO_2, PaO_2 is improved by the administration of supplemental oxygen and initiating therapy for the "removal of CO_2." The following pulmonary changes are almost universally identified in the patient with a low ventilation/perfusion ratio, i.e., perfusion of nonventilated alveoli.

—Increased extravascular lung water (interstitial-alveolar edema) secondary to increased pulmonary capillary permeability (low pressure, noncardiogenic pulmonary edema)

—Decreased pulmonary compliance

—Decreased lung volumes (functional residual capacity, FRC)

The primary therapy of hypoxia secondary to low ventilation/perfusion relationships is reexpansion of the alveoli and restoration of the functional residual capacity toward normal. The low ventilation/perfusion state may be transient (hours to 2–3 days) or protracted (adult respiratory distress syndrome, ARDS).

1. Causes

   a. Impaired excretion of CO_2 (see p. 313)

   b. Low ventilation/perfusion ratio

   (1) Pulmonary contusion

   (2) Aspiration

   (3) Pneumonia

   (4) Mucous plug

   (5) Sepsis

   (6) Fat emboli syndrome

   (7) Profound shock

   (8) Smoke inhalation

   (9) Near drowning

   (10) Cardiogenic pulmonary edema (fluid excess)

2. **Clinical manifestations** The following manifestations in the patient who has a history of trauma are usually suggestive of hypoxia secondary to a low ventilation/perfusion ratio.
   a. Tachypnea
   b. Cyanosis
   c. Out of phase on the ventilator

3. **Objective manifestations**
   a. **Decreased PaO_2/FIO_2** The normal PaO_2/FIO_2 ratio is 500, which compares with a normal pulmonary shunt of 5–6%. That is, the normal PaO_2 is approximately 100 and the normal room air FIO_2 is 0.2. A ratio of approximately 300 is comparable to a 15% pulmonary shunt. A PaO_2/FIO_2 ratio of 200 on supplemental oxygen is comparable to a 20% pulmonary shunt. To use this concept, the FIO_2 must be precisely known. The only time the FIO_2 is of certainty is if the patient is intubated and on a ventilator system or if the patient is breathing room air. The PaO_2/FIO_2 ratio is valid as a **shunt approximation.** Clinically, a PaO_2/FIO_2 ratio of 200–250 or less on supplemental oxygen or a PaO_2 less than 60 on room air implies that the patient has a significant shunt problem and will usually require the administration of positive end-expiratory pressure (PEEP) or continuous positive airway pressure (CPAP).
   b. **Increased pulmonary shunt** If a Swan-Ganz catheter is in place, the pulmonary shunt can be calculated.

   $$\dot{Q}s/\dot{Q}t = \frac{Cc_{O_2} - Ca_{O_2}}{Cc_{O_2} - Cv_{O_2}} \times 100$$

   Cc_{O_2} = pulmonary capillary O_2 content; Ca_{O_2} = arterial content; Cv_{O_2} = mixed venous O_2 content (see p. 337)
   c. **Decreased compliance** The patient with acute respiratory failure secondary to a low ventilation/perfusion ratio will usually have a decrease in the pulmonary compliance. A compliance of 35 cc/cm of pressure, or less, usually implies the need for continued respirator therapy (see p. 321).
   d. **Normocapnia** The $PaCO_2$ is usually normal or low secondary to normal ventilation or hyperventilation. In the preterminal stage, the $PaCO_2$ may rise.
   e. **Chest x-ray** The chest x-ray reveals interstitial and alveolar infiltrates (edema).

4. **Treatment**
   a. **CPAP/PEEP** If the PaO_2/FIO_2 ratio is less than 200–250, the patient will generally need PEEP or CPAP to restore the FRC toward normal, during which time the shunt will generally decrease and the PaO_2/FIO_2 ratio will improve. Oxygen is usually administered at a FIO_2 of 0.40–0.50. An FIO_2 greater than this usually has minimal effect on arterial oxygenation when the pulmonary shunt is elevated. The lowest possible FIO_2 should be used since any elevation in the FIO_2 will tend to cause alveolar collapse and damage and exacerbate the shunt (see p. 319).

b. **Management of cardiac insufficiency**   Cardiac failure (cardiogenic pulmonary edema) may contribute to arterial hypoxemia due to an increase in interstitial and alveolar edema. Decreased left ventricular performance (hypoperfusion) may result in an increased $A-VO_2$ content which, in the patient with an increased pulmonary shunt, will contribute to arterial hypoxemia. The patient may have cardiac insufficiency (hypoperfusion) secondary to a decreased preload (decreased venous return) or increased right ventricular afterload secondary to "supraphysiologic levels" of PEEP. In other words, if PEEP is significantly elevated, i.e., greater than 10 cm, venous return may be impaired and cardiac output will fall. Elevated levels of PEEP (>10 cm) may impair ventricular contractility, thus causing hypoperfusion. A Swan-Ganz catheter is necessary to assess the cardiovascular status during acute respiratory failure. Indications for insertion of a Swan-Ganz catheter are

—Levels of PEEP greater than 10 cm

—Overt manifestations of hypoperfusion or pulmonary congestion

See p. 335.

c. **Optimal PEEP**   Ideally, PEEP is increased until the pulmonary shunt is 15%, i.e., a PaO_2/FiO_2 ratio of approximately 300. If the level of PEEP must be increased to greater than 10, a Swan-Ganz catheter should be inserted to evaluate the effect of PEEP on cardiac output. Tissue oxygen delivery equals cardiac output $\times$ arterial O_2 content. Arterial O_2 content is affected by the hemoglobin, the percentage of oxygen saturation, and the PaO_2. PEEP may improve the percentage of oxygen saturation and PaO_2, yet it may impair cardiac output, which may result in a depression in oxygen transport. It is not in the best interest of the patient to increase PEEP to a level which markedly impairs cardiac output. If the cardiac output diminishes and cardiac output can be supported easily with fluids and inotropic agents, PEEP is increased until the shunt is approximately 15%. On the other hand, if cardiac output is significantly impaired and cannot be supported with fluids and/or inotropic agents, PEEP is administered at a level that will result in a PaO_2 of approximately 75–80 on an FiO_2 of 0.5.

d. **Fluids**   Since a major component in acute respiratory failure is increased extravascular lung water, fluids should be judiciously administered to minimize the formation of extravascular lung water. If the patient has isolated pulmonary dysfunction, fluid restriction may be more intense; however, the clinician must be more cautious with aggressive volume restriction in the multiple trauma patient who is at increased risk for the development of acute renal failure.

e. **Albumin**   The administration of albumin may be beneficial in mobilizing pulmonary interstitial edema after initial stabilization is obtained. There is concern that during the first few days colloid **may** leak into the interstitial-alveolar space and increase extravascular lung water. We are not certain when albumin can be optimally administered.

f. **Steroids** Methylprednisolone, 30 mg/kg, q6h × 4, may be helpful **early,** when there is an acute elevation of the pulmonary shunt, in order to prevent a protracted course.

g. **Management of sepsis** Pulmonary or extrapulmonary sepsis must be aggressively controlled to reverse the pathology of acute respiratory insufficiency. Sputum should be monitored every other day since changes on the chest x-ray which may reflect pneumonia are difficult to appreciate on an abnormal film.

h. **Tracheobronchial toiletry** The following measures are beneficial in minimizing the effects of secretions:
   (1) Airway suctioning
   (2) Hyperinflation of the lungs
   (3) Humidification of inspired gases
   (4) Postural drainage
   (5) Chest physiotherapy
   (6) **Mobilize the patient into a chair and institute ambulation as soon as possible.**
   See p. 323.

i. **Management of a pneumothorax** The lung should be reexpanded if the patient is on a ventilator in order to
   (1) Minimize restrictive lung pathology
   (2) Prevent the development of a tension pneumothorax

   > Note A chest tube does not protect the patient from a tension pneumothorax if it is occluded or isolated by visceral-parietal pleural adhesions.

j. **Management of a hemothorax** A chest tube should be inserted to evacuate blood from the pleural space to minimize restrictive lung pathology.

k. **Management of fat emboli syndrome** There is no specific therapy indicated for respiratory failure secondary to the fat emboli syndrome. Fracture fragments should be stabilized and steroids may be beneficial.

l. **Management of aspiration** See p. 323.

m. **Monitoring** The following parameters should be monitored daily:
   (1) Pulmonary shunt; PaO_2/FIO_2 ratio
   (2) Compliance
   (3) Cardiovascular assessment
   (4) Chest x-ray (rule out atelectasis, hemothorax, and pneumothorax)
   (5) Sputum examination
   (6) Parameters of sepsis
   (7) Efficiency of CO_2 excretion (dead space)
   (8) Fluid status
   (9) Hemoglobin level

n. **Weaning** When the pulmonary shunt and compliance improve, the patient can be considered for weaning (see p. 321).

C. **Ventilator systems** The appropriate mechanical respiratory support system, CPAP, IMV, or CMV, should be individualized to a given patient's needs. All of these systems require endotracheal intubation or tracheostomy.

1. **CPAP/PEEP** The larynx provides "physiologic PEEP" in the normal patient; therefore, we administer 3–5 cm of PEEP in patients with tracheal tubes. Patients with acute respiratory failure secondary to low ventilation/perfusion ratios generally have an elevated pulmonary shunt, decreased pulmonary compliance, increased extravascular lung water, and a decreased functional residual capacity. PEEP and CPAP minimize the pulmonary shunt by restoring the functional residual capacity toward normal in the patient with acute respiratory failure.

   a. **Initial level of CPAP/PEEP** The system is initially established with an $FIO_2 = 0.5$ and the predicted CPAP/PEEP. Predicted CPAP/PEEP is selected according to the PaO_2/FIO_2 ratio. If the ratio is less than 150, 10–15 cm of CPAP/PEEP is used; 8–10 cm is used if the ratio is 150–200. The gas flow rate is adjusted such that the patient's inspiratory effort does not **decrease** the CPAP level by more than 3 cm of water.

   b. **Complications** The major complication of supraphysiologic levels of PEEP/CPAP is cardiac depression. Cardiac depression is a result of impairment of venous return and impairment of contractility. If patients are on levels greater than 10 cm, a Swan-Ganz catheter should be introduced to monitor the effect on cardiac output (see p. 317).

   c. **Optimum CPAP/PEEP** Ideally, PEEP/CPAP is increased to the point at which the pulmonary shunt is decreased to 15% (PaO_2/FIO_2 ratio, approximately 300). If the cardiac output is depressed and is easily supported with fluids and/or dopamine/dobutamine, PEEP is increased to a point at which the shunt is approximately 15%. If cardiac output cannot be easily supported, a PaO_2 of 70–80 with an $FIO_2 = 0.4–0.5$ is accepted (see p. 317).

   d. **Decreasing CPAP/PEEP** If the PaO_2/FIO_2 ratio increases to 250, decrease the FIO_2 to less than or equal to 0.4 before PEEP/CPAP is decreased. If there is significant cardiovascular instability, PEEP/CPAP is decreased before the FIO_2. If the patient has difficulty with spontaneous respirations at high levels of CPAP, intermittent mandatory ventilation (IMV) is added until the patient is comfortable, i.e., has an intrinsic respiratory rate ≤ 30/min.

2. **IMV/CMV** Patients who need respiratory support to improve both oxygenation and ventilation need ventilator assistance. This includes patients who cannot ventilate well on high levels of CPAP. IMV and CMV (controlled mechanical ventilation) are two ends of a spectrum of mechanical ventilation. When the patient's spontaneous ventilation provides a significant portion of his minute ventilatory requirement (usually at a machine rate < 8/min), the ventilation is considered IMV. When the machine provides most or all of the patient's minute ventilatory requirement, the ventilation is considered CMV. The Engstrom ventilator can only provide CMV, unless modified. The Bourns (Bear I) ventilator provides IMV or CMV and will control patients in

the IMV mode when the respiratory rate is set high. The CMV mode does not allow patients to breathe "through the machine" and can cause "restlessness" in patients who have increased ventilatory drive. IMV is usually preferable to sedation/paralysis to manage a patient.

After deciding to place the patient on a ventilator, an appropriate minute ventilation, FIO_2, and PEEP need to be set. The starting point is to choose a minute ventilation of 150 ml/kg/min, $FIO_2=0.60$, and to adjust the PEEP according to the PaO_2/FIO_2 ratio, as described on p. 319.

The Engstrom ventilator is used by setting up the minute volume at the appropriate FIO_2 on the flow meters. The nomogram on the machine describes the ratio of O_2:air necessary to achieve the desired FIO_2. The rate is set from 12–36. The tidal volume is determined by the minute ventilation divided by the rate. The Engstrom works most efficiently in the 12–24 breaths/min range. The Bourns is initiated by setting the FIO_2 dial, the tidal volume, the frequency, and the level of PEEP. The minute ventilation is the product of the tidal volume and the frequency. The inspiratory flow rate is set to give an inspiratory-expiratory (I:E) ratio of 1:2–1:4, since the flow rate changes the inspiratory time required to achieve the desired tidal volume and the respiratory rate control fixes the length of time for each breath.

In general, patients with obstructive airway disease prefer low frequency and high volumes, and patients with restrictive disease prefer high frequency and low volumes. To minimize barotrauma in patients with adult respiratory distress syndrome (ARDS), a severe restrictive disease, the tidal volumes are set low in the 5–10 cc/kg range so that the peak airway pressure is ≤ 70 cm H_2O. The Bourns tapering flow wave helps reduce high peak pressures. Respiratory rate and peak flow rate are adjusted to provide adequate minute ventilation for CO_2 removal and a 1:1.5 to 1:2 I:E ratio. PEEP should be added using the same criteria described for CPAP, i.e., by keeping the $PaO_2/FIO_2 \geq 250$. The FIO_2 should be reduced to 0.50 or less as rapidly as possible, since prolonged ventilation with a high FIO_2 (≥ 0.60) leads to decreased pulmonary compliance (oxygen toxicity) and adsorption atelectasis. It is usually best to decrease the FIO_2 before PEEP is decreased. When the patient is ready for weaning, the ventilator is adjusted to decrease the IMV frequency, until ventilator support is no longer needed.

Patients with normal lungs and whose need for ventilation is relatively brief usually wean very rapidly from mechanical ventilation. Patients whose lung pathology is extensive and who require prolonged ventilation usually are candidates for a slowly decreasing IMV rate until they are weaned. Respiratory rate, FIO_2, and PEEP should be weaned to achieve the extubation criteria discussed in the weaning protocol. In general, the FIO_2 should be weaned first, then the IMV rate, and then the PEEP.

In general, a ventilator rate greater than 6–8/min increases the patient's dead space. The more ventilator breaths/min the greater the impairment of venous return. For these reasons, it is ideal to decrease the ventilator rate toward zero, **when possible** (see p. 321).

D. Weaning from respiratory support Assessment and correction of neurologic, metabolic, electrolytic, septic, cardiovascular, and renal abnormalities are influential in weaning a patient from respiratory support.

1. **Patients on CMV** The patient should have a $FIO_2 \leq 0.40$ and a PEEP ≤ 5 cm H_2O before considering weaning.
   a. **Mechanical criteria**
      (1) MIF (maximum inspiratory force) ≤ -20 cm H_2O
      (2) VC (vital capacity) ≥ 15 cc/kg or 1,000 cc
   b. **Shunt criteria**
      (1) $PaO_2/FIO_2 \geq 250$
      (2) $\dot{Q}s/\dot{Q}t$ via Swan-Ganz catheter $\leq 15\%$
   c. **Ventilatory criteria**
      (1) VD/VT (dead space) ≤ 0.55

$$VD/VT = \frac{PaCO_2 - P\bar{E}CO_2}{PaCO_2}$$

$P\bar{E}CO_2 = $ mixed expired CO_2
      (2) TLTC (total lung-thorax compliance) ≥ 35 cc/cm H_2O

$$Compliance = \frac{TV - (\text{compression factor} \times \text{plateau pressure})}{\text{Plateau pressure} - PEEP}$$

Compression factor is the milliliters of air compressed in the ventilator tubing/cm of plateau pressure: Engstrom, 4.5 cc/cm; Bourns (Bear), 5 cc/cm.

Patients on CMV who meet all the above criteria can be placed on CPAP with 40% O_2. They should be monitored every 30 min for respiratory rate (RR), level of consciousness, blood pressure, pulse, and arterial blood gases (ABG). If after 1 hr the patient can maintain a $PaO_2 \geq 100$ torr, a $PaCO_2 \leq 45$ torr, and RR < 30 without changing the other parameters, extubation is accomplished. Meeting these criteria does not always guarantee that the patient will be successfully weaned. Reintubation is considered if
   —The respiratory rate increases to a rate of 40/min or 5 breaths/min/hr for 3 consecutive hr or 10 breaths/min/hr for 2 consecutive hr.
   —The $PaCO_2$ increases to 50 torr or pH < 7.35.
   —There is a deterioration of consciousness.

Patients unable to clear or protect their airway should have a tracheostomy before weaning off respiratory support.

2. **Patients on IMV**
   a. **Ventilation** The IMV rate can be decreased if
      (1) $PaCO_2 \leq 45$
      (2) pH > 7.35
      (3) Intrinsic respiratory rate ≤ 30/min

    b.   **Oxygenation**   Maintain the $PaO_2/FiO_2 \geq 250$ **at all times.**
        (1)   The FiO_2 should be lowered to ≤ 0.4 if the PaO_2/FiO_2 can be maintained.
        (2)   PEEP is reduced to 5 cm, when possible.

        An arterial blood gas should be obtained 30 min after each ventilator change. If the patient at any point meets the CMV weaning criteria, the patient can be weaned and extubated with the same monitoring care. The goal is to decrease ventilatory support until the patient is on an $FiO_2 \leq 0.4$ and CPAP of 5 cm with a $PaO_2/FiO_2 \geq 250$.

  3.   **Patients on CPAP**   A patient is ready for removal from the CPAP system when
    a. $FiO_2 \leq 0.4$
    b. $PEEP \leq 5$ cm H_2O
    c. $PaO_2/FiO_2 \geq 250$
    d.   Respiratory rate ≤ 30
    When the patient meets the criteria for weaning from CPAP, the patient is extubated to utilize the physiologic PEEP of the larynx.

          | Note | Patients with neuromuscular diseases, COPD, and quadriplegia will be evaluated separately and a weaning program established.

  4.   **Extubation**   Once the patient is considered to be able to maintain oxygenation and ventilation spontaneously, extubation is considered. Extubation is then performed if the following criteria are met
    a.   The patient is alert enough to protect the airway from aspiration and spontaneously mobilize secretions.
    b.   There will be a patent airway after extubation.
    c.   The patient is systemically stable (no sepsis, cardiovascular instability, etc.)

II. **Complications**   Multiple trauma patients commonly develop respiratory complications both early and late in the course of their illness.

  A. **Early respiratory complications**   Pulmonary contusion, flail chest, rib fractures, pneumothorax, hemothorax, ruptured diaphragm, and laryngotracheobronchial injuries are respiratory complications which occur at the time of injury. These problems are discussed elsewhere in the manual.

  B. **Late respiratory complications**   Late complications include retained secretions, aspiration, respiratory insufficiency, pulmonary infections, pulmonary emboli, fat emboli syndrome, and complications associated with tracheal tubes and barotrauma.

1. **Retained secretions**   Impaired clearance of tracheobronchial secretions with resultant atelectasis is one of the most common respiratory complications seen in the trauma intensive care unit. Trauma victims frequently have depressed levels of consciousness and impaired cough reflexes, become immobilized and splint their chest due to pain, all of which contribute to retained secretions. Indiscriminate use of diuretics and inadequate humidification lead to a propensity for infection of retained secretions, which accentuates the pathophysiologic consequence of retained secretions. (See p. 106 for atelectasis.)
   a. **Manifestations**
      (1) Dyspnea
      (2) Tachypnea
      (3) Rales or wheezing during auscultation
      (4) Elevated temperature
      (5) Difficulty "controlling patients" during mechanical ventilation
      (6) Atelectasis on chest x-ray

   b. **Treatment**
      (1) Frequent postural changes
      (2) Adequate humidification of inspired gases
      (3) Adequate hydration of the patient
      (4) Chest physiotherapy with appropriate position for maximal drainage of each pulmonary segment
      (5) Frequent manual hyperinflation of the trachea and lavage with 2–4% sodium bicarbonate
      (6) Intermittent positive pressure breathing (IPPB) with bronchodilation and mucolytics for bronchospasm and thick secretions
      (7) Mechanical ventilation where indicated
      (8) Early mobilization
      (9) Incentive spirometry
      (10) Encouragement to cough and deep breathe
      (11) **Early** bronchoscopy is indicated if atelectasis does not clear with chest physiotherapy. Bronchoscopy is for therapeutic and diagnostic purposes.

2. **Aspiration**   Shortly after injury, trauma victims may aspirate food, blood, saliva, and other gastric contents. If aspiration is left untreated, respiratory failure may result. The aspirated material may be present in the lung for a relatively long time if the accident victim is difficult to extract from a vehicle or is found some time after the accident occurred. Aspiration can also occur during intubation of the trauma victim for general anesthesia or airway control. Aspiration of colonized oral secretions may occur during tracheal tube cuff deflation or should the cuff accidentally burst.
   a. **Manifestations**
      (1) Tachypnea
      (2) Dyspnea
      (3) Cyanosis
      (4) Bronchospasm with wheezing and/or rales
      (5) Pulmonary edema

      (6) Blood, oral secretions, and/or gastric contents suctioned through an endotracheal tube

      (7) Acute temperature elevation

      (8) Low pH of the aspirate (if gastric contents are unbuffered)

      (9) Alveolar infiltrate on chest x-ray

b. Prophylaxis

    (1) During intubation

      (a) Awake intubation, if possible, under local anesthesia

      (b) Preintubation oxygenation by **spontaneous** breathing only, because bagging the patient can cause gastric insufflation and vomiting

      (c) Small dose of nondepolarizing muscle relaxant before using succinylcholine for intubation

      (d) Cricoid pressure (Sellick's maneuver)

    (2) Follow tracheal cuff pressures so that the cuff is not overinflated and ruptured.

    (3) If the cuff is to be deflated, suction oral secretions so that they are not aspirated.

c. Treatment

    (1) If the patient is not intubated, perform tracheal intubation.

    (2) Apply PEEP and IMV as indicated (see pp. 319 and 321).

    (3) Steroids **may** be useful; however, there are no clinical data to support this practice.

    (4) Vigorous tracheal suctioning is performed to remove the aspirate.

    (5) Bronchoscopy is indicated for the removal of particulate matter or for an infiltrate on chest x-ray that does not rapidly clear with tracheal suction and chest physiotherapy.

    (6) Bronchodilators may be necessary if bronchospasm does not clear with the removal of the aspirate.

    (7) The sputum Gram stain with cultures is analyzed daily and antibiotics are begun if there is indication of an infection (see p. 418).

    (8) Lavage is not used because it will spread debris peripherally.

    (9) Serial ABG and chest x-ray are indicated.

3. Respiratory insufficiency   See p. 313.

4. Pulmonary infections

   a. Pneumonia

   b. Lung abscess

   c. Empyema

See p. 418.

5. Pulmonary emboli   Pulmonary embolism should be suspected in any multiple trauma patient who develops an unexplained sudden drop in arterial oxygen tension. Bedridden patients, especially those with spinal cord lesions, may develop pulmonary emboli. Clinical evidence of thrombosis of leg and pelvic veins should be sought, but its presence is not necessary to confirm the diagnosis of pulmonary emboli.

a. **Manifestations**
   (1) Tachypnea—acute
   (2) Tachycardia—acute
   (3) Blood-tinged sputum obtained by coughing or tracheal suction if intubated
   (4) Acute onset of fever
   (5) Acute hypoxic episode
   (6) Atrial arrythmia
   (7) Increase in the intensity of the pulmonary component of the second heart sound

b. **Diagnosis**
   (1) Acute onset of right axis deviation on EKG
   (2) Increase in V_D/V_T (dead space)
   (3) Acute rise in the right-sided cardiac pressures ($\overline{PA}$ and CVP) without a rise in the wedge
   (4) Acute reduction in end tidal carbon dioxide tension
   (5) Increase in $PaCO_2$ if on controlled ventilation
   (6) $PaCO_2$ may fall if there is spontaneous breathing.
   (7) A normal chest x-ray and an abnormal perfusion scan are suggestive.
   (8) A defect on perfusion scanning without an associated defect on ventilation scanning is highly suggestive of pulmonary embolization.
   (9) A normal perfusion scan essentially excludes the diagnosis of a significant pulmonary embolus.
   (10) If there is a question regarding the diagnosis after scanning and/or there is a contraindication to the use of heparin, a pulmonary arteriogram is advisable.

c. **Prophylaxis** We urge the use of intravenous dextran 40 in high-risk patients who are
   (1) More than 50 years old with a pelvic, hip, or leg fracture
   (2) Bedridden and obese
   (3) Bedridden with congestive heart failure
   (4) Bedridden with a history of venous thrombosis and/or pulmonary embolus

d. **Treatment** Appropriate treatment is well described in standard medical and surgical texts. The major question we must address is "when is it safe to administer heparin in the multiple trauma patient who has a confirmed or likely diagnosis of pulmonary embolism?"

   If it is felt by the clinician that there is a contraindication to heparinization, caval interruption (ligation or screen) must be considered. Each case must be treated individually.

Perspective

We do not find clinically significant pulmonary emboli to be common. We have not aggressively used prophylaxis for patients for pulmonary emboli except for the high-risk patient, for whom we feel intravenous dextran 40 is relatively safe (see p. 239).

6. **Fat emboli syndrome** The fat emboli syndrome (FES) usually develops in a relatively young patient (≤ 30 years old) within 12–24 hr following injury. There are usually lower extremity fractures present. It is uncertain whether this is a systemic stress response or actual fat embolization from the marrow of the fractured extremity, or both. The patient usually presents with a respiratory, cerebral, and/or febrile response.

   a. **Manifestations**
      (1) Tachypnea
      (2) Agitation
      (3) Fever
      (4) Upper chest and axillary petechia

   b. **Diagnosis** There is no diagnostic finding in FES.
      (1) Chest x-ray may be normal, initially, and progress to the development of interstitial and alveolar infiltrates.
      (2) $PaO_2/FiO_2 < 300$ and a normal or low $PaCO_2$ (see p. 316).
      (3) A Swan-Ganz catheter may reveal acute pulmonary arterial hypertension.

   c. **Treatment** See p. 316.

7. **Tracheal tube complications**
   a. **Tracheomalacia** is the softening of tracheal cartilages.
      (1) **Etiology**
         (a) Ischemia to tracheal mucosa and tracheal cartilages secondary to overdistention of the cuff of the tracheostomy or endotracheal tube, which exceeds capillary perfusion pressure (25 mm Hg)
         (b) Pressure necrosis from excessive movement or angulation of either endotracheal or tracheostomy tubes
         (c) Prolonged tracheal intubation, especially if high airway pressures are present
         (d) Contributory factors
            i. Poor nutrition
            ii. Steroid use (head and spine injuries)
            iii. Infectious tracheitis
            iv. Drying of the airway
            v. Excessively large endotracheal or tracheostomy tubes
      (2) **Prophylaxis**
         (a) Do not overinflate tracheal tube cuffs. Hyperinflation is prevented by measuring pressures which should not rise above 25 mm Hg. The AP chest x-ray should be observed for evidence of cuff hyperinflation. If the diameter of the cuff is ≥ 1.5 times the diameter of the trachea, the cuff is excessively inflated. If cuff pressures are high in a patient with poor pulmonary compliance, a small air leak should be allowed in order to prevent excessive tracheal cuff pressures.
         (b) Use a tracheostomy tube or endotracheal tube with a safety valve venting system which prevents overinflation.
         (c) Avoid angulation and properly anchor tracheal tubes.

(d) Provide good nutritional support.

(e) Discontinue steroid use as soon as possible.

(f) Provide proper humidification of all inspired gases.

(g) Use aseptic technique while suctioning the airway.

(h) Use corrugated ventilation tubes to prevent excessive tug on endotracheal tube or tracheostomy tube; relieve tension on ventilator tubing while turning the patient.

(i) Use proper size tubes.

(j) Use high-volume, low-pressure cuffs.

(k) Adjust the ventilator to allow the lowest reasonable peak airway pressures.

(3) **Diagnosis**

(a) Excessive volume of air needed to inflate the cuff to occlude tracheal air leak

(b) Chest x-ray showing marked overdistention of the tracheal cuff

(c) Endoscopic evidence of erythema, edema, and tracheal collapse during spontaneous inspiration

(4) **Management**

(a) **Prevention is of the utmost importance.**

(b) Once established, remove the nasogastric (NG) tube to reduce the risk of tracheoesophageal fistula. Perform a gastrostomy, if necessary.

(c) Lower the tidal volume to reduce the airway pressure.

(d) The cuff of the tracheal tube should be placed below the area of tracheomalacia and a small leak allowed around the cuff.

(e) Administer antibiotics, as necessary, to treat tracheitis.

(f) If respiratory distress secondary to tracheomalacia develops after extubation, the patient is reintubated. The tracheomalacia will usually disappear as the trachea "stiffens" by fibrosis. The patient should be endoscoped in about 10 days and decannulated if stenosis is not severe and the tracheomalacia has disappeared. The cuff should be below the involved area, if possible.

| Note | The major problem with tracheal cuff complications arises in the patient with very poor pulmonary compliance, who requires high airway pressures to provide adequate alveolar ventilation.

b. **Tracheal stenosis** is the narrowing of the trachea secondary to the presence of exuberant granulation tissue and/or cicatrix.

(1) **Location**

(a) At the site of the tracheostomy stoma

(b) At the site of the tracheal cuff

(c) At the tip of the tracheal tube

(2) **Etiology**

(a) Same as for tracheomalacia

(b) Improper stoma made during tracheostomy

(c) Direct trauma from original injury

(3) **Prophylaxis**
  (a) Avoid tracheomalacia (see p. 326).
  (b) Do not remove large segments of tracheal wall when performing tracheostomies (see p. 481).

(4) **Diagnosis**
  (a) **Clinical** Acute or chronic obstruction of airway after extubation
  (b) **Radiographic** Narrowed tracheal air shadow
  (c) **Endoscopic** Direct visualization of stenosis

(5) **Management**
  (a) Ear, nose, and throat (ENT) and/or thoracic surgical consultant should adopt a treatment plan based on the diagnostic evaluation.
  (b) PO zinc sulfate to reduce granulation tissue
  (c) Steroids
  (d) Perform tracheostomy or replace tracheostomy tube below stenotic segment.
  (e) Montgomery tracheal stent
  (f) Removal of exuberant granulation tissue
  (g) Tracheal dilation
  (h) Tracheal resection electively, if necessary

c. **Tracheoesophageal fistula** is an anatomical communication between the trachea and esophagus.

(1) **Etiology**
  (a) Tracheomalacia
  (b) Esophageal necrosis
  The mechanism is basically the same as for tracheomalacia; in addition, an esophageal tube is usually in place. The result is a common erosion of the anterior wall of the esophagus and the posterior wall of the trachea.

(2) **Prophylaxis**
  (a) Avoid tracheomalacia by minimizing tracheal cuff hyperinflation.
  (b) Avoid esophageal necrosis by removing esophageal tubes if the tracheal cuff must be hyperinflated.

(3) **Diagnosis**
  (a) **Clinical**
    i. Abdominal distention secondary to insufflation of the gastrointestinal tract.
    ii. NG tube bubbles in synchrony with the inspiratory cycle of the ventilator.
    iii. Methylene blue placed down the tracheostomy or endotracheal tube returns through the NG tube.
    iv. Aspiration of tube feedings or gastric contents via tracheal suctioning.

        (b)   **Radiographic** Barium swallow

        (c)   **Esophagoscopy** and visualization of the tracheal tube

        (d)   **Tracheoscopy** and visualization of esophageal mucosa or tube

  (4) **Management**

        (a)   Prevention yields the best prognosis.

        (b)   Place the tracheal tube cuff below the fistula.

        (c)   Cervical esophagostomy prevents oral secretory contamination of the trachea.

        (d)   Occlusion of the gastroesophageal juncture, by ligature or stapling device to prevent gastric reflux

        (e)   Gastrostomy allows gastrointestinal decompression and the institution of feedings when peristalsis begins.

        (f)   Tracheobronchial toiletry

> | Note | Definitive repair cannot be performed until the patient is ready for extubation; the above steps are to prevent soilage of the lungs until the respiratory failure resolves, i.e., until pulmonary compliance and oxygenation improve.

d. **Tracheo-innominate artery fistula** is the abnormal communication between the trachea and the innominate artery.

  (1) **Etiology** Low placement of tracheostomy (usually through the fourth or fifth tracheal ring). The fistula may occur at the level of the stoma or at the cuff level.

  (2) **Prophylaxis** Do not place a tracheostomy lower than the fourth tracheal ring.

> | Note | These fistulas can occur as soon as 24 hr after tracheostomy.

  (3) **Diagnosis**

        (a)   Excessive pulsation of the tracheostomy tube may be a warning sign.

        (b)   There may be sentinel, minimal bleeding around the tracheostomy tube or into the trachea.

        (c)   Endoscopy after sentinel bleeding may reveal bleeding into the trachea from the stoma. The absence of a tracheal lesion increases the likelihood of an extratracheal source of hemorrhage into the stoma. There is no characteristic endoscopic finding to secure the diagnosis. There may be an erosion identified in the anterior trachea at the cuff level.

        (d)   The first sign may be massive hemorrhage around the tracheostomy tube, into the trachea, or out the mouth and nose.

  (4) **Differential diagnosis**

        (a)   Tracheitis with bleeding from the mucosa

        (b)   Bleeding from soft tissues around the tracheal stoma

(5) **Management**
   (a) **Temporary control of hemorrhage**
      i. Overinflation of the tracheal cuff
      ii. If overinflation fails, remove the tracheostomy tube and insert a translaryngeal tube; the cuff is inflated at the level of the fistula to control bleeding into the trachea.
      iii. If the above does not control the hemorrhage, the cuff of the translaryngeal tube is advanced below the fistula and digital control is obtained by advancing the finger along the anterior surface of the trachea and compressing the innominate artery against the sternum.
   (b) **Definitive control**   Surgical division of the innominate artery with oversew of the ends is performed through a median sternotomy. A translaryngeal tube with the cuff below the tracheal defect is left in place.

   | Note | Mediastinitis is the major complication of this procedure (see p. 141).

e. **Subglottic stenosis** is a granulomatous/cicatricial narrowing below the cords.
   (1) **Etiology**
      (a) Tracheolaryngomalacia secondary to translaryngeal intubation
      (b) High tracheostomy
      (c) Direct trauma from the original injury
      (d) Cricothyroidotomy
   (2) **Prophylaxis**
      (a) Same general measures as for preventing tracheomalacia
      (b) "Control" the agitated or spastic patient with a translaryngeal tube or perform an early tracheostomy to prevent "tugging" on the translaryngeal tube.
      (c) Convert cricothyroidotomy to a standard tracheostomy as soon as feasible.
      (d) Avoid "high" tracheostomies.
   (3) **Diagnosis**
      (a) **Clinical**   Acute or chronic obstruction of the airway after extubation
      (b) **Radiographic**   Narrowed air column through the stenotic area
      (c) **Endoscopic**   Direct visualization of the stenosis
   (4) **Management**
      (a) Zinc sulfate to prevent granulation tissue formation
      (b) Steroids
      (c) Perform tracheostomy or replace the tracheostomy tube, but below the stenotic segment.
      (d) Removal of exuberant granulation tissue
      (e) Montgomery tracheal stent
      (f) Elective tracheal resection, if necessary

f. **Vocal cord injury** may include ulceration, edema, exuberant granulation tissue, and/or stenosis (fibrosis).
  (1) **Etiology**
    (a) Prolonged use of a translaryngeal tube
    (b) Direct trauma from original injury
  (2) **Prophylaxis**
    (a) Avoid prolonged translaryngeal intubation (14 days is our maximal limit).
    (b) Prevent tension on the translaryngeal tube while moving the patient.
  (3) **Diagnosis**
    (a) **Clinical** Voice changes or airway obstruction after extubation
    (b) **Endoscopic** Direct visualization of pathology
  (4) **Management**
    (a) Racemic epinephrine inhalations for edema
    (b) Steroids for edema
    (c) Tracheostomy if the airway is compromised
    (d) Surgical removal of exuberant granulation tissue
    (e) Antibiotics
    (f) Elective surgical repair, if necessary
g. **Peristomal sepsis** may include cellulitis, abscess formation (superficial and deep), and/or mediastinitis.
  (1) **Contributing factors**
    (a) All tracheostomy stomas are colonized with bacteria.
    (b) Poor host defenses
    (c) Excessive immobilization in the supine position, which causes poor peristomal drainage
    (d) Poor wound care
    (e) Poor technique during tracheostomy
    (f) "Tugging" on the tracheal tube
    (g) Use of steroids (head and spine injuries)
  (2) **Prophylaxis**
    (a) Optimum general supportive care
    (b) Aggressive mobilization of the patient
    (c) Local wound care with povidone-iodine (Betadine) and dilute acetic acid
    (d) Avoid tugging and pulling on the tracheal tube.
    (e) Meticulous technique during tracheostomy
    (f) Discontinue steroids as soon as possible.
  (3) **Diagnosis**
    (a) **Clinical** Erythema, induration, suppuration, fever, leukocytosis, "septic"
    (b) **Laboratory** Gram stain and culture
    (c) **X-ray**
      i.   Air fluid level in the neck or mediastinum
      ii. Displacement of the trachea or esophagus
      iii. Mass effect in soft tissues

                    iv. Widening of the mediastinum
                    v. Pneumomediastinum
        (4) **Management**
            (a) Local wound care
            (b) Antibiotics
            (c) Surgical drainage
            (d) Replace the transtracheal tube with a translaryngeal tube if treatment is refractory to (a) through (c).

    h. **Retropharyngeal laceration**
        (1) **Etiology**   The oropharynx may be lacerated during a difficult emergency oral translaryngeal intubation. A superimposed abscess may occur.
        (2) **Diagnosis**
            (a) Pharyngeal laceration may be noted during endoscopy.
            (b) Abscess
                    i. Fever and leukocytosis
                    ii. Oral-nasal purulent drainage
                    iii. Soft tissue x-ray of the neck may reveal gas and/or a mass effect.
        (3) **Management**
            (a) Remove the translaryngeal tube.
            (b) Administer systemic antibiotics if an abscess has formed.
            (c) Drain the abscess.
            (d) Rule out mediastinitis.

8. **Barotrauma (Macklin phenomenon)**   Alveolar air disperses into the interstitium, pleural space, mediastinum, subcutaneous tissues, and/or peritoneal cavity.
    a. **Etiology** (increased airway pressure causing alveolar rupture)
        (1) Blunt chest trauma with a closed glottis
        (2) Out of phase on the ventilator
        (3) "Overventilation"
        (4) Decreased pulmonary compliance
    b. **Prophylaxis**
        (1) The patient must be in phase during controlled ventilation.
            (a) Adequate sedation and analgesia
            (b) Paralyze patient if unable to keep in phase with other methods.
            (c) Adequate minute ventilation to induce slight hypocarbia (helps keep the patient in phase)
            (d) Remove endobronchial secretions
        (2) Ventilator may be adjusted to obtain the lowest effective airway pressure.
        (3) Use IMV instead of CMV, when possible.
        (4) Use the lowest effective PEEP.

c. **Diagnosis**
    (1) **Clinical**
        (a) Subcutaneous emphysema, local or widespread
        (b) Tension pneumothorax
            i.   Decreased breath sounds
            ii.   Tracheal shift
            iii. Hyperexpansion of the hemithorax
            iv.   Resonance to chest percussion
            v.   Acute elevation of peak airway pressure
            vi.   Out of phase on the ventilator
            vii. Deterioration of ABGs
    (2) **Radiographic**
        (a) Pneumothorax
        (b) Pneumomediastinum
        (c) Pneumoperitoneum
        (d) Interstitial emphysema of the lung
        (e) Air in soft tissues

d. **Management**
    (1) Insert bilateral chest tubes, prophylactically, when using super PEEP (25 cm H_2O).
    (2) Chest tube for pneumothorax—If the patient develops findings consistent with a tension pneumothorax and is hypotensive, a needle should be inserted into the midaxillary line, fifth intercostal space, for immediate decompression, followed by a chest tube. If the blood pressure is stable, a chest x-ray should be obtained first, unless there will be an inordinate delay.
    (3) Make a collar incision in the base of the neck if superior vena caval compression syndrome is suspected, i.e., if there is excessive tension in the mediastinum.
    (4) Lower PEEP, if possible.
    (5) Lower airway pressures by manipulation of the tidal volume, if possible.
    (6) Induce mild hypocapnia, sedation, and analgesia, if tachypneic.
    (7) Paralyze the patient, if unable to keep in phase with other modalities.
    (8) If the patient develops subcutaneous emphysema, observe for the manifestation of a tension pneumothorax.

> Note | We are not certain whether prophylactic chest tubes are indicated when subcutaneous emphysema develops secondary to barotrauma. The purpose of the tube is to prevent the development of a tension pneumothorax; however, we have seen numerous complications from these prophylactic tubes (see p. 471).

(9) Maximize pulmonary compliance.

(10) Rule out sepsis.

(11) Clear the tracheobronchial tree of secretions.

e. **Complications** A persistent bronchopleural air leak may develop secondary to barotrauma (see p. 138).

19
CARDIAC INSUFFICIENCY

I. Cardiac Assessment and Failure

A. Goal of cardiac function The goal of cardiac function is to maintain oxygen delivery to the tissues to satisfy their demand for oxygen. If tissue oxygen demands are not met, anaerobic metabolism ensues. Anaerobic metabolism creates cellular dysfunction, which will ultimately lead to cellular death if hypoxia continues. **Oxygen demand** is the amount of oxygen needed to furnish energy efficiently for cellular function. **Oxygen delivery** is the amount of oxygen made available to the cells for utilization. **Oxygen consumption** is the amount of oxygen utilized by the cell. Oxygen consumption depends upon oxygen demand and the capability of oxygen delivery to supply the tissues with oxygen.

B. Determinants of tissue oxygen delivery

Tissue oxygen delivery = cardiac output × arterial O_2 content
(flow)   (O_2 carrying capacity)
Arterial oxygen content = Hb gm/100 cc × 1.34 cc O_2/gm × % O_2 sat
+ 0.003 × PO_2
(cc O_2/100 cc blood)

Hemoglobin appears to be optimal at a level of approximately 12–13 gm/100 cc of blood. The PO_2 and % O_2 sat are determined by the pulmonary shunt and the FIO_2, i.e., pulmonary function. If hemoglobin is 12–13 gm % and pulmonary function is normal, tissue oxygen delivery is primarily determined by flow (cardiac output).

C. Determinants of cardiac output Cardiac output = heart rate × stroke volume. The **heart rate** is the number of systolic ejections/min. **Stroke volume** is the amount of blood the heart ejects during systole. In general, if the heart rate decreases significantly, cardiac output will fall. If the heart rate rises, cardiac output will rise until there is a heart rate of approximately 150, at which point diastole is so brief that there is inadequate filling of the heart, with a resultant fall in cardiac output.

Stroke volume is determined by preload, contractility, and afterload. **Preload** is related to the muscle fiber length of the ventricle. In general, the greater the length of the fiber prior to contraction, the greater the muscle will contract; therefore, the greater the stroke volume. However, if the fiber is stretched too much, stroke volume will fail to rise. If the muscle fiber is not stretched with an adequate intraventricular volume (left ventricular end-diastolic volume), the stroke volume will fall. Clinically, the left ventricular end-diastolic volume cannot be easily measured, but the next order of estimation, the left ventricular end-diastolic pressure (LVEDP), can be approximated by the pulmonary wedge pressure. LVEDP is affected by

—Intravascular volume
—Ventricular contractility and compliance
—Vascular tone

If the LVEDP is too low, the cardiac output will also be low. The range of the normal LVEDP is 5–12 mm Hg and of the normal right ventricular end-diastolic pressure (RVEDP), estimated by the CVP, is 5–10 mm Hg.

Contractility is the ability of the heart to alter its contractile force and velocity, independent of the fiber length. The greater the force and velocity of contraction, the greater the cardiac output. If contractility is normal, cardiac output is determined by preload and resistance to ventricular ejection (afterload). Contractility is expressed as a given cardiac output for a given left ventricular end-diastolic pressure. If cardiac output is lower than expected at a given LVEDP, contractility is depressed. The patient's relative ventricular contractile state can be determined by plotting a ventricular function curve. Fluid is administered and the change in LVEDP and cardiac output is noted:

—If fluid is administered and the LVEDP rises minimally, but there is a significant rise in the cardiac output, contractility is good.
—If the LVEDP rises significantly and cardiac output changes minimally, the state of contractility is poor.

Causes of elevated LVEDP (> 15 mm Hg)
—Hypervolemia
—Decreased ventricular contractility/compliance
—Vascular constriction
—PEEP

Causes of low LVEDP (< 8 mm Hg)
—Hypovolemia
—Hyperdynamic ventricular contraction (sepsis)
—Vascular dilatation

Afterload is the resistance to ventricular ejection. The afterload governs the amount of intraventricular tension that must be generated to produce a given stroke volume. Clinically, **systemic vascular resistance** (SVR) is the best reflection of afterload.

$$\text{Systemic vascular resistance} = \frac{\text{MAP} - \text{CVP}}{\text{CO}} \times 80$$

Systemic vascular resistance and mean arterial pressure (MAP) are directly proportional; that is, as aortic pressure rises, resistance rises, and ventricular tension must rise to maintain flow (cardiac output). The systemic vascular resistance is usually elevated due to an increase in the mean arterial pressure and/or a fall in the cardiac output.

—If the mean arterial pressure is increased, ventricular tension must rise to maintain cardiac output; if mean arterial pressure is markedly elevated, the ventricle may not be able to generate the appropriate level of tension and cardiac output may fall.

—If cardiac output falls, there is a reflex outflow of catecholamines, which may cause a rise in the mean arterial pressure and, therefore, a rise in the systemic vascular resistance.

Each component of systemic vascular resistance must be analyzed to decide which is primary and which is secondary.

Pulmonary vascular resistance is the afterload on the right ventricle.

$$\text{Pulmonary vascular resistance} = \frac{\overline{PA} - \text{wedge pressure}}{CO} \times 80$$

The normal pulmonary vascular resistance is less than 200.

D. Arterial venous O_2 content difference

$$\text{Oxygen content} = \text{Hb gm/100 cc} \times 1.34 \text{ cc } O_2/\text{gm} \times \%O_2 \text{ sat}$$
$$+ 0.003 \times PO_2$$
$$(\text{cc } O_2/100 \text{ cc blood})$$

The normal arterial PO_2 is approximately 98 mm Hg, percent oxygen saturation is approximately 98, and the oxygen content is about 20 cc of O_2/100 cc of blood if the hemoglobin is 15 gm %. As the oxygenated blood passes through the tissues, oxygen is extracted. Venous blood has a PO_2 of 35–40, a percent oxygen saturation of 75, and an oxygen content of about 15 cc/100 cc of blood. Therefore, the normal arterial venous oxygen content difference is 5 cc of oxygen/100 cc of blood. The Fick Equation states that

$$CO = \frac{\text{oxygen consumption}}{A - V O_2 \text{ content}}$$

Normal cardiac output is 5 liters/min, oxygen consumption is approximately 250 cc of oxygen/min, and arterial-venous O_2 content is 50 cc of oxygen/1,000 cc of blood. If cardiac output falls, oxygen consumption frequently remains normal because of increased extraction of oxygen from the hemoglobin. Increased oxygen extraction will lead to a fall in the $P\overline{v}O_2$ and venous O_2 saturation, which causes a fall in the venous O_2 content. An $A - V O_2$ content is considered elevated when it is greater than 5 cc of oxygen/100 cc of blood. If the $A - V O_2$ content is greater than 5, this implies that the heart is providing "inadequate" flow relative to the tissue oxygen needs. Since there is a limit to oxygen extraction, oxygen consumption may fall if cardiac output falls significantly. The oxygen demand of the tissues may not be met if demand is markedly elevated as may be seen in stress, fever, shivering, or sepsis. In this case, oxygen consumption may be less than oxygen demand if cardiac output (oxygen delivery) is relatively low.

E. Myocardial oxygenation

Myocardial oxygen consumption depends upon the work that the heart must perform. Clinically, this is reflected in the heart rate × systolic blood pressure product. The normal value is about 12,000. If the heart rate-systolic blood pressure product rises, myocardial oxygen consumption or work is elevated.

Myocardial oxygen supply is reflected by the transmyocardial gradient. The transmyocardial gradient is the difference in the systemic diastolic blood pressure and the left ventricular end-diastolic pressure (wedge). Coronary flow is determined primarily by the diastolic blood pressure. If the diastolic blood pressure and the LVEDP are relatively normal, there is a "normal" myocardial perfusion gradient from the epicardium to the endocardium. If the LVEDP is elevated due to hypervolemia and/or decreased contractility, or diastolic pressure falls, the gradient decreases and myocardial perfusion is impaired.

Note | The EKG should be closely followed for evidence of myocardial ischemia.

Commonly used cardiovascular formulas and their normal values are listed in Table 1.

F. **Goal of cardiovascular assessment**

1. Determine if oxygen consumption is optimal.

2. Assess myocardial work and oxygen supply.

    An isolated cardiac output may be absolutely or relatively low. The endpoint of manipulating cardiac output is to "optimize" oxygen consumption, i.e., we must make certain that oxygen delivery has satisfied the systemic oxygen demand.

G. **Classical manifestations of cardiac insufficiency**   Classical manifestations of cardiac insufficiency are **hypoperfusion** or **congestion.** Hypoperfusion implies an inadequate cardiac output; congestion refers to an elevation in the pulmonary venous pressure, usually secondary to an elevation in the LVEDP. An elevated LVEDP is usually secondary to hypervolemia and/or impairment of ventricular contractility. Because of an increase in pulmonary venous pressure, water accumulates in the alveolar and interstitial spaces of the lung (pulmonary edema).

1. **Hypoperfusion**
    a. Oliguria
    b. Pallor
    c. Cool extremities
    d. Decreased sensorium
    e. Diaphoresis
    f. Decreased capillary refill
    g. Metabolic acidosis (lactic)

2. **Congestion**
    a. Gallop
    b. Distended neck veins
    c. Pulmonary edema ("tracheal froth")
    d. Rales
    e. Peripheral edema
    f. Chest x-ray which reveals cardiomegaly, hilar engorgement, and/or interstitial-alveolar edema

Table 1. Cardiovascular parameters in the hemodynamically stable, unstressed patient

Cardiac output (5–6 liters/min)

$$\text{Cardiac index} = \frac{CO}{BSA} \quad (3.5\text{–}4 \text{ liters/min/m}^2)$$

Heart rate (60–100 beats/min)

$$\text{Stroke index} = \frac{CO}{HR \times BSA} \quad (35\text{–}45 \text{ ml/beat/m}^2)$$

Wedge pressure (5–12 mm Hg)

Mean pulmonary arterial pressure (10–18 mm Hg)

Central venous pressure (5–12 cm H_2O)

Mean systemic arterial pressure (85–95 mm Hg)

$$\text{Systemic vascular resistance} = \frac{MAP - CVP \times 80}{CO} \quad (800\text{–}1{,}200 \text{ dynes} \cdot \text{sec} \cdot \text{cm}^{-5})$$

$$\text{Pulmonary vascular resistance} = \frac{\overline{PA} - \text{wedge} \times 80}{CO} \quad (150\text{–}250 \text{ dynes} \cdot \text{sec} \cdot \text{cm}^{-5})$$

Left ventricular stroke work index
$$SI \times (MAP - \text{wedge}) \times 0.0136 \quad (35\text{–}40 \text{ gm} \cdot \text{m/m}^2)$$

Right ventricular stroke work index
$$SI \times (\overline{PA} - CVP) \times 0.0136 \quad (3\text{–}5 \text{ gm} \cdot \text{m/m}^2)$$

Arterial O_2 content   (20 cc O_2/100 cc blood; depends on the Hb)

Mixed venous O_2 content   (15 cc O_2/100 cc blood; depends on the Hb)

Arterial-venous O_2 content   (4–5 cc O_2/100 cc blood)

Oxygen consumption
$$\dot{V}O_2 = CO \times A - V\ O_2 \text{ content}^a \quad (130\text{–}140 \text{ cc } O_2/\text{min/m}^2)$$

Transmyocardial gradient
$$\text{Systemic diastolic pressure} - \text{wedge pressure} \quad (70 \text{ mm Hg})$$

Myocardial oxygen consumption
$$HR \times \text{systemic systolic blood pressure} \quad (12{,}000)$$

Abbreviations used in Table 1 are: BSA, body surface area; CO, cardiac output; HR, heart rate; MAP, mean arterial pressure; PA, mean pulmonary arterial pressure; SI, stroke index; CVP, central venous pressure.
[a] A – VO_2 content is measured in cc O_2/1,000 cc blood.

Most commonly, hypoperfusion is present in the trauma patient with only minimal or absent manifestations of congestion. The manifestations of hypoperfusion in the trauma patient may be similar to those seen in classic heart failure or they may be subtle. Manifestations of hypoperfusion in the unstable high-risk patient (Table 2) are often subtle.

H. Patients who should be evaluated regarding cardiovascular function

1. Patients with obvious manifestations of hypoperfusion or congestion

2. High-risk, unstable patients with or without obvious manifestations of cardiac insufficiency.

Table 2. High-risk situations in which hypoperfusion is common

Decreased preload
  PEEP
  Hypovolemia
	Increased afterload Postresuscitative hypertension

Impairment of contractility
  Hypoxia
    Near drowning
    Cardiopulmonary arrest
    Pulmonary contusion
    Aspiration
    Pneumothorax
    Hemorrhagic shock
    Smoke inhalation
      Carbon monoxide
      Cyanide
      Plastics
  Cardiac contusion
  Infarction (uncommon)
  Cardiomyopathy
  Tamponade
  Drugs
    EtOH
    Barbiturates
    Valium
    PCP (large dose)
    Anesthetics
  Sepsis
  Propane inhalation
	Tachycardia
	    Supraventricular tachycardia
	    Ventricular tachycardia
	
	Bradycardia
	    Quadriplegia
	    Heart block
	    Intracranial hypertension
	    Hypoxia

After resuscitation and operative procedures, the trauma victim's myocardial performance is affected by the metabolic state, need for mechanical ventilation, associated injuries, and administered drugs.

I. **Cardiac Catherization**

1. **Central venous catheterization**   The central venous pressure reflects the right atrial pressure which reflects the right ventricular end-diastolic pressure. The RVEDP is a reflection of the preload of the right heart. RVEDP frequently reflects LVEDP, but there is often a discrepancy in patients with pulmonary disease and/or on ventilators.

2. **Swan-Ganz catheterization**   The Swan-Ganz catheter is a balloon-tipped catheter, which passes through the right heart and enters the pulmonary arterial circulation. When the balloon is inflated, the tip of the catheter reflects the pulmonary venous, left atrial, and left ventricular end-diastolic pressures. In other words, the "wedge" pressure is a reflection of the preload of the left ventricle. In addition, cardiac output and $A - VO_2$ content can be determined.

J. **Approach to evaluating cardiac insufficiency**

1. The patient who has overt symptoms may be followed by
   a. Clinical examination
   b. Central venous pressure
   c. Swan-Ganz catheter determinations

2. High-risk patients without overt manifestations of cardiac insufficiency should be monitored by
   a. Central venous pressure
   b. Swan-Ganz catheter

> **Note** Multigated radionuclide examination is a noninvasive tool for evaluating the ejection fraction of the heart (stroke volume/LVEDV). Normal left ventricle ejection fraction is 0.55–0.78. If there is a question regarding ventricular performance and the patient has difficult venous access (Swan-Ganz catheter), radionuclide evaluation is helpful. A value less than 0.55 implies impaired contractility (ventricular dilation).

K. **Conceptual approach to the manipulation of cardiovascular parameters**

   1. **Hypoperfusion without congestion**
      a. Fluids are administered to improve the preload and cardiac output. If the patient responds clinically, the clinician may stop at this point or elect to insert a central venous or Swan-Ganz catheter.
      b. If the patient does not respond to a bolus of fluid, a central venous line is needed to evaluate right ventricular preload. If the patient does not respond to fluid administration and the central venous pressure rises 5 cm, a Swan-Ganz catheter is needed to evaluate preload, cardiac output, systemic vascular resistance, etc.

   2. **Congestion without hypoperfusion**
      a. Digoxin may be administered to improve ventricular contractility.
      b. Lasix may be administered to decrease the preload.
      c. If the patient does not respond, a Swan-Ganz catheter should be inserted.

   3. **Hypoperfusion and congestion** A Swan-Ganz catheter should be inserted to accurately monitor the patient; this is not a common situation in the trauma patient.

   4. **High-risk patient** A Swan-Ganz catheter is advisable since there may be only nebulous clinical manifestations of cardiac insufficiency; this will allow the clinician to assess cardiac output, preload, oxygen consumption, systemic vascular resistance, etc.

L. **Using the Swan-Ganz catheter data**

   1. If the patient has congestion and/or hypoperfusion, the abnormal parameters of cardiac output are manipulated to reverse the signs and symptoms.

   2. If the patient has nebulous clinical manifestations, such as those in a high-risk patient, the clinician must assess cardiovascular parameters, which may be abnormal, but not apparent on physical examination.

M. Manipulating cardiac output parameters

1. **Preload and contractility** are considered together by constructing a ventricular function curve. The wedge pressure and cardiac output (LVSWI) are recorded. The patient is administered a 250-cc bolus of plasmanate **over 5 min.** Immediately after the fluid is infused, the wedge pressure is recorded. Five min following infusion, the cardiac output and wedge pressure are recorded.

   Likely responses include

   —**Hypovolemia** If the wedge pressure does not rise during fluid administration or afterward, especially if the cardiac output rises, a further rise in cardiac output may be obtained by fluid administration.

   —**Euvolemia** If the wedge pressure rises during fluid infusion and falls to preinfusion levels 5 min after infusion, the patient is considered to be euvolemic, especially if cardiac output does not rise. If further improvement in cardiac output is needed, contractility or afterload therapy must be initiated.

   —**Hypervolemia** If the wedge pressure rises during volume infusion and fails to decrease with time (5 min), further improvement in cardiac output is obtained with agents that improve ventricular contractility or reduce the afterload.

   | Note | A significant change in wedge pressure is 3–5 mm Hg.

2. **Contractility therapy** (for euvolemic or hypervolemic patients)

   a. **Dobutamine** (Dobutrex) If the systemic vascular resistance is elevated (decreased cardiac output/increased mean arterial pressure), dobutamine is used. Dobutamine is a beta-1 agonist which improves cardiac contractility with little peripheral effect. The dose is 1–20 μg/kg/min.

   b. **Dopamine** (Intropin) If the systemic vascular resistance is low (e.g., with sepsis), dopamine is used. Dopamine has a beta-1 agonist effect which stimulates cardiac contractility and a peripheral alpha effect which induces vasoconstriction. The alpha effect is dose-related. The specific effect on a given patient must be evaluated after administration. The dose is 1–20 μg/kg/min.

   If dobutamine or dopamine fail to improve contractility, consideration for the addition of an afterload reducing agent must be made. The effect of dopamine and dobutamine must be monitored by following cardiac output, systemic and pulmonary vascular resistance, oxygen consumption, transmyocardial gradient, and myocardial oxygen demand.

   c. **Digoxin** Digoxin is a useful drug for the elderly patient with poor left ventricular reserve. Unlike dopamine or dobutamine, should complications arise from the drug, it cannot simply be "turned off."

3. **Afterload reduction** Afterload reducing agents are vasodilators. Agents that induce venous dilatation cause a decrease in the preload and, therefore, a decrease in propensity to cause pulmonary congestion. Vasodilators which dilate the arterial tree produce a decreased resistance to ventricular ejection

and usually improve cardiac output. Vasodilators, in general, should only be used if the wedge pressure is 15 mm Hg or greater, since a drop in the wedge pressure may cause a fall in cardiac output.

a. **Nipride** (sodium nitroprusside) Nipride is a venous and arterial dilator. Venous dilatation tends to drop the wedge pressure and arterial dilatation tends to decrease the afterload and improve cardiac output. The dose range of Nipride is 0.5–8 μg/kg/min. Indications for the use of Nipride are
   (1) Significantly elevated mean arterial pressure and low cardiac output
   (2) Low cardiac output which is not responsive to fluids, dopamine, or dobutamine

Note Young patients who are hypovolemic may have a significant outflow of catecholamines and become hypertensive. In this case, fluid administration is the treatment of choice, not Nipride.

b. **Nitroglycerin** Intravenous nitroglycerin in low doses (20–40 μg/min) is a venous dilator which tends to drop the wedge pressure. Decrease of an elevated wedge pressure tends to improve coronary flow, i.e., myocardial oxygen availability. In higher doses (50–250 μg/min), nitroglycerin is an arterial dilator which tends to decrease resistance to ventricular ejection and improve cardiac output. Intravenous nitroglycerin is indicated for patients who have an elevated wedge pressure with or without an EKG that reveals myocardial ischemia and who have
   (1) Significant elevation in mean arterial pressure and a low cardiac output, and/or
   (2) Cardiac output which is not responsive to fluids, dopamine, or dobutamine.

During afterload reduction, the wedge pressure, mean arterial pressure, cardiac output, transmyocardial gradient, heart rate × systolic blood pressure, and electrocardiogram must be monitored. If the wedge pressure precipitously drops, cardiac output may fall. If mean arterial pressure precipitously falls, tissue perfusion may fall. If diastolic pressure precipitously falls, there may be a decrease in coronary flow. The optimal effect of a vasodilating agent is to decrease the afterload (SVR), increase cardiac output, decrease myocardial oxygen demand, and improve myocardial oxygen supply. Afterload reduction is not commonly used in the trauma patient except for
   —Post injury/operative hypertension
   —An elderly patient with cardiac failure

4. **Heart rate**
   a. If the cardiac output is decreased secondary to bradycardia (less than 60), the patient may need a pacemaker. If severe bradycardia is transient, isoproterenol (Isuprel) or atropine are appropriate.
   b. If the heart rate is too fast, cardiac output may fall. If the heart rate exceeds 150 beats/min, diastole is so short that the ventricle fails to ade-

quately fill. This reduces preload, thus reducing cardiac output.

    c. **Treatment**
        —**Supraventricular tachycardia**
           Inderal
           Digoxin
           Cardioversion
        —**Ventricular tachycardia**
           Cardioversion
           Lidocaine (Xylocaine)

N. **Intra-aortic balloon pump**

    1. May improve cardiac output

    2. May improve coronary perfusion

The intra-aortic balloon pump is not commonly used in the trauma patient, unless the patient is elderly and has primary cardiac failure.

O. **Conclusion**   To optimally manipulate cardiac performance, we must know what parameters, if manipulated and "improved," will correlate with survival. Unfortunately, we do not know what these parameters are.

When we perform a manipulation of cardiac output, we must ask

    1. What is the indication?

    2. Will manipulation of this parameter affect survival?

    3. Did the manipulation improve the "abnormal" parameter?

    4. Did "cardiac performance" improve?

    5. Was oxygen consumption improved?

    6. What was the effect on myocardial oxygen consumption (work)?

    7. What was the effect on myocardial oxygen availability?

Ideally, the treatment should improve cardiac output, oxygen consumption, and myocardial oxygen availability, and should decrease myocardial work (oxygen consumption).

The ultimate question that the clinician must ask is, **"Did I help the patient with this manipulation?"**

When the clinician considers assessment of cardiovascular performance, he must remember that patients may have overt signs and symptoms of cardiac insufficiency; therefore, it is "apparent" that therapy is needed. On the other hand, high-risk patients may not express classical overt manifestations of cardiac insufficiency, yet may require cardiovascular assessment and manipulation.

II. Cardiac Arrhythmias

A. Arrhythmias associated with inadequate cardiac output

In general, the recommendations of the American Heart Association as given in Advanced Cardiac Life Support are followed. Two major differences in trauma patients compared to patients with only myocardial disease should be remembered:

1. **Hypovolemia** may be a major problem and the circulatory volume status of any patient with electromechanical dissociation should be critically evaluated and volume deficiencies quickly repaired.

2. **Open cardiac massage** is very often employed as part of resuscitation. Because of the possibility of cardiac perforations or pericardial tamponade, this maneuver may be diagnostic and lead to immediate therapy, as well as the only effective supportive measure.

B. Arrhythmias associated with adequate or borderline cardiac output

These arrhythmias pose less of an immediate threat to the patient and usually treatment may be delayed while attention is given to the cause of the arrhythmia. In this regard, certain problems are fairly common in trauma patients. **Sinus bradycardia** in a patient with a head injury may indicate dangerous elevation of the intracranial pressure. The same rhythm in a patient with a high spinal injury may be the result of unopposed vagal activity. Causes of sinus bradycardia encountered in post-trauma patients are listed in Table 3.

Sinus tachycardia may indicate hypovolemia, inadequate sedation, anoxia, or a pharmacologic response to pancuronium bromide (Pavulon) or a catecholamine. Other causes are listed in Table 4.

Premature ventricular contractions (PVCs) may be the result of enhanced sympathetic activity either from drugs or anxiety and pain, electrolyte imbalance or anoxia, myocardial contusion, or may indicate the improper placement of a central venous catheter (within the right ventricle). In all cases, it is best to search for the primary cause of the arrhythmia rather than to rush for some pharmacologic means of suppressing the abnormality. If no "primary cause" can be determined and it is established that the arrhythmia is harmful, the first approach is usually that advocated by the American Heart Association. In trauma patients, PVCs do not seem to have the same ominous significance as those seen in patients after myocardial infarctions. More often than not, they can be eliminated by maneuvers such as pulling back a central line. The automatic use of lidocaine should be

---

Table 3.   Causes of sinus bradycardia

Drugs
    Atropine (low dose)
    Digitalis compounds
    Cimetidine (Tagamet)

Hyperbilirubinemia

Increased cerebral pressures (Cushing reflex)

High spinal cord injury (interrupted sympathetic pathways)

Table 4. Causes of sinus tachycardia

Lack of sedation; pain

Hypovolemia; hypervolemia

Anoxia

Hyperdynamic states
    Large heat loss; burns
    Fever
    Sepsis
    Anemia

Drugs
    Atropine
    Aminophylline
    Pavulon
    Sympathomimetic agents

resisted until the possible etiologic factors are explored. During this period, the patient should be carefully monitored. Only then should suppression with lidocaine be considered. Causes of PVCs encountered in post-trauma patients are listed in Table 5.

III. **Hypertension**   Hypertension in the trauma victim may represent a pre-injury problem that may cause a potassium deficiency induced by diuretic treatment. Causes of trauma-induced hypertension are listed in Table 6. The primary decision is whether or not to reduce the blood pressure. This decision depends upon the etiology and/or presence of cardiac failure. Vascular overload may be treated with diuretics and/or fluid

Table 5. Causes of PVCs

Hypoxia

Electrolyte imbalance (particularly low potassium and low calcium)

Drugs
    Aminophylline
    Digitalis preparations
    Beta-sympathomimetics
    Dobutamine
    Dopamine
    Epinephrine
    Isoproterenol

Vagal stimulation

Psychic stimulation (lack of sedation; pain)

Sepsis

Intracardiac lines

Cardiac contusion

Pulmonary embolus

Myocardial ischemia

Table 6.   Causes of trauma-induced hypertension

Hypervolemia; hypovolemia

Inadequate sedation; pain

Hypoxia

Drugs
    Pavulon
    Tricyclic antidepressants with alpha-sympathomimetics

Head injury

Cushing reflex

Compensatory response to cerebral arterial spasm

Hypothermia

restriction. Heart failure associated with hypertension may be treated with an arteriolar dilator such as nitroprusside (Nipride), phentolamine (Regitine), hydralazine (Apresoline), or minipress (Prazosin), or with combined arteriovenous dilators such as nitroglycerin, given either i.v. or by skin paste. Nitroprusside and phentolamine are particularly useful in that they may be regulated by intravenous drip to produce the desired response.

Hypertension associated with head injury or intracerebral bleeding is a dilemma. The high pressure may be viewed as a contributor to increased intracranial pressure or as a risk factor for intracerebral bleeding. On the other hand, the high pressure may represent a response that is necessary to produce adequate cerebral perfusion. The usual compromise is to leave moderate hypertension untreated and to cautiously reduce severely elevated blood pressure to a high, normal range. The neurosurgeon plays the leading role in this decision.

Hypovolemia may cause hypertension secondary to a catecholamine response. The therapy, in this case, is volume expansion, not an anti-hypertensive medication.

Hypothermia may cause significant hypertension (see p. 375).

20
RENAL INSUFFICIENCY

I. **Renal Failure**   The major causes of posttraumatic renal insufficiency are relatively few and consist of
   —Shock
   —Sepsis
   —Drug toxicity
   —Hemoglobinuria
   —Myoglobinuria
   —Obstruction

Renal insufficiency becomes apparent in one of three ways. In order of increasing subtlety, the clinical manifestations of renal failure are
   —Anuria
   —Oliguria
   —Nonoliguric renal failure

The mortality following oliguric posttraumatic renal failure is about 80–90% and that following nonoliguric posttraumatic renal failure is about 50%. The high mortality associated with any form of renal failure justifies vigorous therapeutic efforts aimed at the prevention of the problem in any form, even at the risk of producing pulmonary congestion. The difference in mortality between oliguric and nonoliguric renal failure justifies vigorous efforts to prevent conversion of nonoliguric renal failure to oliguric renal failure.

A. **Manifestations of Renal Failure**

   1. **Anuria**   Total cessation of urine production (anuria) usually results from obstruction of the renal excretory system or of the renovascular system. Obstruction in the Foley catheter, bilateral ureteral obstruction, or bilateral renal arterial obstruction are typical causes. The Foley catheter may be checked by irrigation or replacement. The possibility of bilateral ureteral obstruction may be evaluated by ultrasound. The presence of arterial occlusion can be verified or excluded by radioactive hippurate renal scan or arteriography. Should none of these conditions be present, acute renal parenchymal failure is the likely diagnosis.

   2. **Oliguria**   If the patient is oliguric, the clinical and investigative approach changes. Obstruction is no longer the chief reversible etiology. Hypovolemia (prerenal failure), sepsis, and drug toxicity become the major concerns. Attention is directed to ensuring normal plasma volume and cardiovascular function, withdrawal of drugs known to be nephrotoxic, and consideration of

trials of osmotic agents (mannitol) or diuretics such as furosemide (Lasix) and ethacrynic acid (Edecrin). If the patient's volume status is unknown, it is usually necessary to insert a central venous line or Swan-Ganz catheter and conduct a formal fluid challenge (see p. 342). If inotropic support is considered, the agent is usually either dopamine or dobutamine. Advantages of dopamine lie in its dopaminergic action, increasing renal blood flow and urine volume. Dobutamine, on the other hand, lacks dopaminergic and alpha effects, but increases tissue perfusion by its effect on myocardial contraction. A Swan-Ganz catheter is invaluable in managing these medications. Finally, a consideration of sepsis as the etiology of acute renal failure is always indicated.

The major nephrotoxic drugs encountered in an intensive care unit are the aminoglycoside antibiotics. These drugs may cause an elevation of the blood urea nitrogen (BUN) and creatinine and a decrease in the creatinine clearance. The onset of the toxic effect on the kidney is usually gradual and may appear after cessation of antibiotic use. Most often the damage clears spontaneously if further exposure to the offending drug is avoided. Aminoglycosides can be monitored by blood level determinations and, if levels are restricted to therapeutic ranges, toxicity is very uncommon.

Other drugs may be associated with renal damage. The penicillins, particularly methicillin, may lead to interstitial nephritis and progressive renal failure. This entity is frequently associated with eosinophilia and eosinophiles in the urinary sediment. Cephalosporins, vancomycin, sulfonamides, and amphotericin B all have renal toxicity.

When oliguria is persistent and cannot be explained other than by the supposition of the appearance of renal failure, an attempt often is made to see if the kidneys are capable of producing a greater urine flow by a test dose of mannitol (100 ml of a 20% solution i.v.) and/or furosemide (40–80 mg i.v., initially, followed by geometrically increasing doses in rapid succession to a total of 320 mg). The theory is that the flow will lead to a better prognosis, converting the patient from oliguric renal failure to nonoliguric renal failure. The danger in this approach is that any diuresis provoked by these agents may lead to worsening of existing hypovolemia and prerenal failure. There may be a further nephrotoxic insult to the kidneys if furosemide is administered. Usually, a response to furosemide implies oliguria, which is usually secondary to decreased renal blood flow. Failure to respond to furosemide implies renal parenchymal dysfunction. Renal function parameters may help to define prerenal and renal parenchymal failure (see p. 352).

3. **Nonoliguric renal failure** The evaluation of nonoliguric renal failure is a controversial area. The problem lies in the definition of renal dysfunction. The presence of a renal problem is obvious to all if, in spite of a good urine output, there is a steadily rising serum creatinine (**azotemia**) and a falling creatinine clearance. It is less obvious if the sole difficulty is inability to concentrate the urine, i.e., a free water clearance that approaches zero. Usually urinary output is "normal," yet there is glomerular and tubular dysfunction. The causes of nonoliguric and oliguric renal failure are the same.

4. **Hemoglobinuria—myoglobinuria** Hemoglobinuria most commonly is the result of a hemolytic transfusion reaction. Myoglobinuria most commonly results from ischemic and/or contused muscle. Urine for hemoglobin or myoglobin should be checked in patients with transfusion reactions or muscle ischemia or damage. If there is difficulty in obtaining a urinary hemoglobin or myoglobin level, the urine can be checked with a dipstick for blood. If the dipstick test is positive and there are no red blood cells seen on microscopy, this suggests myoglobinuria or hemoglobinuria.

Therapy is directed at maintaining a urinary output of about 100 cc/hr with crystalloids and/or colloids. Mannitol may be used if brisk diuresis does not follow an appropriate volume infusion. Intravascular volume expansion and left ventricular performance should be optimal to maintain renal blood flow. If the urine is acidic, the patient should be administered bicarbonate to prevent pigment precipitation in the tubules. Serial creatinine and free water clearance determinations should be followed. See pp. 41 and 277.

B. **Diagnosis** Most renal function tests evaluate glomerular and/or tubular function. Creatinine clearance is the clinical test that primarily reflects glomerular function. Tubular function is primarily reflected by urinary sodium and osmolality.

Glomerular function may deteriorate secondary to a decrease in renal blood flow or renal parenchymal failure. This is reflected as a decreased **creatinine clearance**, an elevated serum creatinine, and/or a fall in urine creatinine excreted each 24 hr.

If the tubules are damaged, as in renal parenchymal failure, they lose their ability to concentrate. Loss of concentrating ability results in isosthenuria, i.e., the urinary osmolality approaches that of the serum. If the patient has decreased renal blood flow and the tubules are intact, the urine is concentrated. If the urine is concentrated, the urine osmolality is significantly higher than the plasma osmolality. If the tubules are intact and the patient has decreased renal blood flow, sodium is usually conserved. The **sodium fractional excretion** is used to look at glomerular and tubular function to discern the presence of prerenal versus renal parenchymal failure in oliguric patients.

$$\text{Sodium fractional excretion} = \frac{\text{U/P Na}}{\text{U/P Creat}} \times 100$$

Free water clearance (FWC) is a reflection of the tubule's ability to concentrate urine. Normally, FWC is more negative than -30. If FWC becomes less negative than -30, or approaches zero, tubular dysfunction secondary to renal parenchymal failure may be present. If FWC is more negative than -30, tubular function is generally normal. Diabetes insipidus, mannitol, radiographic contrast dye, and "polyuria of recovery" may cause the FWC to approach zero, yet tubular function is not defective.

Free water clearance is calculated as UOP − (U/P osmolality × UOP), where UOP is urine output in cc/hr.

Index	Prerenal failure	Renal failure
U/P osmolality	>1.5	<1.2
Urinary sodium	≤ 20 mEq/liter	>20 mEq/liter
U/P creatinine	>20	<20
Free water clearance	−30 to −60	0 to −30
Sodium fractional excretion	<1	>1
Creatinine clearance	↓	↓

The urine in prerenal failure appears relatively normal, while the urine frequently reveals casts in renal failure.

C. **Management of acute renal failure** In general, the oliguric phase lasts from 1–5 weeks. The urinary output during this phase is approximately 10–50 cc/day. The diuretic phase manifests with a gradual increase in urinary volume. This is followed shortly by a fall in the serum creatinine, an increase in the excretion of waste products, and restoration of concentrating ability of the tubules. The management of nonoliguric failure is simpler than the oliguric form, since fluid administration may be more liberal and hyperkalemia occurs less frequently.

1. **Fluid balance** The objective of fluid administration is to provide adequate cellular hydration without inducing fluid overload (congestive heart failure). The insensible losses of water per day are approximately 1,000 cc. Endogenous metabolism supplies about 400 cc of water/day. Therefore, there is a necessity to administer approximately 500–600 cc of fluid/day plus ongoing losses. Ongoing losses consist of urinary volume, sweating, nasogastric output, etc. Frequently, there is significant hemodynamic instability secondary to third-space losses, septic vasodilation, etc., and intravascular volume will have to be more liberal.

2. **Sodium** Forty-five to 75 mEq of sodium should be administered per day. There is a greater need for sodium infusion if there are concomitant gastrointestinal losses. The serum sodium level should be sequentially followed.

3. **Potassium** Hyperkalemia is the most frequently occurring and life-threatening electrolyte abnormality in acute renal failure. The major concern is ventricular fibrillation. Continuous cardiac monitoring and frequent determinations of serum potassium levels are indicated. EKG changes frequently reveal peaked T-waves and/or flat P-waves. Treatment is dictated by the serum potassium level and consists of the following: removal of potassium from intravenous fluids; use of exchange resins; dextrose-insulin infusion; administration of bicarbonate if the patient is acidotic; administration of calcium if hyperkalemia becomes severe; and dialysis for recalcitrant hyperkalemia.

4. **Calcium** The patient usually has hypocalcemia secondary to hyperphosphatemia. Hypocalcemia may be exacerbated if there is infusion of bicar-

bonate with a subsequent rapid change in the pH toward a more alkaline level.

5. **Phosphate** Usually the phosphate level is elevated secondary to inadequate renal excretion. Administration of Amphojel (aluminum hydroxide) with enteric feedings will decrease the amount of phosphorous absorption from the GI tract.

6. **Magnesium** Patients with acute renal failure tend to develop hypermagnesemia with resultant hypotension and cardiac blocks. The majority of antacids contain magnesium. If an antacid is indicated, it should be administered as Amphojel, since it contains no magnesium.

7. **Platelet dysfunction** With a BUN greater than 100, there is frequently an associated platelet defect. Many of these patients are under stressful situations and prone to upper gastrointestinal stress bleeding. If a patient develops a coagulation problem and the BUN is greater than 100, dialysis should be considered.

8. **Nutritional support** The objective, as with any nutritional support, is to maintain visceral protein compartment expansion. The goal in the patient with renal failure is to maintain visceral proteins without exacerbating azotemia. Calories are required to minimize protein breakdown and, consequently, azotemia. Since there is a need for fluid restriction, calories must be administered in a concentrated fashion. Calories are primarily administered as hypertonic glucose either PO or parenterally, if the GI tract does not work. Essential amino acids are primarily administered with a maximum of about 40 gm of protein/day to minimize azotemia (see p. 447).

   Patients with acute renal failure tend to develop hypermagnesemia, hyperkalemia, and hyperphosphatemia. With administration of carbohydrates and the induction of anabolism, these values tend to decline. The serum magnesium, phosphorus, and potassium levels need to be frequently evaluated with administration of carbohydrates (glucose).

9. **Dialysis** The primary indications for dialysis are
      —Pulmonary edema
      —Hyperkalemia
      —Metabolic acidosis
      —Uremic encephalopathy (seizures)
      —Coagulopathy (thrombasthenia)

The choice between hemodialysis and peritoneal dialysis is often determined by the patient's general condition. Hemodynamic instability and/or a bleeding tendency would favor the use of peritoneal dialysis. Peritoneal dialysis is less effective per unit of time than hemodialysis, but requires less technically trained staff for administration. Hemodialysis is more effective than peritoneal dialysis per unit of time, but is more difficult to administer from the technical standpoint. With hemodialysis, there is less ability to control rapid fluid shifts from the patient. This is a detriment to the hemodynamically unstable patient. Hemodialysis does require some degree of anticoagulation. Even if regional heparinization is used, there is poor ability to control systemic anticoagulation; therefore, a potential danger to the multiple trauma patient may exist. Hypoxia and hypovolemia commonly occur during hemodialysis. Arterial blood gases and intravascular monitoring should be considered during hemodialysis. A very unstable patient may need Swan-Ganz catheter monitoring and/or consideration for peritoneal dialysis. All medication orders should be reviewed and dosages adjusted on a daily basis in accordance with renal excretory function (see Table 1).

Many antibiotics require modification during renal insufficiency. The following is a recommendation for antibiotic supplementation during or following peritoneal dialysis or hemodialysis.

a. Peritoneal dialysis

(1) **Aminoglycosides** The patient receives the estimated dose/24 hr based on his creatinine clearance. The aminoglycoside may be added to the dialysis fluid at a concentration equal to the desired serum level. Frequent serum aminoglycoside levels must be obtained to accurately dose the patient.

(2) **Flucytosine** Dosage modification is necessary, but the exact dosage is unknown.

(3) **Cephalothin** 1 gm q12–24h, plus 1 gm q6–12h during dialysis

(4) **Carbenicillin** 2 gm i.v. during dialysis

(5) **Penicillin** Dosage modification is necessary, but the exact dosage is not known.

(6) **Ticarcillin** 2 gm q12h, plus 3 gm q12h during dialysis

(7) **Vancomycin** Dosage is governed by the serum levels and those recommendations made for the aminoglycosides.

b. Hemodialysis

(1) **Aminoglycosides** One-half of the entire usual single dose is given after dialysis and supplemented, if necessary, depending on a 1-hr post-dialysis serum aminoglycoside level, which is obtained post-aminoglycoside infusion.

(2) **Flucytosine** 25–50 mg/kg after dialysis. Monitor the serum levels frequently and supplement, if necessary.

(3) **Cephalothin** 1 gm q12–14h, plus 1 gm before and after each dialysis

(4) **Ampicillin** 0.5–1 gm q24h, with an additional 500 mg after dialysis

(5) **Carbenicillin** 2 gm q12–24h, plus 2 gm after dialysis

(6) **Penicillin** Modification is necessary, but the exact dosage is not known.

(7) **Ticarcillin** 2 gm q12h, plus 3 gm after each dialysis

(8) **Cefoxitin** 1 gm q24–48h, plus 1–2 gm after each dialysis

(9) **Vancomycin** Doses subsequent to dialysis must be governed by serum levels.

10. **Drug modification** All medication orders should be reviewed and dosages adjusted on a daily basis in accordance with renal excretory function (see Table 1). A useful source of information regarding the use of drugs in the patient with renal insufficiency is Bennett, W. M. (1977) *Annals of Internal Medicine* 85:754.

Perspective

The multiply injured patient is at risk for the development of oliguric or non-oliguric renal failure. The patient is monitored with a 2-hr creatinine clearance and free water clearance each morning. The young trauma patient normally has a creatinine clearance of 140–200 ml/min during the first 3–5 days post-injury. A low creatinine clearance may be an indication of inadequate cardiac output, i.e., decreased renal blood flow. Renal failure will usually be detected prior to oliguria if a daily creatinine clearance is performed. During the first 3–5 days post-injury, a low creatinine clearance implies inadequate cardiac output or renal parenchymal insult from the initial "shock" state. A fall in creatinine clearance after the first 3–5 days is likely to reflect inadequate cardiac output, sepsis, or nephrotoxicity from drugs.

Great care should be devoted to minimizing sepsis in patients with acute renal failure, since **sepsis is the major cause of death in these patients.** Vascular catheters should be minimized and Foley catheters removed, if possible.

II. **Syndrome of inappropriate secretion of antidiuretic hormone** (SIADH) is diagnosed by the discovery of a low serum sodium concentration, a low serum osmolality, and an inappropriately concentrated urine, i.e., a urine osmolality greater than plasma

Table 1. Commonly used drugs requiring dosage reduction in renal failure

Antibiotics
  Penicillin, except nafcillin
  Cephalosporins, cephamycins
  Aminoglycosides
  Tetracyclines, except doxycycline
  Nalidixic acid (NegGram)
  Nitrofurantoin (Furadantin)
  Sulfonamides

Cardiac drugs
  Digoxin
  Nitroprusside (Nipride)
  Procainamide (Pronestyl)

Miscellaneous
  Acetylsalicylic acid (aspirin)
  Dilantin (phenytoin sodium)
  Pavulon (pancuronium bromide)
  Phenobarbital (Luminal)

osmolality. A urine sodium of greater than 40 mEq/liter is usually present. Since myxedema, adrenal insufficiency, and some chronic infections may produce this picture, these entities must be ruled out. If the serum sodium drops rapidly to levels below 120 mEq/liter, SIADH may result in mental confusion, vomiting, muscle twitching, or convulsions. Many drugs have been associated with the appearance of the syndrome (see Table 2). The treatment consists of withdrawing any suspect medication and restricting fluid intake. Hypertonic saline is employed only as a desperate measure.

A low serum sodium may suggest the diagnosis of SIADH, but it is not sufficient by itself. There are other causes of hyponatremia, which are excluded by measuring serum osmolality and evaluating the urine osmolality and sodium. For example, a markedly increased serum osmolality associated with an elevated serum blood glucose or BUN, excessive water loading, and chronic diuretic therapy may result in hyponatremia.

III. **Diabetes insipidus** in the trauma patient is almost always associated with severe head injury and a dismal prognosis. The diagnosis is usually suggested by marked polyuria. Other conditions in the trauma victim may lead to polyuria. A **nonphysiologic diuresis** (polyuria) usually results in hypernatremia, hyperosmolar serum, and an elevated BUN. A **physiologic diuresis** (polyuria), i.e., which maintains homeostasis, usually results in a normal or slightly low serum sodium, osmolality, and BUN. This physiologic diuresis usually results when stress abates and antidiuretic hormone (ADH) and aldosterone normalize or when excess fluids are administered. The etiology of polyuria in the head-injured patient is often a difficult diagnosis to make since a given patient may have hyperglycemia, may have received mannitol, or have diabetes insipidus. If the polyuria is an osmotic diuresis, the urine osmolality is generally ≥ 300; if the polyuria is due to diabetes insipidus, the urine osmolality is usually ≤ 150 mOsm. Certain drugs may cause a nephrogenic diabetes insipidus (see Table 3). Polyuria may occur secondary to hypercalcemia and/or hyperkalemia (Table 4).

The management of a patient with a severe head injury and diabetes insipidus can be quite a challenge because of the need to titrate the circulating volume to a level needed to support tissue perfusion, yet not so great as to elevate intracranial pressure. A Swan-Ganz catheter and an intravenous drip of vasopressin (Pitressin) (5 units of vasopressin in a liter of 0.22% saline) are usually required to control both circulatory volume and intracranial pressure. The ideal replacement fluid for hypernatremia is usually one-quarter normal saline, since the total body sodium is usually low or normal and the

Table 2. Commonly used drugs associated with hyponatremia

Barbiturates
Chlorpropamide (Diabinese)
Carbamazepine
Isoproterenol (Isuprel)
Mellaril (thioridazine)
Opiates
Tolbutamide (Orinase)
Thiazide diuretics
Tricyclic antidepressants

Table 3. Commonly used drugs associated with nephrogenic diabetes insipidus

High dose lithium
Methoxyflurane (Penthrane)
Declomycin (demeclocycline hydrochloride)
Phenytoin sodium (Dilantin)
Acetohexamide (Dymelor)
Tolazamide (Tolinase)
Propoxyphene (Darvon, Wygesic)

patient requires increased amounts of water and maintenance amounts of sodium. The fluid should not contain dextrose if large volumes are being administered, since hyperglycemia may occur and result in glycosuria, causing an osmotic diuresis.

Table 4. Common causes of polyuria

Physiologic
    Fluid excess
    Polyuria of recovery

Nonphysiologic
    Osmotic diuresis
        Mannitol
        Hyperglycemia
        Contrast dye
    Diabetes insipidus
    Sepsis

21
HEPATIC DYSFUNCTION

I. **Etiology** Hepatic dysfunction following major trauma is a relatively common problem. The epidemiologic setting of severe automobile accidents suggests a predisposing factor, since many accidents are associated with alcohol and other drug intoxications. However, the chief predisposing factors appear to be shock, anesthesia, massive blood transfusion, and prolonged operations. Clinically, the problem is the development of jaundice after trauma. The following is a list of common etiologies:

—Shock liver
—Benign postoperative cholestasis
—Hepatic venous congestion
—Increased pigment load
—Sepsis
—Drug induced
—Major hepatic resection
—Miscellaneous

A. **Shock liver** The hypoxic insult to the liver, secondary to hypotension, is probably the most significant factor contributing to the development of jaundice in the trauma patient.

Only occasionally does the investigation of posttraumatic jaundice lead to the identification of a single cause. Usually, several of the conditions listed above are present. Almost always, the hypotensive patient has received multiple blood transfusions, drugs, has had one or more operations and one or more bouts of hypoxia. Yet, shock alone leads to hepatic mitochondrial swelling and centrilobular necrosis. In the typical patient, the serum bilirubin rises to 5–20 mg % within 2–10 days after resuscitation, while the serum glutamic oxaloacetic transaminase (SGOT) ranges from 100–500 units/ml and the alkaline phosphatase increases to 2–3 times normal. The treatment of shock liver consists of supportive measures and the avoidance of drugs known to be dependent on hepatic mechanisms for inactivation or excretion. A partial list of such drugs commonly employed in intensive care units is given in Table 1. With these general measures, most patients with shock liver do well and appear to recover completely.

B. **Benign postoperative cholestasis** A second type of liver injury is associated with shock and coincident hypoxia, benign postoperative cholestasis. Patients with this condition have obstructive liver chemistries with bilirubins in the 10–40 mg % range and markedly elevated alkaline phosphatases. SGOT levels are usually less than 200 units/ml. Uneventful recovery is the rule.

Table 1. Drugs to avoid in liver disease

Sedatives—narcotics
  All narcotics, including fentanyl
  Most benzodiazepines   (The metabolism of lorazepam (Ativan) is probably not impaired with hepatic dysfunction.)
  Phenothiazines
  Some barbiturates, e.g., pentobarbital (Nembutal)

Analgesics
  Aspirin
  Acetaminophen

Antibiotics
  Chloramphenicol
  Nafcillin, oxacillin
  Erythromycin estolate
  Tetracyclines
  Clindamycin (?)

Antiarrhythmics—local anesthetics
  Lidocaine (Xylocaine)

Miscellaneous
  Aminophylline
  Dilantin
  Hyperalimentation solutions   (Modified solutions containing less aromatic amino acids, more arginine, and more branched chain amino acids seem better.)
  Intralipid   (Some claim that this triggers fatty metamorphosis of the liver. We have found it, in moderation, to be a useful source of calories in treating advanced liver disease.)
  Halothane

C. **Hepatic venous congestion** A third type of hypoxic liver damage is related to prolonged venous congestion of the liver. Usually this condition is called cardiac jaundice and occurs in patients with mitral stenosis and constrictive pericarditis. Centrilobular necrosis and hemorrhage result from the elevated venous pressure and presumed anoxia. A bilirubin up to 8 mg %, alkaline phosphatase twice normal, and SGOT greater than 400 units/ml have been observed. This same condition has been suspected to occur in persons on prolonged mechanical ventilation, particularly those with high values of PEEP. Hypervolemia and massive crystalloid infusion may contribute to hepatic edema.

D. **Increased pigment load** Overt jaundice following a hemolytic reaction is uncommon without hepatic parenchymal dysfunction. The usual response to intravascular hemolysis is a decrease in the haptoglobin level, the appearance of free hemoglobin in the blood and urine, and an increased unconjugated (indirect) bilirubin. Since unconjugated bilirubin is strongly protein-bound, it is limited to the vascular space, does not appear in the interstitial fluid, and is not filtered by the kidney. Massive hemolysis may saturate both the reticuloendothelial system (with red blood cell debris) and the bilirubin excretory system, allowing conjugated (direct) bilirubin to reflux into the blood. Since conjugated bilirubin is more soluble and less strongly protein-bound than unconjugated bilirubin, it diffuses into the interstitial fluid and appears in the urine. Following a hemolytic episode, conjugated bilirubin levels greater than 15% of the total bilirubin concentration indicate hepatic dysfunction. A serum bilirubin greater than 5 mg % usually implies some element of hepatic parenchymal dysfunction.

Posttraumatic hemolysis usually results from the destruction of transfused red blood cells which have a shortened life span because of senescence during storage, mechanical damage during transfusion, or immunologic reactions. Large quantities of blood may be hemolyzed during the reabsorption of a large hematoma. Sometimes hemolysis may be triggered by drugs, such as aspirin, chloramphenicol, sulfonamides, or nitrofurantoin in glucose-6-phosphatase-deficient individuals. Other drugs, such as high doses of penicillin or alpha-methyl-dopa, may cause hemolysis by immunologic mechanisms.

E. **Sepsis** Sepsis is not infrequently associated with jaundice. The mechanism is uncertain. The bilirubin may be elevated as an isolated finding or accompanied with an elevation of the hepatocellular and/or alkaline phosphatase enzymes. When infection is superimposed on the shocked liver, the prognosis is grave.

F. **Drug induced** Various drugs may cause jaundice by allergic or idiosyncratic reactions. A patient with such a reaction may present with a picture of cellular hepatitis, as with halothane (Fluothane) or isoniazid (INH) toxicity, or cholestatic jaundice, as with erythromycin estolate (Ilosone), chlorpromazine (Thorazine), or chlorothiazide (Diuril) toxicity. Narcotics such as morphine cause an intrahepatic cholestasis secondary to an increase in biliary ductal pressure. Table 1 lists drugs that produce or exacerbate hepatic dysfunction.

G. **Major hepatic resection** Major liver resections may be associated with jaundice, since the hepatocellular mass has been decreased. Frequently, there has been a significant period of ischemia, i.e., "shock liver."

H. **Miscellaneous** A number of miscellaneous conditions may present as jaundice. Surgical misadventures may result in hepatic dysfunction. Ligation of the hepatic artery or of the biliary duct are examples. Hepatic artery ligation may have been undertaken deliberately to control severe hepatic bleeding encountered during abdominal exploration. Interestingly, the degree of hepatic necrosis following a deliberate hepatic artery ligation is often surprisingly small. Acute pancreatitis may result in obstructive jaundice. The patient may have had a pre-injury disease, such as hepatitis. Excess carbohydrate calories may cause liver dysfunction (see p. 436).

II. **Manifestations**

A. Jaundice

B. Encephalopathy

C. Hepatomegaly

D. Acholic stools

III. **Laboratory**

  A. Hyperbilirubinemia

  B. Elevated SGOT, SGPT, LDH, or alkaline phosphatase

  C. Elevated BSP

  D. Elevated prothrombin time

  E. Elevated ammonia

  F. Hypoalbuminemia

IV. **Management** In general, the approach to a patient who develops postoperative jaundice consists of

  A. Determination of any history of prior liver disease or predisposing factors

  B. Determination of whether the disorder is primarily hepatocellular or obstructive

  C. **Evaluation of the possibility of sepsis**

  D. Review of all medications and anesthetics with hopes of identifying an offending agent and to exclude all drugs requiring hepatic metabolism

  E. Assessment of the role of hemolysis in the appearance of the jaundice

  F. Ensuring that PEEP is at minimal values compatible with adequate oxygenation and pulmonary function

  G. Support of the patient while investigations are made to identify a specific etiology, i.e., maintenance of tissue oxygen delivery

  H. Adjustment of hyperalimentation fluids   Current thinking favors reducing aromatic amino acids and supplying extra arginine and branched chain amino acids in patients with liver dysfunction. These alterations appear to minimize the changes in liver function tests that may be provoked by hyperalimentation. Careful monitoring of the serum ammonia level is indicated since it usually reflects excess nitrogen administration.

  Hepatic glucose intolerance (steatosis) is often encountered in patients with liver dysfunction. Caution must be exercised regarding the amount of carbohydrate calories that is administered. Either cyclic alimentation or the cautious substitution of lipid calories for glucose calories is favored over the use of large doses of insulin. Careful attention to blood glucose and, if Intralipid is used, to lipid levels is required. Hepatic steatosis is usually manifest by major elevations in the bilirubin, alkaline phosphatase, and hepatocellular enzymes. (See p. 448.)

I. Management of hepatic encephalopathy

1. Eradicate blood from the GI tract if hemorrhage has taken place.

2. Minimize drugs requiring hepatic metabolism.

3. Minimize protein intake; consider use of branched chain amino acids.

4. Clean out the colon to minimize the nitrogenous load.

5. Administer neomycin to decrease urease-producing bowel flora.

6. Lactulose appears to minimize encephalopathy.

7. **Vigorously evaluate the patient for a septic focus.**

8. Prevent hypokalemic alkalosis, which increases encephalopathy, with KCl infusion and intravascular expansion by albumin infusion.

Perspective

In survivors, hyperbilirubinemia generally clears by 10–14 days after injury. A progressive rise in the bilirubin level is likely to be associated with sepsis and/or subsequent death.

22

STRESS GASTROINTESTINAL
ULCERATION

Acute gastric and/or duodenal ulceration may develop following "stress insults." These stress states are
  —Shock
  —Sepsis
  —CNS trauma
  —Hypoxia
  —Multiple organ failure
  —Multiple trauma
  —Combinations of these factors

Hemorrhage is the most frequent complication that occurs. Perforation occurs, but is less frequent than bleeding. Usually the ulcerations are located in the body and fundus of the stomach, but occasionally the duodenum or both regions are involved. The lesions are usually multiple and superficial, but occasionally single, large ulcerations occur in the stomach and/or duodenum. Clinical and subclinical lesions are very common in the patient who has incurred one of the above stress states.

I. Manifestations

  A. Signs

    1. Hemorrhage
       a. Blood from the nasogastric tube (varies from minimal guaiac positive results to gross, bright, red bleeding)
       b. Melena
       c. Shock ±

    2. Perforation
       a. Peritonitis
       b. Free air ± (x-ray)
       c. Abdominal distention
       d. "Septic" (fever, tachycardia)

  B. Symptoms Epigastric pain

C. **Laboratory data**

1. Falling hematocrit

2. Coagulopathy

3. Leukocytosis

D. **Diagnosis** Endoscopy is the means by which the extent and location of the gastric and/or duodenal lesions are identified.

II. **Treatment**

A. **Prophylaxis** The optimal therapy for stress gastrointestinal ulceration is prophylaxis. The primary mode of prophylaxis against stress gastrointestinal ulceration is by vigorously monitoring and controlling the gastric pH within a range of 4–5 during the above-mentioned stress states.

1. Antacid is titrated to whatever rate is required to control the gastric pH. This appears to be the most efficacious method of prophylaxis against stress gastrointestinal ulceration.

2. Cimetidine appears to be effective in prophylaxis against stress gastrointestinal ulceration, but does not appear to be as effective as antacid therapy. Cimetidine may occasionally need to be added to the antacid regimen to control the gastric pH.

3. Tube feedings supply the patient with nutritional support and buffer the gastric acid. If the patient will tolerate tube feedings, antacids are added only if necessary to maintain the gastric pH between 4 and 5.

B. **Medical therapy**

1. **Hemorrhage**
   a. Antacids
   b. Cimetidine
   c. Gastric lavage Lavage with ice saline primarily monitors the rate of hemorrhage, but may be of some therapeutic benefit.
   d. Instillation of Levophed by gastric lavage may be beneficial.
   e. Replace coagulation factors, if necessary (fresh frozen plasma; platelets)
   f. Maintain cardiovascular function.
   g. Consider vasopressin (Pitressin) infusion via the left gastric artery or by the i.v. route.
   h. **Remove stress insults, if possible.**

2. **Ulceration without hemorrhage**
   a. Control gastric pH (antacids, cimetidine, and/or feedings)
   b. **Remove stress insults, if possible.**

C. **Surgery**

1. **Hemorrhage**   Considerations for surgical intervention are
    —Elderly patient (tend toward early surgery)
    —Requirements for 6 units of blood within a 24-hr period without a major decrease in the rate of hemorrhage
    —Control the septic process surgically, if indicated; this may control the hemorrhage without a specific gastrointestinal procedure.
    —Bleeding in a patient who has a history of an ulcer diathesis
    —If the patient has stress bleeding and an underlying pathologic process which is not correctable, it is unlikely that the bleeding will be controlled medically.

    It is important to control any underlying septic process; otherwise, the gastrointestinal procedure is doomed to failure. A vagotomy is indicated in virtually 100% of the cases since it will decrease gastric mucosal blood flow at the time of the surgical procedure and will decrease acid production in the postoperative period.

    a. **Duodenal ulceration**
        (1)   Oversew the ulcer and perform a vagotomy and pyloroplasty, or
        (2)   Perform a vagotomy and antrectomy with oversew of the ulcer.
    b. **Solitary gastric ulceration**
        (1)   Perform a vagotomy and pyloroplasty with oversew or excision of the ulcer, or
        (2)   Perform a vagotomy and antrectomy with oversew or excision of the ulcer.
    c. **Multiple gastric ulcerations**
        (1)   Perform a vagotomy and pyloroplasty with oversew of the ulcers, or
        (2)   Perform a vagotomy and antrectomy with oversew of the ulcers, or
        (3)   Perform a total gastrectomy.

    In essence, a vagotomy is almost always indicated; the ulcer is usually oversewn or excised; the vagotomy is accompanied by a pyloroplasty or antrectomy, or a total gastrectomy is performed. Indications for antrectomy or total gastrectomy are more appropriate when ulceration is diffuse and bleeding is profuse.

2. **Perforation**
    a. **Duodenal**
        (1)   Vagotomy and pyloroplasty, or
        (2)   Duodenal patch with omentum, or
        (3)   Vagotomy and antrectomy with Billroth II anastomosis (if the patient is diagnosed **early** after perforation and there is a history of ulcer diathesis)

    The duodenal perforation is usually amenable to vagotomy and pyloroplasty; this is considered to be the optimal intervention in most cases.
    b. **Gastric**
        (1)   Vagotomy and pyloroplasty with ulcer excision, or
        (2)   Vagotomy and antrectomy with ulcer excision

23

MULTIPLE SYSTEMS FAILURE

Multiple systems failure is a not infrequent clinical entity which is seen in the patient who incurs a "major systemic insult." Clinically, these major insults are
—Shock
—Sepsis
—"Surgical misadventure"
—Major operative insult
—Multi-systems trauma
—Prolonged hypoxia, e.g., near-drowning

Cellular hypoxia and loss of cellular integrity in major organ systems is the common denominator in these conditions. Initially the patient may manifest with "obvious" renal insufficiency, cardiovascular insufficiency, and/or pulmonary insufficiency, or when considering the initial systemic insult, the patient may appear to be "relatively stable." After a couple of days, a major organ system begins to deteriorate. This single system failure may then stabilize and result in a gradual improvement over several days to several weeks. On the other hand, major deterioration in the single organ system may be followed by sequential multiple system deterioration and death.

Major clinical dysfunction is most apparent in pulmonary, cardiovascular, and renal function. Other physiologic systems which may deteriorate or be stressed include: coagulation, metabolism, hematology, gastrointestinal function, liver, immune system, nutrition, and central nervous function. Failure in these systems is usually more subtle.

I. **Manifestations** The following is a list of systems involved in the maintenance of homeostasis. Listed under each system are "clinical markers" of dysfunction or stress.

A. **Pulmonary**

1. $PaO_2/FiO_2 < 200$

2. Requirement of > 5 cm of PEEP

3. Mechanical ventilation for > 24 hr

4. Total compliance < 35 ml/cm H_2O

B. **Cardiovascular**

1. Hypotension (90 mm Hg or less systolic pressure)

2. Left ventricular stroke work index < 35

3. Pulmonary artery occluded pressure (wedge) > 20 mm Hg

4. Ventricular arrhythmias

C. **Renal**

1. Creatinine clearance < 75

2. Urine to plasma osmolarity ≤ 1.2

3. Oliguria with urinary sodium > 40 mEq/liter

D. **Coagulation**

1. Increased PT

2. Increased PTT

3. Platelet count $< 100,000/mm^3$

4. Increased fibrin split products

5. Requirement of > 3 units of FFP in 24 hr

E. **Metabolic**

1. Electrolytes
   a. Sodium < 130 or > 150 mEq/liter
   b. Potassium < 2.8 or > 6.0 mEq/liter

2. Glucose < 70 or > 300 mg %

3. pH < 7.3 or > 7.55

4. Inability to maintain body temperature, i.e., temperature $< 35°C$ or $> 39°C$

5. Lactate > 2.5 mEq/liter

F. **Hematologic**

1. WBC $< 5,000/mm^3$

2. Hematocrit < 33 (without blood loss)

3. Bone marrow depression, reticulocytes $< 1\%$ of RBCs

G. **Gastrointestinal**

1. Ileus (nasogastric output $> 1,000$ cc/day and/or inability to institute tube feedings)

2. Stress ulceration

3. Pancreatitis

H. Liver

1. Bilirubin ≥ 5 mg %

2. Elevated LDH, SGOT

3. PT elevation without an associated requirement for RBC transfusion

4. Albumin < 3 gm % with "adequate" nutritional support

5. Hyperammonemia

I. Immune system

1. Anergy—relative anergy

2. Sepsis (bacteremia)

3. Abscess

4. WBC $> 20,000/\text{mm}^3$

J. Nutrition

1. $> 10\%$ weight loss

2. Hypocaloric input > 7 days total (< 30 cal/kg/day)

3. Albumin < 3.0 gm %

4. Inadequate protein input (< 1 gm/kg/day)

K. Central nervous system

1. Unable to follow commands

2. Quadriplegic

3. Paraplegic

4. Sustained intracranial pressure > 15 mm Hg

II. **Treatment**   Inadequate perfusion, tissue hypoxia, and/or sepsis appear to be the three most common factors that incite or perpetuate sequential systems failure. The therapy is primarily directed toward the eradication of a septic process, if present, and support of the systems that are in failure. Necrotic tissue may cause multiple systems failure in the absence of frank suppuration.

Specific therapy includes
- —Eradicate the septic process with appropriate antibiotics and/or adequate external drainage.
- —Provide cardiovascular support by maintenance of a cardiac output (tissue perfusion) which meets the tissue oxygen demand.
- —Provide ventilatory support to minimize pulmonary shunt and correct any anemia to maintain arterial O_2 content.

—Provide nutritional support to supply adequate calories, protein, vitamins, water, minerals, and trace elements.

—Support specific failing systems as covered in other areas of this manual.

Perspective

Organ systems function and stress offers a clinical means of evaluating the patient's progress. If a patient has a fever and leukocytosis, but no system instability, it is most likely that the patient has either a nonseptic process or a "controlled" infectious process. If the PaO_2/FiO_2, creatinine clearance, level of consciousness, etc., are improving or stable, it is unlikely that further therapy is necessary. On the other hand, if there is system dysfunction and/or stress, the clinician must look vigorously for a septic process or necrotic tissue and "control it." In other words, if organ function is stressed and/or deteriorating, qualitatively or quantitatively, an aggressive posture must be adopted. A more aggressive approach usually entails a change in antibiotics, drainage of a septic process, or debridement of necrotic tissue.

24
NEAR DROWNING, HYPOTHERMIA, AND SMOKE INHALATION

As a part of the Emergency Medical Systems of Maryland, MIEMSS is frequently referred patients who have various emergent problems which may be isolated or associated with trauma. Since MIEMSS possesses a hyperbaric chamber and because of its position in the Emergency Medical System, patients who are subjected to near drowning, hypothermia, and smoke inhalation are frequently seen. The common denominator among these three entities is that they tend to produce multiple systems dysfunction. Near drowning usually causes multiple systems dysfunction secondary to hypoxia and pulmonary aspiration. Hypothermia affects all physiologic systems; its effects include metabolic depression and/or systems alterations such as arrhythmias and interstitial edema. Smoke inhalation frequently affects multiple physiologic systems secondary to hypoxia and the inhalation of combustion products. The sequel to these diseases may be minimal physiologic derangement, or the insult may lead to death within minutes to weeks.

I. **Near Drowning**   Near drowning refers to an initial recovery following immersion. There was previously felt to be a pathophysiologic difference between fresh and salt water drowning. The major physiologic alterations in drowning are usually secondary to hypoxia. Since aspiration is usually minimal, the type and amount of pulmonary aspirate is infrequently a significant factor. The following systems are frequently involved:
   —**Pulmonary**   Hypoxia is the primary factor which leads to multiple systems deterioration. Hypoxia occurs secondary to aspiration, laryngospasm, bronchospasm, and interstitial pulmonary edema.
   —**Cardiovascular**   Fluid shifts are variable and hypovolemia may result. Cardiac output may be impaired by hypovolemia and/or myocardial depression secondary to hypoxia. Atrial fibrillation and premature ventricular contractions are relatively common.
   —**Central nervous system**   Hypoxic encephalopathy is relatively common.
   —**Renal**   Transient azotemia may occur secondary to hypoxia, shock, and/or hemoglobinuria. Occasionally, the patient will develop acute renal failure.
   —**Electrolytes**   Electrolytic abnormalities are usually not clinically significant.
   —**Acid-base balance**   Acidosis is common and may be respiratory and/or metabolic.
   —**Hematologic**   Fresh water drowning may be associated with a hemolytic process. Hemolysis usually implies significant aspiration.

Note Hypothermia may contribute to central nervous system and cardiac depression if immersion took place in a cold environment (see p. 376).

A. Manifestations

1. **Pulmonary** The patient may be apneic, dyspneic, or spontaneously breathing without difficulty. Physical examination may reveal rales, rhonchi, or wheezing.

2. **Central nervous system** CNS manifestations are variable. The patient may be alert, lethargic, decorticate, or flaccid. Seizure activity is not uncommon.

3. **Cardiovascular** Due to hypoperfusion, the patient may be cool, tachycardic, oliguric, and/or may show pallor.

B. Diagnosis

The following evaluations are recommended to completely evaluate the near drowning victim: chest x-ray (serial), arterial blood gases (ABG), EKG, electrolytes, CBC, plasma hemoglobin, BUN, creatinine, creatinine clearance, urinalysis, temperature, and cervical spine film (if diving accident).

C. Treatment

1. The patient may need only supplemental oxygen or intubation and administration of IMV-PEEP or CPAP (see p. 316).

2. The patient may need bronchodilator therapy for bronchospasm.

3. If the patient has a decreased level of consciousness and history of trauma, a CAT scan should be considered to rule out intracranial trauma. Steroids and hyperventilation may be helpful if the patient has significant cerebral edema (see p. 222).

4. Arrhythmias are treated in a manner nonspecific for drowning.

5. The patient should have at least a central venous pressure line. A Swan-Ganz catheter may be needed for persistent hypotension, severe metabolic acidosis, persistent oliguria, or a large pulmonary shunt (hypoxia requiring greater than 8 cm of PEEP) (see p. 341).

6. If hemoglobinuria is present, urinary output should be maintained at approximately 100 cc/hr. Serial creatinine clearance determinations should be performed (see p. 351).

7. If the patient is hypothermic, rewarming should be instituted (see p. 377).

8. Metabolic acidosis usually responds to restoration of the cardiac output; however, bicarbonate administration may be necessary.

Perspective

In general, aggressive therapy is advisable in all cases of near drowning victims, especially if immersion has taken place in a cold environment. It is very difficult to evaluate the patient and predict eventual neurologic function.

II. **Hypothermia**   Hypothermia, defined as a core temperature of 95°F (35°C) or less, is relatively common in trauma victims during the winter. In addition to prolonged exposure to the elements caused by time delays in locating and extracting the victim from the scene of injury, other factors predispose to hypothermia: alcohol ingestion; other drugs, the most common being barbiturates and phenothiazines; old age; and hypothyroidism. Severe hypothermia produces a clinical picture that may be confused with myxedemic coma. The signs of coma are edema, hoarseness, lethargy, and diminished deep tendon reflexes. A number of other disease states predispose to hypothermia: diabetic ketoacidosis; myocardial infarction; sepsis; hypoglycemia; parkinsonism; anorexia nervosa; cerebral vascular disease; cerebral trauma; spinal cord injuries; burns; and malnutrition.

Note   Prolonged exposure to the elements (e.g., if trapped in a vehicle) not infrequently coupled with alcohol abuse is the most common trauma-related setting. Appropriate investigation should define causes of hypothermia other than exposure.

The diagnosis of hypothermia is made by taking the patient's temperature. Standard glass thermometers do not record temperatures below 94°F (34°C); hence, temperatures recorded at the lower limits of a standard thermometer require the use of a low reading glass thermometer or rectal thermocouple probe.

A. **Manifestations**

1. **Neuromuscular**   Shivering is a normal response to heat loss. Below 91.4°F (33°C), the beneficial effects of shivering are inhibited by progressive muscle rigidity. Muscle tone is lost below 80.6°F (27°C). Some shivering may occur down to 75.2°F (24°C). At low temperatures, shivering may only be detectable as EKG artifacts.

2. **Vascular**   If not impaired by drugs or vascular disease, the initial, normal peripheral response to cold is vasoconstriction which may cause significant hypertension. At about 89.6°F (32°C), arteriolar paralysis occurs and peripheral pallor changes to erythema; further heat loss then occurs. At this temperature, capillary permeability increases and edema results.

3. **Central nervous system**   As the core temperature decreases, mentation progressively deteriorates. Mood alterations, amnesia, impaired motor function, and diminished deep tendon reflexes are seen. Below 86°F (30°C), loss of consciousness with unreactive dilated pupils is seen. Loss of sensation, which

precedes loss of consciousness, may result in a feeling of well-being and lead to unprotective activity.

4. **Cardiac** The initial response to cold is tachycardia. Below 89.6°F (32°C), bradycardia is noted. Initially, the blood pressure rises, but it subsequently falls with cooling. As the core temperature drops, there is a progressive depression of the cardiac output. When the core temperature drops below 82.4°F (28°C) atrial or ventricular fibrillation or asystole can occur. EKG changes in hypothermia include prolongation of the QT interval and the QRS complex, and the classic J (Osborn) waves. J waves are a positive reflection appearing after the QRS complex before the S-T segment. They are best seen in the lateral precordial leads (V_4–V_6). The amplitude of the J wave is proportional to the degree of hypothermia.

5. **Respiratory** The initial response to cold is tachypnea. Deepening hypothermia results in a decrease in the respiratory rate. At lower temperatures, respirations may be infrequent enough to appear as apnea. Severe bronchorrhea coupled with a diminished cough reflex, caused by hypothermia, can result in partial or complete airway obstruction. For this reason, aspiration and pneumonia are not unusual complications of hypothermia.

> | Note | The CNS, cardiovascular, and respiratory manifestations of severe hypothermia may produce a clinical picture compatible with death, i.e., the patient may be unconscious, have fixed dilated pupils, absent deep tendon reflexes, undetectable pulse, and "apnea." **Remember, a cold patient cannot be declared dead.**

6. **Renal** A diuresis may be associated with hypothermia when peripheral vasoconstriction occurs. The diuresis can lead to hemoconcentration and hypovolemia. As the patient is rewarmed, the peripheral vascular bed dilates, and the true hypovolemic state of the patient may become evident. If appropriate fluid therapy is not administered, hypovolemic shock may result.

7. **Hematologic** The hematocrit may rise due to hemoconcentration. An increase in blood viscosity below 80.6°F (27°C), a decreased leukocyte and platelet count, a decreased platelet adhesiveness, and increased fibrinolytic activity may be seen. Disseminated intravascular coagulopathy has been described in hypothermia.

8. **Gastrointestinal** At 93.2°F (34°C) gastrointestinal mobility is affected and an ileus may be seen. The ability of the liver to detoxify and metabolize substances is diminished.

Hypothermia inhibits the pancreatic release of insulin and inhibits the peripheral utilization of glucose, resulting in hyperglycemia. Exogenously administered insulin may not be active and is slowly metabolized; hence, insulin therapy for hyperglycemia must be prudently monitored. When rewarming occurs, large amounts of administered insulin which become biologically active can result in hypoglycemia. As with insulin, all drugs given during hypothermia must be given cautiously because high blood levels may be inadvertently attained due to a decrease in metabolism. Gastrointestinal bleeding and pancreatitis have been described in hypothermia.

B. Management

1. **Temperature monitoring** This should be done with a rectal thermometer or probe. Insertion of an esophageal probe could result in cardiac arrhythmias.

2. **Vital signs**

3. Continuous **EKG monitoring**

4. Catheterization of the urinary bladder and monitoring of **urinary output.**

5. Admitting and serial **chest x-rays**

6. **Laboratory data** (serial determinations)
   a. Hb/Hct
   b. Glucose
   c. Coagulation profile
   d. Amylase
   e. Renal function
   f. ABG

> **Note** Uncorrected arterial PO_2 and PCO_2 are higher than the true corrected values. Consistent acid-base abnormalities are not the rule. However, the patient is best managed by interpretation of uncorrected arterial blood gases. Monitoring of the arterial pH is particularly important as rewarming occurs. As the peripheral vasculature dilates and stagnant acidotic products are mobilized into the general circulation, profound acidosis may be seen. Bicarbonate should be given judiciously.

7. **General support**
   a. Minimal handling of the patient is necessary to prevent cardiac arrhythmias, particularly ventricular fibrillation.
   b. Deliver O_2 via face mask or endotracheal tube and controlled mechanical support. Endotracheal intubation must be done cautiously in an attempt to avoid ventricular fibrillation. Endotracheal suctioning of secretions should be done only when necessary.
   c. Administer warm i.v. solutions.
   d. Use a CVP line to monitor volume status. The heart should not be entered by the catheter, to avoid precipitation of cardiac arrhythmias.
   e. Generally, cardiac arrhythmias such as atrial disturbances and bradycardia do not require specific treatment, since they revert to normal upon rewarming. The cold heart is not responsive to atropine, pacing, or coun-

tershock. Ventricular fibrillation is usually refractory to countershock until the core temperature is increased to about 82.4°F (28°C). External cardiac massage is necessary until a temperature is reached at which the ventricular fibrillation can be successfully treated by countershock.

f. All drugs should be given judiciously. Accumulated nonactive, and non-metabolized drugs in the hypothermic state may result in inadvertent overdosing on rewarming. Insulin, particularly, must be given with caution. Usually only extreme hyperglycemic states require treatment.

g. Should ventricular fibrillation occur, an initial countershock should be tried. If not effective, external cardiac massage is performed until a core temperature of approximately 82.4°F (28°C) is reached. Countershock is tried again; if still not effective, cardiac massage and rewarming should continue until a core temperature is reached at which countershock is effective.

h. When a core temperature of approximately 90°F (32°C) is reached, placement of a Swan-Ganz catheter is indicated if hemodynamic stability is not easily maintained by fluid administration. Prior to this temperature, placement of such a catheter may precipitate cardiac arrhythmias. Also, information gained (such as a cardiac output) is difficult to interpret clinically at low temperatures.

8. **Rewarming** The ultimate goal in the treatment of hypothermia is to safely rewarm the patient. The initial goal should be to rapidly attain a core temperature of 86°F (30°C) to prevent cardiac arrhythmias, including ventricular fibrillation and asystole. Rewarming can be accomplished using internal (central) or external methods. "Cold shock" can occur if only external methods are used. As the peripheral vascular bed opens up, a centrally depressed cool heart may be unable to respond with an appropriate cardiac output. In addition, acidemia resulting from the release of stagnant metabolic products from the periphery may precipitate ventricular fibrillation. The following measures are recommended to accomplish central rewarming:

a. If the patient is intubated, a cascade humidifying device is added to the ventilator, allowing for the delivery of heated air at 104°F (40°C).

b. Plasma expanders and crystalloids are run through a warming coil and warm water bath set ideally at 104°F (40°C). Banked blood should be administered through a warming coil about 95°F (35°C). If rapid fluid administration is required to treat shock, crystalloid i.v. fluids warmed to a temperature of 110°F (43.3°C) are delivered rapidly without passage through a coil.

c. Many trauma patients require peritoneal lavage to rule out intra-abdominal injury. This procedure can be used as a diagnostic and therapeutic modality in the hypothermic patient. When used therapeutically for rewarming, 1 liter of potassium-free normal saline is run rapidly into the peritoneal cavity. Ideally, the fluid should be 110°F (43.3°C). If a standardized water heating bath is not available, the fluid should be heated by flowing tap water or by some other method until it feels like it is about 4–5°F above body temperature. Once the fluid is run in, it should be

Table 1. Temperature conversions

37°C = 98.6°F
35°C = 95.0°F
33°C = 91.4°F
31°C = 87.8°F
29°C = 84.2°F
27°C = 80.6°F
25°C = 77.0°F
23°C = 73.4°F

Temperature conversion formulas
$$°C = 5/9 \, (°F - 32)$$
$$°F = (9/5 \times °C) + 32$$

siphoned off and the process repeated until the core temperature reaches 90°F (32°C).

| Note | Placing the patient on an extracorporeal circulation unit with a heat exchanger is another method of central rewarming. This process is usually not practical or available in many institutions.

    d. Throughout the period of central rewarming the patient is covered with blankets.

    e. When the core temperature reaches approximately 90°F (32°C), warm blankets or a hyperthermia blanket may be used to slowly warm the patient.

Perspective
The diagnosis of hypothermia is made with an appropriate recording device. Optimal therapeutic management involves rapid central rewarming to 90°F in an attempt to avoid serious cardiac arrhythmias. Vital signs, cardiograms, arterial pH, arterial blood gases, blood glucose, and electrolytes must be monitored throughout the rewarming process. Prevention and recognition of complications of hypothermia such as pneumonia, renal failure, pancreatitis, etc., is important.

III. Smoke Inhalation Smoke is defined as all products of combustion or pyrolysis. This includes all of the gases and particulates that are both normal products of combustion and unique to a particular material being pyrolyzed.

Components of inhalation injury may include
    —Constituents of smoke, e.g., carbon monoxide and cyanide
    —Thermal effects
        Dry heat—Damage is rare
        Wet heat (steam)—Airway burns
    —Small airway and/or alveolar disease
    —Large airway disease (laryngotracheobronchitis)

—Pneumonia 5–7 days after inhalation
—Acute and long-term CNS sequelae (carbon monoxide, hypoxia)
—Myocardial depression (carbon monoxide, hypoxia)

A. Manifestations

1. Burns to the face and/or upper airway

2. Carbonaceous sputum

3. Smell of smoke on breath

4. Altered level of consciousness

5. Bronchospasm with wheezing and/or rhonchi

6. Intercostal or supraclavicular retraction, stridor, or hoarseness

7. Dyspnea

8. Hypotension

9. Cherry red color (in the presence of carbon monoxide inhalation)

B. Diagnosis

1. Signs of pulmonary edema, loss of volume or "whiteout" on chest x-ray

2. Elevated CO-Hb levels

3. Elevated Met-Hb levels

4. ABG
   a. PaO_2 is usually normal unless there is an acute intrinsic restrictive disease (interstitial edema) producing a shunt.
   b. Arterial O_2 saturation is decreased if the CO-Hb or Met-Hb levels are significantly elevated or PaO_2 is low.
   c. Arterial O_2 saturation will be "normal" if it is derived from a PO_2 nomogram in a patient with a normal shunt.
   d. Hypocarbia may be present if the patient is hyperventilating.
   e. Metabolic acidosis is not infrequent.

5. Frequently, other drugs are present (toxicology screen).

6. Bronchoscopy reveals laryngotracheobronchial pathology.

C. Management

1. Cerebral edema   Prevent hypoxia, hypercapnia, and cardiac failure.

2. Cardiac failure   Dobutamine or dopamine is usually the drug of choice for cardiac failure (see p. 342).

3. Obtain ABG and specifically ask for CO-Hb and Met-Hb levels and a **measured** arterial O_2 saturation.

4. Frequent ABG are obtained for shunt evaluation.

5. Give 100% oxygen until the diagnosis of carbon monoxide poisoning is ruled out (see p. 508).

6. See p. 313 on respiratory insufficiency.

7. Use bronchodilators as necessary (i.v. and nebulized).

8. Steroids are advised for severe bronchospasm, not for routine use.

9. Sputum Gram stain and cultures should be obtained serially to monitor for the development of pneumonia.

10. Vaponefrin may be required for laryngeal edema.

11. Pathophysiology and treatment of the specific constituents of smoke are as follows:
    a. Carbon monoxide causes asphyxia and interferes with peripheral oxygen utilization—100% oxygen; hyperbaric oxygen if CO-Hb > 25%.
    b. Hydrogen cyanide interferes with oxygen utilization—Thiosulfate i.v., amyl nitrate inhaled, and hyperbaric oxygen.
    c. Antimony, zinc, and lead particulates—Pulmonary toilet.
    d. Polychlorinated biphenyls (PCBs) cause enzyme induction—avoid halogenated hydrocarbons.
    e. Halogenated hydrocarbons cause arrhythmias and renal failure—Monitor renal function and hydration and treat arrhythmias.
    f. Aldehydes (acrolein) cause pulmonary edema—Intubate and use PEEP.
    g. Benzene causes CNS depression (effects may appear late)—Treat as an anesthetized patient.
    h. Acids (HCl, H_2SO_4) cause mucosal damage and edema—Treat with aerosol and/or ventilation with PEEP.
    i. Chlorine causes pulmonary edema—Use PEEP.

Perspective

Smoke inhalation produces direct damage from the particulates and temperature of the smoke. It also produces immediate and delayed toxicity from the constituents in smoke; therefore, it is necessary to know what material was burning.

25

ALCOHOL AND OTHER DRUG-INDUCED PROBLEMS

Drugs can be dangerous as well as beneficial. During treatment of the trauma patient, multiple drug therapy is the rule, and this compounds the incidence of drug-induced problems. Included in these problems are side effects and interactions with other medications. Below is a list of the most commonly used drugs utilized in the trauma patient, with some adverse drug reactions and the more common metabolic complications characteristic of these drugs. The trauma patient is different from any other patient facing surgery or medicine. Not only are this patient's metabolic demands extremely variable, but the clinical picture can change hourly. This makes diagnosing and evaluating problems secondary to drug therapy even more challenging.

Past medical history is important in the care of the trauma patient. Communication with the patient, family members, or family physician is necessary to glean information concerning concurrent drug therapy by the patient. Not only will this information allow the physician to continue critical treatment of ongoing disease, but it will also allow avoidance of drug interactions which otherwise might be blindly encountered.

I. **Ethyl Alcohol**

   A. **Acute ingestion** prior to the trauma

      1. The patient may present with a depressed core temperature.

      2. Alcohol has an anticonvulsant action because of its central nervous system depressant properties. Any anticonvulsant action is followed by a period of hyperexcitability, which may precipitate seizures.

      3. Acute ingestion produces variable degrees of CNS depression.

   B. The patient who is a **chronic alcohol abuser**

      1. May be able to metabolize a variety of drugs faster than a patient who does not consume large amounts of alcohol (e.g., pentobarbital)

      2. May have an undiagnosed folate deficiency

   C. **Alcohol withdrawal** Sudden abstinence from alcohol can precipitate a wide range of withdrawal symptoms. Whenever the daily routine of a patient is interrupted by trauma, a period of regular alcohol use may also be interrupted. The natural history of alcohol withdrawal begins with minor symptoms and progresses as a continuum to more intense and severe symptoms. Within 8–10 hr of forced abstinence, the patient may show signs of mild tremor, complaints of insomnia, mild disorientation, intermittent hallucinations, or a slight rise in temperature, blood pressure, pulse, or respiratory rate. After 48–72 hr, signs and symptoms may intensify. The patient may experience seizures.

1. **Prophylactic treatment** should be considered in a patient with suspected or documented history of regular alcohol use. Avoiding the symptoms of alcohol withdrawal may make the difference between a complicated and an uncomplicated course of treatment post-trauma. The patient should be monitored closely for signs of withdrawal. The prophylactic treatment of choice is oral or intravenous alcohol. Fifteen milliliters of bourbon or vodka may be given orally each hour for 48–72 hr, if needed. **The goal is to produce a manageable patient. Do not induce stupor with excess alcohol administration.** The patient may require as little as 30 cc qid. Consider the possibility of alcoholic gastritis if large doses are administered. If the patient is unable to tolerate oral alcohol, intravenous alcohol is indicated. Five percent alcohol in 5% dextrose is given i.v. Two hundred milliliters contains 10 ml of alcohol. The first 200 ml of solution is given rapidly over 1 hr. Thereafter, a continuous infusion is titrated to produce a manageable patient. The patient is monitored at frequent intervals for signs of euphoria, analgesia, inebriation, or over-sedation. If these signs are observed, the infusion rate must be slowed.

2. **Treatment of severe alcohol withdrawal** (hallucinations, pulse over 120, and temperature over 100°F)   Ten milligrams of diazepam (Valium) is given every 4–6 hr i.v. If the patient is able to tolerate oral medication, the diazepam may be given orally. Begin intravenous or oral alcohol, as outlined above. Subsequent doses of diazepam must be given judiciously, keeping in mind the synergism between sedatives and alcohol.

3. **Treatment of repeated seizures** (status epilepticus)   Repeated seizures occasionally occur in the syndrome of alcohol withdrawal. The mild, self-limited "withdrawal seizures" are usually seen within the first 24–48 hr of withdrawal and may be accompanied by hyperventilation and photophobia. Repeated seizures are treated as a neurologic emergency and phenytoin (Dilantin) is administered i.v. The dosage is 12 mg/kg given at a rate not exceeding 25 mg/min. Seizures that occur from withdrawal usually require no specific therapy. Repeated seizures should hasten an evaluation for a cause other than alcohol withdrawal.

4. **Medical considerations in the patient with alcohol withdrawal**
    a. Water balance with close attention to electrolytes (sodium, potassium, phosphorus, magnesium, calcium)
    b. Thiamine hydrochloride, 100 mg daily
    c. Multiple vitamins daily

d. Magnesium sulfate, 8–15 mEq i.v. daily for 72 hr

e. Serum glucose to rule out hypoglycemia

Note Hypoxia, head injury, and sepsis must always be excluded before treating the patient for a presumed diagnosis of alcohol withdrawal.

II. Phenobarbital

A. Phenobarbital is a well known enzyme inducer, e.g., the metabolism of warfarin (Coumadin) is enhanced.

B. Phenobarbital enhances the metabolism of phenytoin in low doses. In higher doses, it will compete for the metabolism of phenytoin resulting in higher levels of phenytoin and possible toxicity.

III. Phenytoin

A. **Cardiac** Phenytoin will cause a decreased PR interval and functions as an antiarrhythmic agent.

B. **Hypotension** may occur when the drug is given rapidly by the intravenous route. We recommend an i.v. rate of not greater than 25 mg/min.

C. **Hyperglycemia**

D. **Seizures** may result if serum levels exceed 30–35 μg/ml.

E. **Toxicity** may be manifested by ataxia, slurred speech, and nystagmus.

F. **Skin eruptions** (maculopapular and urticarial)

G. **Chloramphenicol** inhibits the metabolism of phenytoin.

IV. Digoxin

A. **Manifestations of toxicity**

1. Nausea, vomiting, anorexia

2. Increasing heart failure

3. Any arrhythmia or conduction block

4. Diarrhea

B. **Importance of serum digoxin level** Toxicity is diagnosed more appropriately by signs and symptoms than by the level. By having a clear idea of the specific indications (signs/symptoms) for administering digoxin, the clinician will have a knowledge of the end points of therapy, i.e., eradication of specific signs and symptoms will dictate the amount needed by a given patient. Hypokalemia and hypercalcemia increase toxicity. Hypothyroidism will result in decreased clearance of digoxin. If the serum potassium is low and thyroid function is depressed, toxicity can be seen at virtually any serum concentration of digoxin. Statistically, 85% of all patients manifesting toxicity to digoxin have serum levels greater than 2.0 ng/ml. Blood for serum digoxin levels should be drawn 6 hr after administration.

V. **Amphotericin B**

    A. Occasional anaphylactoid reaction   A test dose of 1 mg in 250 ml of D5W is given over 2 hr as an initial screening measure.

    B. Anorexia, nausea, vomiting

    C. Headaches

    D. Fever

    E. Thrombophlebitis

    F. Hypomagnesemia

    G. Nephrotoxicity

        1. The BUN will rise predictably in most patients.

        2. Serum creatinine will rise and the concentrating ability of the kidneys will diminish.

VI. **Tricyclic Antidepressants**

    A. Anticholinergic effects   Dry mucous membranes, mydriasis, adynamic ileus, urinary retention

    B. Drowsiness (additive with other sedatives and hypnotics)

    C. Extrapyramidal side effects (common with an overdose)

    D. Cardiac toxicities

        1. Flattened T-waves

        2. Bundle branch block

3. AV blocks

4. Tachycardia

5. Bradycardia

6. Ventricular premature contractions

7. Syncope

8. Convulsions

VII. **Haloperidol**

A. Attenuates dopamine effects

B. CNS depressant activity (may potentiate the action of other CNS depressants)

C. May lower the seizure threshold

VIII. **Chlorpromazine**

A. Potentiates the effect of other sedatives and opiates

1. Respiratory depression

2. Postural hypotension

3. Lethargy or excessive somnolence

B. Extrapyramidal side effects

C. Urinary retention, ileus, mental depression

D. Arrhythmias, conduction defects

E. Cholestatic jaundice

F. Alpha-adrenergic blocking (may induce profound hypotension in bedridden patients)

IX. **Pentobarbital** Significant adverse effects occur when used in high i.v. doses.

A. Hypotension (cardiac depression)

B. Bronchospasm

C. Chronic alcohol ingestion will lead to an increased level of the hepatic enzyme that metabolizes pentobarbital.

D. When used in high i.v. doses over a prolonged period, pentobarbital will stimulate its own metabolism and increase its clearance by the end of day 7 of continuous infusion.

E. Blisters on the skin

F. Withdrawal syndrome (possible in a patient chronically ingesting high doses of pentobarbital or in a patient receiving high doses of pentobarbital therapeutically for longer than 7 days)

   1. Symptoms usually appear after 8–12 hr of abstinence.

   2. Symptoms vary from mild symptoms (anxiety or tachycardia) to convulsions.

   3. Withdrawal manifestations may occur as early as 6 hr or as late as 5 days post-withdrawal.

X. Penicillins

A. Anaphylaxis (rare)

B. Cutaneous effects

   1. Morbilliform eruptions are most common.
      a. Occur after approximately 1 week of therapy
      b. More irritating to the patient than life-threatening

   2. Check for penicillin allergy history.

   3. Cross-resistance exists for penicillin and cephalosporins.

   4. With the exception of nafcillin, penicillins are excreted by the kidney; dosage adjustments are necessary in patients with impaired renal function.

   5. Hypokalemic, metabolic alkalosis may occur secondary to urinary potassium excretion (ticarcillin and carbenicillin).

   6. Interstitial nephritis is often reported with methicillin. Nafcillin appears to be less likely to cause interstitial nephritis.

   7. Convulsions or hyperreflexia may occur due to exceedingly high doses reaching the brain:
      a. High doses (greater than 20 million units/day)
      b. Administering standard doses to patients with impaired renal function

8. Hypernatremia as well as hyperkalemia or hypokalemia may occur with penicillin therapy. Carbenicillin and ticarcillin contain significant amounts of sodium. Penicillin is supplied as a sodium or potassium salt.

9. Hematologic changes
   a. Thrombocytopenia, leukopenia, and agranulocytosis can occur.
   b. Coagulation abnormalities (decreased platelet aggregation)

10. Diarrhea (Ampicillin is the most common penicillin associated with diarrhea or pseudomembranous colitis.)

XI. Antacids

A. Causing diarrhea (Maalox and Mylanta)

B. Constipating (Amphojel)

C. All antacids effect an increase or decrease in the rate or extent of absorption of concomitantly administered drugs by changing the gastrointestinal transit time or by binding and chelating enterically administered drugs.

XII. Cimetidine

A. Hemodialyzable

B. Mild and transient diarrhea

C. Small increases in serum creatinine

D. Mental confusion

E. Neutropenia, thrombocytopenia

F. Arrhythmias

XIII. Diazepam

A. Hypotension

B. Respiratory depression

C. The total body clearance of diazepam is inversely proportional to the age and directly proportional to the liver function of the patient. (As a rule of thumb, the half-life of diazepam in hours is roughly equal to the patient's age in years.)

XIV. Theophylline

A. Gastrointestinal irritant

    1. Nausea and vomiting

    2. Epigastric pain and abdominal cramps

    3. Anorexia

B. Headache, irritability, nervousness

C. Convulsions

D. Sinus tachycardia with or without premature ventricular contractions

E. Clindamycin decreases theophylline clearance.

XV. Aminoglycoside Antibiotics

A. The major aminoglycoside toxicities are vestibular, auditory, renal, and neuromuscular blocking.

    1. Auditory nerve toxicity is more common when potent diuretics are given and in patients with renal failure.

    2. Early signs of ototoxicity include a motion-related headache, dizziness, nausea, or vomiting.

B. Neomycin is considered to be the most nephrotoxic aminoglycoside.

    1. When neomycin is used as an irrigant or in dressings saturated with 1% concentrations, systemic absorption is very good and may result in toxic serum concentrations (trough level greater than 5 μg/ml).

    2. Neomycin is the most potent neuromuscular blocker among the aminoglycoside antibiotics: the neuromuscular blockade of pancuronium bromide may be potentiated by neomycin.

XVI. Meperidine

A. Respiratory and CNS depression

B. Hypotension

C. Smooth muscle spasm

D. Either bradycardia or a tachycardia (the latter due to a vagolytic action)

XVII. **Morphine Sulfate**

A. Amnesia (can be of obvious benefit)

B. Respiratory depression

C. Constipation

D. Urinary retention (especially in the elderly)

E. Dependence (various components can be involved)

1. Physical dependence is related to the development of tolerance and withdrawal symptoms.

2. Psychologic dependence is common to most psychoactive drugs.

3. Development of tolerance may require an increase in the dosage to obtain the initial pharmacologic effect.

F. If morphine is used as a respiratory depressant, tolerance to this effect occurs at the same time as tolerance to its analgesic effects.

G. **The abstinence syndrome**

1. Appears within a few hours of the last dose, reaches peak intensity in 24–48 hr, and subsides spontaneously

2. The most severe symptoms usually disappear within 10 days

3. Symptoms
    a. Rhinorrhea
    b. Perspiration
    c. Mydriasis
    d. Piloerection
    e. Hot flushes
    f. Nausea
    g. Emesis
    h. Diarrhea
    i. Fever
    j. Tachypnea
    k. Increased systolic blood pressure
    l. Abdominal cramps
    m. Tachycardia

H. Immediate side effects

1. Hypotension

2. Respiratory depression

3. CNS depression

4. Ileus

5. Increase in the biliary tract pressure (cholestasis and increased serum amylase)

6. ADH-like effect

XVIII. Succinylcholine

A. Malignant hyperthermia

B. Release of intracellular potassium into the plasma (The drug should be used with caution in patients with hyperkalemia.)

C. There is a potentiation of succinylcholine effect with hypermagnesemia or hypocalcemia.

D. Administration may result in fasciculations that could cause additional trauma to patients with fractures or dislocations.

E. A decrease in body temperature will result in an increase intensity and duration of succinylcholine activity.

F. Patients with severe hepatic impairment may have decreased plasma levels of pseudocholinesterase (resulting in increased duration of succinylcholine).

G. Succinylcholine causes a rise in intraocular pressure.

XIX. d-Tubocurarine

A. A release of histamine resulting in hypotension and bronchospasm

B. Hypokalemia, hypermagnesemia, and hypocalcemia potentiate the effects of curare.

C. Hypothermia will result in increased neuromuscular blockade.

D. Hyperthermia will result in decreased intensity and duration.

E. Curare is excreted by the kidneys (caution with renal failure).

XX. Pancuronium Bromide

A. Primarily excreted by the kidney

B. Hypokalemia will potentiate the effects of pancuronium bromide.

C. Hypocalcemia or hypermagnesemia potentiates the effect of pancuronium bromide.

D. Hypothermia will decrease and hyperthermia will increase the blockade effect.

E. Aminoglycoside antibiotics possibly potentiate pancuronium bromide.

F. Quinidine, beta-adrenergic blocking agents, and high doses of lidocaine potentiate pancuronium bromide effects.

G. There is an increase in blood pressure (particularly with higher doses) and pulse rate.

XXI. **Chloramphenicol**

A. Bone-marrow suppression (two forms)

1. Non-dose related, irreversible bone marrow depression resulting in aplastic anemia with a mortality exceeding 50% is rare.

2. Dose-related depression, the more common form, is usually reversible when the drug is discontinued.
    a. Patient presents with anemia, reticulocytopenia, leukopenia, increased serum iron, and increased total iron binding capacity.
    b. Occurs more regularly when plasma concentrations exceed $25\,\mu g/ml$ or when the daily dose exceeds 4 gm/day

B. Chloramphenicol is inactivated in the liver (caution in patients with hepatic impairment).

C. Chloramphenicol interferes with the metabolism of phenytoin.

XXII. **Mannitol**

A. Fluid and electrolyte imbalance (hyponatremia or hypernatremia)

B. Expansion of intravascular fluid if mannitol accumulates due to inadequate urinary output or due to rapid administration of large doses of the drug

C. Osmotic nephrosis due to its action as an osmotic diuretic

D. Extravasation resulting in local edema and skin necrosis

E. Hyperosmolality and an osmolar gap

F. As a rule of thumb, the daily dose of mannitol should not exceed 4 gm/kg/day.

XXIII. **Furosemide**

    A. Hypovolemia

    B. Hyponatremia

    C. Hyperglycemia

    D. Hypomagnesemia

    E. Hyperuricemia

    F. Hypokalemia

    G. Ototoxicity is best avoided by keeping the patient in the proper state of hydration.

    H. Renal toxicities occur when salt and water loss are superimposed upon pre-existing renal insufficiency.

XXIV. **Acetylsalicylic Acid**

    A. Gastrointestinal irritation and possible bleeding

        1. The incidence of gastritis due to aspirin increases with age.

        2. Gastrointestinal bleeding may be painless.

    B. Small doses (1–2 gm/day) cause retention of uric acid

    C. Aspirin inhibits platelet aggregation (This effect lasts up to 5–7 days after the aspirin has been discontinued.)

    D. False negative urine test if Tes-tape is used to measure urine glucose in a patient receiving 2½ to 5½ gm/day

    E. False positive result with Clinitest method for evaluating urinary glucose

XXV. **Radiopaque Organic Iodine Compound**

    A. Liberates histamine when given i.v. and may cause a severe anaphylactic reaction

B. Nausea, vomiting, excessive salivation, pallor, flushing, dizziness, urticaria, sweating

C. Cardiac arrhythmias

D. Nephrotoxic potential Patients given these agents must be adequately hydrated before administration.

E. These agents are hypertonic and will cause significant fluid shifts if present in body cavities for any length of time.

F. Osmotic diuretic when given i.v.

XXVI. **Methyldopa**

A. Drowsiness (may disappear on continued dosing)

B. Mental depression, lapses in memory, profound decrease in mental acuity

C. Sodium and water retention resulting in congestive heart failure in a borderline compensated patient (Treatment with a diuretic is imperative when methyldopa is given.)

D. Nasal stuffiness is common.

E. Impotence

F. Drug fever (manifested within 21 days of therapy)

G. Hypertension during or after dialysis because methyldopa is dialyzable and must be replaced after dialysis

H. Darkened urine if urine is exposed to air

XXVII. **Fentanyl**

A. Depressed renal function (due to decreased renal plasma flow)

B. Dilutional hyponatremia due to stimulation of antidiuretic hormone

C. Skeletal and thoracic muscle rigidity frequently occurs after rapid intravenous administration.

    1. May be associated with decreased pulmonary compliance and/or apnea, laryngospasm, and bronchial constriction

2. Controlled with neuromuscular blocking agent

D. Bradycardia (treat with atropine)

XXVIII. Tromethamine (THAM)

A. Highly alkaline; should be administered via a large needle or indwelling catheter to decrease venous irritation

B. Extravasation results in necrosis

C. If tromethamine must be given in a peripheral vein, the limb should be elevated to increase the venous flow.

D. Transient decrease in blood sugar

E. Respiratory depression

F. Hyperkalemia

G. Accumulation in patients with impaired renal function

H. Has a pH of 10.6 and will inactivate any catecholamine given simultaneously, such as dopamine or dobutamine

XXIX. Droperidol

A. Alpha-adrenergic blockade results in hypotension and tachycardia

B. Attenuates the cardiovascular response to sympathomimetics

C. Potentiates the action of other central nervous system depressants

XXX. Vancomycin

A. Ototoxicity if serum level exceeds 80–95 μg/ml

B. Damage to the auditory branch of the eighth cranial nerve

C. Nephrotoxicity

D. Extremely irritating to the tissues and should never be given intramuscularly

E. A "shocklike state" can occur if given intravenously at a rapid rate. Must be given over a 30-min period.

XXXI. Insulin

A. Overdose can cause acute hypoglycemia. This is especially true if a hypertonic glucose solution such as that used in total parenteral nutrition is discontinued abruptly. The effect of endogenous insulin outflow will decrease in approximately 2½ hr after the glucose load has been changed.

B. When administered with a beta-adrenergic blocker, an enhanced response to insulin can be expected.

XXXII. Clindamycin

A. Most patients that experience diarrhea do so secondary to a change in the bowel flora.

B. The remainder have diarrhea secondary to pseudomembranous enterocolitis.

    1. Discontinue the drug.

    2. Do not administer diphenoxylate

XXXIII. Methylprednisolone and Dexamethasone

A. Glucose intolerance

B. Possible relationship between corticosteroids and pulmonary infections (especially opportunistic infections)

C. Corticosteroids may cause pancreatitis.

D. Acneiform rash will develop on the upper extremities and on the trunk of patients receiving corticosteroids. This is generally related to the dose and duration of therapy.

XXXIV. Heparin

A. Hemorrhage

B. A reversible thrombocytopenia

C. Urticarial rash secondary to hypersensitivity

D. Suppression of aldosterone production with high doses of heparin or administration for extended periods of time.

XXXV. **Beta-Adrenergic Blocking Agents (Inderal)**

    A.   Bronchospasm

    B.   Reduced myocardial contractility

    C.   Hypoglycemia due to impairment of glycogenolysis in the skeletal muscle

XXXVI. **Lidocaine**

    A.   Excess serum levels in patients with liver impairment

    B.   Complete heart block when given to patients with AV conduction disturbance

    C.   Seizures, coma, decerebrate rigidity, or confusion if high serum levels result from excessive dosing or normal dosing in patients with impaired renal function

XXXVII. **Cocaine**

    A.   Dependence (more of a problem in the social setting than in the clinical setting)

    B.   Seizures

    C.   Potentiation of the excitatory and inhibitory responses of organs to endogenous catecholamines by blocking the uptake of catecholamines at the sympathetic nerve endings

    D.   Mild increase in systolic and diastolic blood pressure

XXXVIII. **Phencyclidine**   Phencyclidine (PCP) is discussed not because of its therapeutic value but because as a drug of abuse in the general population there has been a tremendous increase in the number of patients who coincidentally are trauma patients.

    A.   Cardiovascular effects

        1.   Increase in diastolic and systolic blood pressure

        2.   Increase in heart rate

    B.   Drugs that cause hypertension by indirect mechanisms, such as cocaine, are potentiated by phencyclidine.

C. A dose-dependent central nervous system depressant and stimulant

D. Seizures and spasticity

XXXIX. **Dobutamine**

A. Arrhythmias

B. Increase in heart rate or in systolic blood pressure

C. Significant tissue damage if dobutamine should infiltrate

XL. **Dopamine**

A. Increase in pulmonary vascular resistance

B. Tachycardia and ventricular arrhythmias

C. Extensive tissue damage if dopamine should extravasate

D. Peripheral cyanosis of the hands, fingers, feet, or toes due to vasoconstriction (cyanosis can be unilateral and on one digit of an extremity.)

XLI. **Drug Abuse**   Patients whose admission is drug-related or who have a history of chronic drug abuse are to receive a drug abuse consultation before discharge. This will be coordinated by the MIEMSS psychiatrist.

XLII. **Alcohol Abuse Counseling Protocol**

A. **Purpose**   To evaluate and counsel patients with alcohol-related problems.

B. **Criteria**

1. Any patient showing ≥ 150 mg/dl of blood alcohol concentration (BAC) on admission will be evaluated and interviewed.

2. If the Team Leader feels that a patient has an alcohol-related problem, the Alcohol Abuse Service is consulted.

3. The patient must be stabilized and alert.

C. **Procedure**

1. On receipt of the above elevated BAC from the lab, the primary nurse/M.D. obtains a consultation from the Alcohol Abuse Service.

2. The Michigan Alcoholism Screening Test is administered (with the patient's permission) to assess the patient's use of alcohol.

3. If the results are positive and the patient's cooperation is given, the following will take place:
   a. Confront the patient and explain the consequences of alcohol use.
   b. Offer assistance and counseling.
   c. Involve the family.
   d. Initiate a treatment plan.
   e. Initiate follow-up visits, as required.
   f. Assist in arrangements for residential alcoholism treatment center, if needed.

4. For those returning for out-patient clinics, the following will be provided:
   a. Individual counseling
   b. Group counseling
   c. Family counseling

Section VI
INFECTION

INTRODUCTION

Because trauma is the third leading cause of death in the United States, more and more specialty centers are being set up to deal with multiply traumatized patients. Infection is the leading cause of death in patients who survive more than 3 days. There are very few studies from which conclusions can be drawn concerning "appropriate antibiotic use." There are differences of opinion regarding the benefit of prophylactic antibiotics in critically ill, multiple trauma patients.

Infection in the trauma patient is acquired either exogenously or endogenously. Exogenous contamination occurs either at the time of trauma or after admission, as the patient is subjected to the environment of the intensive care unit. In addition to tissue disruption, the presence of devitalized tissue, foreign bodies, hematoma formation, dead space, and shock, therapy frequently impairs the patient's normal defense mechanisms. Invasive foreign bodies, e.g., catheters, provide bacteria in the environment an apperture for invasion. In the effort to save the patient's life, major breaks in surgical technique frequently occur and proper tissue handling, appropriate surgical preparation, obliteration of dead space, and meticulous hemostasis may not take place. Endogenous contamination may result from disruption of the gastrointestinal, genitourinary, or respiratory tract at the time of injury. Inadequate therapy or therapy that is delayed may result in tissue invasion by bacteria.

The majority of infections in the multiple trauma patient are nosocomial and not related to traumatic wounds. The underlying principle of infection control in the shock-trauma patient is that **the patient must be protected from bacterial invasion.** The organisms may originate from the patient, but they may also be carried by the staff, the air, or the equipment. Each careless contact that the staff makes with the patient at the Heliport, at the time of admission, or during recuperation may cause an infection. Aseptic precautions must be taken for all procedures. The thorough cleaning and, whenever possible, sterilization of equipment and fixtures is mandatory. The removal of infected material from the patient care areas and the use of closed collecting systems help minimize airborne infection. The use of an antibiotic may treat or prevent one infection, but allow colonization or superinfection at another site. Antibiotic use must be specific for the organism or organisms isolated and should be used for short periods to treat the infection, yet prevent the emergence of resistant organisms. Unless the patient is unstable, appropriate diagnostic procedures are indicated to determine the site of infection and the specific organism. On the other hand, empiric therapy may be indicated in the unstable patient to prevent deterioration. If the patient is begun on broad-spectrum antibiotics, therapy is reduced to treatment of specific organisms as soon as possible. The continuation of an antibiotic is judged each day based on its risk/benefit ratio.

26

INFECTION CONTROL
AND MANAGEMENT

I. **Definition of Nosocomial Infections** Nosocomial infections are defined as infections developing as a consequence of resuscitative or invasive therapeutic procedures. These infections are not present at the time of admission, nor considered part of the admission diagnosis. Generally, these infections begin to manifest about 3 days following admission and are directly related to an invasive procedure, mechanical support device, or therapeutic measure.

A. **Classification** The following classification has been developed to standardize the identification and documentation of nosocomial infections. The single, most important factor is that a patient manifests the clinical features of an infection, in the eyes of his treating physician.

1. **Bacteremia** A clinical "bacteremic" episode occurs when greater than one blood culture is positive. If only one of two or three blood cultures is "positive," it is usually a contaminant. A primary bacteremia is one in which the source cannot be determined. Secondary bacteremias are those which have an identifiable source.

2. **Phlebitis—catheter-associated**
   a. **Chemical** Signs of inflammation at the catheter insertion site; negative culture at the site
   b. **Suppurative** Signs of inflammation; purulent, culture-positive material from the insertion site; may have secondary bacteremia; may have a palpable cord
   c. **Septic nonsuppurative** Occult bacteremia usually with a member of the klebsiella tribe; does not have purulent material at the insertion site; may not have a palpable cord; may require vein stripping
   d. **Contaminated line** Positive culture of the catheter, no signs of inflammation at the insertion site

3. **Arterial line infection** A positive culture is obtained at the insertion site of an arterial line. There may be a secondary bacteremia or septic emboli distal to the insertion site. Clinical signs of an infection must be present.

4. **Respiratory tract infection**
   a. **Sinusitis** Two of the following three criteria must be present:
      (1) Purulent material aspirated from the involved sinus
      (2) Positive radiologic findings
      (3) Purulent nasal discharge

    b. **Tracheitis** Evidence of inflammation; purulent drainage from the trachea which requires therapy; a negative chest x-ray

    c. **Pneumonia** Production of purulent sputum and an infiltrate on x-ray that does not clear with chest physiotherapy; a significant Gram stain of the sputum, i.e., predominant organism and the presence of polymorphonuclear leukocytes. The patient must have clinical signs of infection.

    d. **Empyema** Purulent, culture-positive material drained from the pleural space either by thoracentesis or material obtained on insertion of a chest tube

5. An **intra-abdominal infection** is defined as nosocomial if an infection is identified after none had originally been found.

6. **Meningitis** is characterized by the presence of appropriate clinical manifestations and at least two of the following:
    a. CSF pleocytosis
    b. Presence of hypoglycorrhachia
    c. Increase in CSF protein that cannot be explained by a noninfectious cause
    d. Isolation of an organism from the CSF

7. A **surgical wound infection** is any surgical wound that drains purulent material, with or without positive culture; any wound with cellulitis and a positive culture; any wound labeled infected by the attending surgeon.

8. **Cutaneous and other superficial infections** are defined as any purulent material exuding from the skin and subcutaneous tissue after admission, e.g., bed sores, conjunctivitis.

9. **Urinary tract infection** is identified by at least two consecutive urine cultures of the same organism with 100,000 pathogens/ml or the presence of visible organisms on a Gram stain of unspun fresh urine with pyuria of ≥ 10 WBC per high power field and clinical signs of infection.

II. Infection Control

A. **The Infection Control and Antibiotic Utilization Committee** has the ultimate authority and responsibility to establish written protocols and procedures for infection control at MIEMSS. The functions of this committee are to ensure compliance with all federal and state regulations and the standards of the Joint Commission on Accreditation of Hospitals, to ensure adequate patient care via bacteriologic surveillance, to implement isolation procedures for communicable infectious hazards to both patients and staff, and to provide infectious disease consultation. Documentation of nosocomial infections are recorded prospectively by the infection control officer and reviewed at least every 2 months by the Infection Control Committee. Assessment of this documentation will provide the identification of an infectious outbreak or epidemic situation as well as monitor the management of infectious complications. This assessment will dictate the need for revision of practice which relates to infectious management.

B. **Principles** The basis of infection control is adherence to a procedural dress code, mandatory hand washing before and after each patient contact, and adherence to strict use of aseptic technique in all invasive procedures. Any physician, nurse, or attendant has the responsibility to remind an individual who does not comply with infection control policy.

1. The **dress code** varies with each unit within MIEMSS and is as follows:
   a. All primary health care personnel entering the **Admitting Area** must wear a clean scrub suit, a cap covering all scalp and facial hair, fresh shoe covers, and a fresh face mask. Every procedure performed in this area should be considered a miniature operation and appropriate attention to hand washing, antiseptic skin preparation, and draping are essential. Consultants in the Admitting Area may wear clean, long sleeved cover gowns, shoe covers, fresh face mask, and a cap covering all scalp and facial hair, for purposes of examining the patient. To perform an invasive procedure, the consultant must wear a clean scrub suit.
   b. All personnel entering the **operating room** must wear a clean scrub suit, a cap covering all scalp and facial hair, clean shoe covers, and a fresh mask. Face mask and shoe covers are applied upon entering the OR and removed after each case.
   c. All health care personnel entering the **Critical Care Recovery Unit** (CCRU), **Intensive Care Unit** (ICU), or the **Neurotrauma Unit** (NTU) must wear either a clean white lab coat and cap, clean scrub suit and cap, or a long sleeve cover gown and cap (caps must cover all scalp and facial hair). Patient procedures performed in these areas require the following modifications in attire:
      (1) **Category A** Sterile gown, cap, sterile gloves and mask for chest tube insertion; Swan-Ganz catheter insertion; total parenteral nutrition (TPN) line insertion; dressing changes on large open wounds or burns; bedside tracheostomy, peritoneal lavage, AV shunt insertion, and vascular cutdowns
      (2) **Category B** Clean scrub attire or cover gown, cap, mask, and sterile gloves for bronchoscopy; central venous and arterial line insertion; arteriography; lumbar puncture; Foley catheterization
      (3) **Category C** Sterile gloves, only, for small dressing changes; insertion of peripheral lines; blood cultures; removal of drains; tracheostomy tube change
      (4) **Category D** Handwashing for percutaneous arterial and venous puncture; suture removal; examining patients
   d. All personnel entering the **Intermediate Care Unit** (IMCU) may wear routine hospital attire; however, performance of a procedure requires adherence to the procedural dress code.

2. **Handwashing** is mandatory. A 20-sec vigorous friction rub of the hands with running water, soap, and shutting off the faucets with the elbows or with paper towels is followed. This precedes and follows any patient contact. All invasive procedures are preceded by a surgical scrub. **Preparation in the Ad-**

mitting Area for an incoming patient includes a full surgical scrub by all team members.

3. **Vascular line management**   Since 40% of our documented bacteremias are related to intravascular lines, it is imperative that all lines be evaluated for infection and/or their continued need by the Team Leader or designate each day. The following guidelines are provided:
   a.   All vascular lines inserted in the Admitting Area should be removed within 24–36 hr. An exception is an arterial line that was inserted with careful, aseptic technique.
   b.   Peripheral i.v. lines should be changed every 48–72 hr or earlier if signs of phlebitis are present.
   c.   Antecubital long lines should be changed every 48–72 hr or earlier if signs of phlebitis or infection are present.
   d.   Subclavian/internal jugular lines must be changed if signs of phlebitis or infection are present. Sterile occlusive dressings should be changed at 48-hr intervals.
   e.   Arterial lines should be removed as soon as feasible. Because the infection rate is lower, placement by percutaneous stick is preferred over a cutdown. The arterial line must be removed if there are manifestations of infection at the puncture site or if there are distal septic emboli. If there are no local signs of infection, yet the patient appears to be septic and there are no other foci of infection, the catheter should be removed.
   f.   Saphenous venous lines are removed as soon as the patient is hemodynamically stable, preferably at the completion of the initial resuscitation/operation.
   g.   Hyperalimentation lines are placed and maintained in accordance with specific guidelines (see p. 441).
   h.   Vascular insertion sites are inspected and cleaned, and iodophor ointment is applied daily.

4. **Respiratory support systems**   Since natural respiratory host defense mechanisms are impaired when the patient is intubated and placed on a mechanical ventilator, the following guidelines have been developed:
   a.   Patients on ventilators receive daily chest x-rays.
   b.   Chest physiotherapy is recommended at 2- to 4-hr intervals, depending upon the clinical conditions of the patient.
   c.   Routine surveillance cultures and Gram stains of sputum are obtained three times weekly.
   d.   All breathing circuits of ventilators and heated humidity set-ups are changed every 24 hr.
   e.   Aseptic technique is used when the trachea is suctioned.
   f.   Lavage fluid for respiratory support equipment is changed every 8 hr.
   g.   The tracheal stoma is cleansed every 4 hr with 0.25% acetic acid.

5. **Foley catheterization**   Indwelling urinary catheters become colonized after 72 hr; therefore, the following guidelines are provided:
   a.   A Foley catheter is placed with strict aseptic insertion technique.

b. Foley catheterization in the Admitting Area is performed by a team of specially trained nurses.

c. A closed system should be maintained and all connections should be taped.

d. Routine surveillance cultures are obtained three times weekly.

e. Foley catheters should never be routinely irrigated.

f. Do not change the Foley catheter if the patient is known to have bacteriuria, but consult the infectious disease service.

g. Do not change the Foley catheter during a "septic crisis."

h. Prevent urine reflux from the drainage bag, especially when moving the patient.

i. The Foley-meatal junction is cleansed and an iodophor solution applied every 8 hr.

j. Remove as soon as possible.

6. **Nasogastric tubes**   The presence of a large bore rigid tube in the nose results in soft tissue swelling. This can result in the obstruction of nasal sinus drainage and the development of a purulent sinusitis. The following guidelines have been developed:

a. Nasogastric tubes should be monitored for the length of time indwelling.

b. Paranasal sinus x-rays should be taken on any patient presenting with cryptic fever or purulent nasal discharge.

c. Nasogastric tubes should be placed orally in all patients with nasal/facial fractures, CSF rhinorrhea, or patients who are immobile.

7. **Intraventricular catheters**   Since intraventricular catheters transverse the skin and subdural/ventricular fluid space, they may be a source of meningitis/ventriculitis. The following guidelines apply:

a. All dressing changes and manipulations are performed with full aseptic precautions and performed by the neurosurgical staff.

b. CSF is obtained daily by the neurosurgical staff and sent for Gram stain and culture, cell count with differential, and glucose. Subarachnoid bolts are infrequently associated with meningitis.

8. **Wound management**   See pp. 191 and 261.

9. **Abdominal drains**   See p. 189.

10. **Chest tubes**   See p. 473.

11. **Isolation**

a. Patients with open wounds that are draining *Staphylococcus aureus* should be placed in isolation.

b. Patients who are hepatitis associated antigen (HAA)-positive should be treated in isolation to protect the staff and other patients.

c. Massive open wounds not draining staphylococci, including clostridial organisms, do not need isolation.

C. **Prophylactic antibiotics**   The usefulness of prophylactic antibiotics in the multiple trauma patient has never been adequately studied. There are, however, several studies from individual disciplines suggesting that, in certain situations, prophylactic antibiotics may be beneficial. Because of the potential complications, specific indications have been devised for the use of prophylactic antibiotics in MIEMSS.

1. **Open fractures** The management of open fractures has been greatly facilitated with the use of external fixation devices, but infection still complicates a substantial number of patients. Since *Staphylococcus aureus* is by far the most common organism infecting open orthopedic wounds, an intravenous anti-staphylococcal antibiotic is used for 5 days following the injury. Usually, cephalothin (Keflin) (1.5 gm q4–6h) or nafcillin (1.5 gm q4–6h) is given for 5 days. If the patient has a CSF leak, prophylactic antibiotics are contraindicated. The effect of these prophylactic antibiotics on other wounds and the flora in the severely traumatized patient is unknown.

2. **Penetrating abdominal injury** Preoperative antibiotics, clindamycin and gentamicin or cefoxitin decrease the septic complications associated with penetrating ileal and colonic injuries. If an ileal or colonic disruption is identified at the time of laparotomy, antibiotics are continued for 3–5 days. If ileal or colonic violation is not identified at surgery, the antibiotics are discontinued.

3. **Maxillofacial trauma** Prophylactic antibiotics are given for maxillary or mandibular fractures which are open intraorally. Penicillin is administered for 3–5 days post-injury (see p. 85).

4. **Vascular prosthesis** Because of the high incidence of staphylococcal bacteremia which occurs in our patients, each patient with a prosthetic heart valve should receive a semisynthetic penicillinase-resistant penicillin for as long as indwelling lines are present. Similarly, each patient with newly inserted vascular or orthopedic prosthetic devices should receive a semisynthetic penicillinase-resistant penicillin for as long as there are indwelling lines.

5. **Penetrating thoracic trauma** The literature suggests that there is very minimal benefit offered to the patient who receives an antistaphylococcal antibiotic soon after penetrating chest trauma. The effect this policy would have on the multiply traumatized patient is not clear. Accordingly, nafcillin or cephalothin for a short period may be useful, and administration is left up to the discretion of the Team Leader.

6. **Cerebrospinal fluid leaks** Infection secondary to cerebrospinal fluid leaks are relatively uncommon, and prophylactic antibiotics make no difference in the incidence of meningitis. On the other hand, prophylactic antibiotics change the patient's flora and lead to Gram-negative colonization, which makes it likely that if meningitis develops it will be due to a more resistant Gram-negative rod. If a patient has a CSF leak, yet has another indication for prophylactic antibiotics, the prophylactic antibiotic is not administered. Nasal tubes should not be inserted in patients with possible CSF rhinorrhea.

7. **Penetrating head injuries** With penetrating injuries of the cranial vault, foreign matter is brought into the wound; this requires meticulous surgical

debridement. There are no well controlled studies which show that antibiotics in a properly debrided wound have a beneficial effect; therefore, we do not use prophylactic antibiotics in these injuries. The patient must be watched closely for the development of brain abscess or meningitis.

III. **Infection Management**

A. **Evaluation of the febrile trauma patient**   Temperature elevations in the traumatized patient may be due to numerous metabolic/physiologic causes. The diagnosis of fever due to noninfectious origin is one of exclusion, and sepsis must be vigorously searched for in all cases. When a patient develops fever, the history should be reviewed regarding the length of time the patient has been hospitalized, the specific injuries incurred, and post-injury complications which have ensued. A detailed physical examination is required to elucidate the cause of the temperature elevation, i.e., foci of infection. The multiply traumatized patient is usually difficult to examine because of the many devices used to monitor him and the bandages and other apparatus necessary to secure the wounds. Both the source and the organisms should be sought. The following is a compilation of sources of sepsis and/or fever which are commonly encountered in the trauma patient:
   —Pneumonia
   —Lung abscess
   —Empyema
   —Phlebitis
   —Arterial line infections
   —Meningitis—brain abscess
   —Wound infection
   —Urinary tract infection
   —Sinusitis
   —Pancreatitis
   —Abdominal abscess
   —Acalculous cholecystitis
   —Endocarditis
   —Osteomyelitis
   —Vascular prosthesis infection
   —Atelectasis
   —Large hematoma
   —Subarachnoid hemorrhage
   —Drug fever

Table 1 is a compilation of the infections that have occurred in our trauma patients over a 2-yr period. Each site must be assessed.

The following guidelines assist in ruling in or out specific infectious complications:

1. **Bacteremia**   Obtain two sets of aerobic and anaerobic blood cultures.

Table 1. Distribution of infections and bacteremia occurring in 639 infections in multiply traumatized patients

	Infection %	Bacteremic infection %
Primary bacteremia (probable vascular lines)	10	21
Vascular		
Phlebitis	12	17
Arterial line	2	4
Sinusitis	5	0
Lower respiratory		
Pneumonia	15	19
Empyema	11	11
Urinary tract	18	3
Central nervous system	7	5
Intra-abdominal	8	11
Surgical wound	10	8
Other	3	1
Total no. bacteremias	284 44%	
Total no. infections	639	

2. **Pneumonia–Lung abscess**
    a. Sputum for Gram stain and culture
    b. Chest x-ray
    c. Arterial blood gases

3. **Empyema**
    a. Chest x-ray
    b. Thoracentesis of undrained pleural fluid for Gram stain, culture, protein, pH, and cell count
    c. Culture and Gram stain of chest tube drainage, if present (caution: **must be interpreted carefully**)

4. **Phlebitis**
    a. Examine present and previous venous line sites.
    b. Note the length of time the present venous lines have been indwelling.
    c. Chest x-ray for evidence of septic pulmonary emboli
    d. Culture suspected lines by rolling most proximal 4 inches over a blood agar plate.

5. **Arterial lines**
    a. Examine present and previous arterial line sites.
    b. Note the length of time the present arterial line has been indwelling.
    c. Evaluate the extremity for evidence of peripheral emboli.

6. **Meningitis—brain abscess**
    a. History of cerebrospinal fluid leak, craniotomy, intraventricular catheter, or penetrating cranial wound (very rare without this history)

b. Change in the level of consciousness, new focal neurologic deficit, or a change in motor response to pain in the presence of high fever
   c. Nuchal rigidity may or may not be present.
   d. Discuss with the neurosurgeon and infectious disease consultant the need for obtaining a CSF specimen.

7. **Wounds**
   a. Evaluate accidental and surgical wounds for the presence of infection.
   b. Obtain a culture and Gram stain of wound drainage.

8. **Urinary tract**
   a. Urine culture and sensitivity and urinalysis
   b. Examine the patient for
      (1) Urethral discharge
      (2) Suprapubic pain
      (3) Costovertebral angle pain
      (4) Epididymitis
      (5) Prostatic tenderness, bogginess, or nodule

9. **Sinusitis**
   a. Evaluate for the presence of a nasal discharge and, if this is present, obtain Gram stain and culture of sinus aspirate.
   b. Sinus x-rays
   c. History of nasal trauma or nasal intubation

10. **Pancreatitis**
    a. Evaluate for the presence of epigastric pain.
    b. Serum/urine amylase
    c. Serum lipase

11. **Abdominal abscess**
    a. Presence of an ileus
    b. Abdominal x-ray (ileus, extraluminal gas, displacement of viscera)
    c. Rectal mass
    d. Chest x-ray ("elevated" diaphragm, pleural effusion)

12. **Cholecystitis**
    a. Right upper quadrant tenderness
    b. Consider hepatobiliary scanning and/or ultrasonography

13. **Endocarditis**
    a. Auscultate for a cardiac murmur.
    b. Evaluate chest x-ray for the presence of pulmonary emboli.
    c. Examine the patient for evidence of peripheral emboli.
    d. Echocardiogram if the diagnosis is likely

14. **Osteomyelitis**
    a. Examine the patient for evidence of infection in a wound that is associated with a fracture.
    b. Obtain x-ray of open fractures or fractures that have been treated surgically.

    c. Examine the patient for change in "fracture site" pain.

    d. Obtain a culture and Gram stain of wound drainage.

15. **Vascular prosthesis infection**

    a. Examine the patient for associated wound infection.

    b. Examine the patient for evidence of hematoma or hemorrhage.

    c. Evaluate the patient for evidence of graft thrombosis.

    d. Evaluate the patient for the presence of septic emboli.

B. **Systemic stress response** Certain parameters may reflect an "overwhelming" stress to the patient. This overwhelming stress frequently represents an underlying septic process (see p. 372). **Manifestations of stress** include

1. Leukocytosis or leukopenia

2. Thrombocytopenia

3. Glucose intolerance

4. Hypo- or hypernatremia

5. Hypotension and/or tachycardia

6. Increased pulmonary shunt, tachypnea, hypocapnia

7. Oliguria, decreased creatinine clearance

8. Decreased level of consciousness and/or confusion

9. Hyperbilirubinemia

10. Ileus, stress gastrointestinal bleeding

11. Elevation of the prothrombin and/or partial thromboplastin times

C. **Fever protocol** With any temperature spike of 102°F or greater or any temperature increase of greater than 2°F, the following should ensue:

1. Two blood cultures at 10-min intervals (aerobic and anaerobic)

2. WBC with differential

3. Urine cultures with stat smear

4. Urinalysis with microscopy

5. Do not change the Foley catheter, but establish the necessity for continuation of Foley catheterization.

6. Sputum or tracheal culture with a stat smear which must be looked at immediately

7. Change all i.v. lines that are in longer than 24 hr.

8. Chest x-ray

The culture part of the above protocol is instituted by writing Fever Protocol and telling the nurse.

D. **Culture guidelines** It is imperative that any fluid aspirated from a closed body space (pleural, peritoneal, meningeal, surgical incision, joint space, or pericardial cavity) be sent to the laboratory for appropriate chemical evaluation and immediate Gram stain and cultures, whether or not infection of this space is considered to be present. The importance of the Gram stain cannot be overemphasized. Detailed instructions as to how the fluid will be handled are available in manuals in patient care areas.

   The following points must be observed to ensure proper processing of specimens in the microbiology lab:

   1. Blood cultures must go to the laboratory immediately, may not be refrigerated, and no stat smears may be requested.

   2. Blood culture bottles **must be labeled.**

   3. Care must be taken not to inject air into anaerobic vials.

   4. All slips must be punched and filled out correctly.

   5. All cultures must be transported to the laboratory without undue delay.

   6. Stool, urine, and sputum cultures never go in anaerobic containers.

   7. There must be two swabs for each wound (one for culture, one for Gram stain).

   8. Sites must be labeled correctly, such as "wound, left knee," not "wound, pus, abscess, suture line."

   9. Only blood is sent in the blood culture bottles.

   Questions regarding the proper procedures may be answered by referring to the Infection Control Guideline Booklet or by contacting the Infection Control Officer.

E. **Antibiotic therapy for the febrile patient** If the patient's clinical status is stable, it is advisable to withhold antibiotics and to reevaluate the patient frequently for manifestations of an infection process. If there are signs of sepsis as revealed by the patient's systemic stress response, antibiotics which are directed at the most likely sources of infection are instituted. Since bacteria causing infection have previously colonized the patient, surveillance cultures should be considered in selecting antibiotics. It is helpful to identify the site (source) and the probable organisms to appropriately choose antibiotics.

   The following clinical situations occur frequently:

   1. The laboratory may report a **positive blood culture for a Gram-positive coccus.** Determine the length of time between the culture becoming positive and the time it was drawn. In general, coagulase-positive staphylococci, which are much more significant, will become positive within 48 hr of the culture being

drawn. Coagulase negative staphylococci, which are usually contaminants, will usually take greater than 48 hr before becoming "positive." In general, coagulase-positive staphylococci will be positive in all bottles, while contaminating coagulase-negative staphylococci will be sporadic and may have only one bottle positive. If the report is likely to be a coagulase-positive staphylococcus, the most likely sources in our unit are the vascular lines, wounds, and the chest. These areas must be inspected and the patient must be recultured and started on nafcillin (1.5 gm) i.v. every 4 hr. This will cover all other Gram-positive cocci, with the notable exception of enterococcus. Enterococcus is usually not the cause of sepsis; it is usually either a contaminant or signifies an intra-abdominal abscess and this is the only organism that "made it into the blood."

2.   The laboratory may report a **positive blood culture for a Gram-negative rod.** This should always be considered a true infection, since Gram-negative rod contaminants may occur but are extremely rare. A thorough search must be made for the source, and surveillance cultures are reviewed. If no source is found, institute a cephalosporin, usually cephalothin, and an aminoglycoside as empiric treatment. The aminoglycoside of choice in our unit is gentamicin, if the patient has been in the unit less than 10 days and has not been on other antibiotics. If the patient has been in the unit more than 10 days or has been on antibiotics, amikacin is administered. If surveillance cultures reveal that the patient is colonized with pseudomonas, ticarcillin and an aminoglycoside are administered.

3.   Lab report of a **specific organism growing in a blood culture**
     a.   **Streptococcus** (pneumococcus, beta-hemolytic streptococcus, enterococcus)
          Source: respiratory tract; wound; abdominal abscess
          Antibiotic regimen: penicillin; ampicillin and gentamicin if enterococcus is significant
     b.   **Staphylococcus**
          (1)   Coagulase-positive
                Source: lines, wounds, chest
                Antibiotic regimen: nafcillin, 1.5 gm i.v. q4h
          (2)   Coagulase-negative
                Source: usually contaminant
                Antibiotic regimen: usually none required
     c.   **Klebsiella**
          Source: lines, respiratory tract, wounds
          Antibiotic regimen: aminoglycoside, cephalosporin (use both for synergy)
     d.   **Enterobacter**
          Source: lines, abdomen, wounds
          Antibiotic regimen: aminoglycoside plus cephalosporin or trimethoprim sulfamethoxazole

e. **Acinetobacter**
Source: water, respiratory tract, respiratory equipment
Antibiotic regimen: ticarcillin and/or tobramycin

f. **Pseudomonas**
Source: respiratory tract, wounds
Antibiotic regimen: ticarcillin plus aminoglycoside

g. <u>**Escherichia coli**</u>
Source: urinary tract, abdominal cavity
Antibiotic regimen: ampicillin or aminoglycoside

h. <u>**Haemophilus influenzae**</u>
Source: lower respiratory tract, meningitis
Antibiotic regimen: ampicillin, chloramphenicol, may use cefamandole if there is no meningitis

i. **Proteus**
Source: urinary tract, abdomen
Antibiotic regimen: ampicillin or aminoglycoside

j. **Bacteroides**
Source: lower respiratory tract, upper respiratory tract, abdominal cavity
Antibiotic regimen: penicillin for respiratory tract bacteroides; clindamycin, chloramphenicol, or cefoxitin for bacteroides below the diaphragm

k. **Polymicrobial bacteremia**
Source: urinary or biliary tract
Antibiotic regimen: cephalosporin plus aminoglycoside

4. Suggested antibiotics for the **patient who is "acting septic" without a known source or a positive blood culture.**
   a. Indications
      (1) Increasing white count
      (2) Fever
      (3) Decreasing PaO_2
      (4) Shock
      (5) Decreasing mental status
      (6) Decreasing platelets
      (See pp. 372 and 414.)
   b. Antibiotic regimen In addition to the administration of steroids and complete culture evaluation, antibiotics must be selected to cover a wide range of organisms, since both Gram-negative and Gram-positive organisms can present, as described above. A cephalosporin and aminoglycoside are administered. Gentamicin is begun if the patient has been hospitalized for less than 10 days or has not been on other antibiotics. In other patients, amikacin is used because of the increasing probability of gentamicin resistance in these patients. If pseudomonas has been previously isolated, ticarcillin is added. If the abdomen is a likely source of sepsis, clindamycin should be added to cover *Bacteroides fragilis.*

F. **Management of specific complications** The following represents the common sources of fever and/or sepsis in the post-trauma patient. The Infectious Disease Service is always available and is consulted prior to instituting antibiotic therapy.

1. **Pneumonia** is a common source of infection due to contamination of the tracheobronchial tree by tracheal tubes, aspiration, and superimposition on atelectatic processes or pulmonary contusions.

   a. **Manifestations**
      (1) Leukocytosis
      (2) Fever
      (3) Deterioration of arterial blood gases
      (4) Sputum examination   The sputum usually reveals moderate to large amounts of polymorphonuclear leukocytes and a predominant bacterial organism.
      (5) Chest x-ray reveals an interstitial and/or alveolar process. There may be difficulty in appreciating a pneumonic infiltrate in a patient who has this process superimposed on a previous chest x-ray abnormality such as pulmonary contusion, adult respiratory distress syndrome (ARDS), atelectasis, aspiration, etc. A patient with a new infiltrate receives intensive physical therapy directed to the involved area and a repeat x-ray is taken. If there is a significant improvement in the x-ray, the patient probably does not have pneumonia.

   b. **Treatment**
      (1) Humidification of secretions
      (2) Chest physiotherapy
      (3) Postural drainage
      (4) Tracheobronchial suctioning to remove excess secretions
      (5) **Antibiotics** are indicated if the above manifestations are present; the patient reveals signs of systemic stress and a repeat chest x-ray shows that an infiltrate has failed to improve with vigorous chest physiotherapy.

         Antibiotics are selected on the availability of previous cultures and **current Gram stain.** If the present Gram stain suggests organisms not previously cultured, infectious disease consultation should be sought for help on antibiotic selection. The following guidelines are offered:
         —**Staphylococcus:** nafcillin
         —**Pneumococcus:** penicillin
         —Mixed flora: clindamycin
         —Gram-negative rods This usually necessitates broad-spectrum antibiotics, usually a cephalosporin and an aminoglycoside. If the patient has previously had pseudomonas isolated, an aminoglycoside and ticarcillin are chosen.

2. **Lung abscess** is not common; however, it is not rare in the trauma patient. Lung abscess is more likely to be seen in the patient who has sustained CNS

trauma and is on steroids. The lung abscess usually follows an aspiration process or previous pneumonia.

a. **Manifestations**
   (1) Fever (may be low grade)
   (2) Leukocytosis
   (3) Chest x-ray—pulmonary infiltrate ± an air fluid cavity
   (4) Sputum may reveal the presence of infection if the process is draining into the tracheobronchial tree; usually has mixed flora.

b. **Treatment**
   (1) **Medical**
       (a) Antibiotics are selected on the basis of previous cultures and a current Gram stain. If the present Gram stain suggests organisms not previously cultured, an infectious disease consultation should be sought for help on antibiotic selection. The following guidelines are offered:
           —**Staphylococcus:** nafcillin
           —**Pneumococcus:** penicillin
           —Mixed flora: clindamycin, since this most likely is an anaerobic infection
           —Gram-negative rods usually necessitate broad-spectrum antibiotics, a cephalosporin and an aminoglycoside. If the patient has previously had pseudomonas isolated, ticarcillin is added.
       (b) Chest physiotherapy and postural drainage
       (c) Bronchoscopy Remove secretions and rule out bronchial plugging
   (2) **Surgical** Patients who manifest rapid, clinical deterioration, despite medical treatment, should be considered for lobectomy.

3. **Empyema** is an infectious process within the pleural space which may or may not be loculated. The following events are associated with empyema in the post-trauma patient:
   —Contamination associated with a chest tube
   —Contamination associated with a pneumonic process
   —Barotrauma which contaminates the pleural space
   —Hematogenous seeding of a previously sterile pleural effusion
   —Superimposition on an unexpanded pneumothorax
   —Contamination by penetrating chest trauma
   —Transdiaphragmatic extension from an abdominal abscess
   —Post-thoracotomy

a. **Manifestations**
   (1) Fever and/or leukocytosis
   (2) Chest x-ray
       (a) Pleural fluid, free or loculated
       (b) Loculated "air pockets"
       (c) Pleural air-fluid levels

(d) "Pleural thickening"

    (3) Thoracentesis or chest tube drainage may reveal a positive Gram stain and/or culture. Send the specimen for a white blood count, protein, and pH.

    (4) The CAT scan may suggest an empyema and/or may locate these lesions in difficult cases.

b. Treatment

    (1) Antibiotics   The antibiotic regimen is based on the Gram stain and culture. The flora associated with empyema is often mixed. Coagulase-positive staphylococcus is the organism most commonly isolated in our unit. Anaerobes are implicated in about one-third of the patients. (See p. 418.)

    (2) Adequate drainage and lung expansion must be obtained with either thoracentesis or, in most cases, the insertion of a chest tube.

    (3) Operative intervention   Surgical intervention is indicated when the patient fails to respond to antibiotic therapy and drainage of the pleural space. Medical failure manifests as "uncontrollable" infection, inability to expand the lung, or extrinsic pulmonary restriction, i.e., deterioration of pulmonary function secondary to decreased lung volume.

    (a) Rib resection is indicated for an isolated loculation.

    (b) Decortication is indicated for multiple areas of pleural loculations.

> **Note** The chest tube should not be suddenly withdrawn following its use in a patient who has sustained an empyema; otherwise, a drain tract abscess will form. After the chest tube has been in the pleural space for 10–14 days, the chest tube is severed approximately 4–5 cm from the skin level. The chest tube is slowly withdrawn over several days to several weeks until it is removed.

4. Phlebitis is a relatively common source of fever and bacteremia in the multiple trauma patient. The incidence of phlebitic infection relates to the length of the catheter and the dwell time. In other words, the longer the catheter and the longer it has been in place (exceeding 72 hr), the greater the likelihood of infection. Septic complications also relate to

    —The lack of use of aseptic technique at the time of insertion

    —The care of the line following insertion

    —The number of manipulations after the insertion

    —Difficulty in inserting the line

    —Drugs infused through the lines

Infection is more common following cutdown technique than after percutaneous technique.

a. Manifestations

    (1) Fever and/or leukocytosis

    (2) The catheter site may reveal no gross evidence of infection; only the history of the length of time the catheter has been in place and the

technique in which it was inserted may reveal that this is a likely source of infection.

(3) Induration
(4) Suppuration
(5) Erythema

b. **Prophylaxis**
(1) Admission lines should be changed within 24–48 hr depending on
    (a) Technique at the time of insertion
    (b) The length of the line
    (c) Cutdown versus percutaneous technique
    (d) Vascular access availability
    (e) Difficulty with initial insertion
(2) Nonadmission venous catheters should be changed every 48–72 hr, when possible.

c. **Treatment**
(1) Remove the venous catheter when there are manifestations of infection.
(2) Remove venous lines when the patient has fever and/or leukocytosis if the catheter has been in place for more than 48 hr, despite the absence of local signs, especially if no other septic foci are identified.
(3) Apply warm compresses
(4) Elevate the extremity
(5) Antibiotics are administered if systemic manifestations are significant, since phlebitis is frequently the source of positive blood cultures. Suppurative phlebitis is almost always caused by staphylococci; frank suppuration is usually found with milking of the vein or aspiration of the vein. Nonsuppurative thrombophlebitis is commonly caused by klebsiella, enterobacter, or serratia. A Gram stain should be obtained from fluid which is expressed from the venous catheter puncture site. There is usually no fluid available in nonsuppurative phlebitis. The presence or absence of gross pus and the Gram stain are usually helpful in deciding the antibiotics to use, as is the presence of positive blood cultures. Candida is occasionally seen with hyperalimentation therapy. A candidemia usually resolves when intravenous lines are removed. If the candidemia persists, the patient may need amphotericin B therapy.
(6) Vein stripping
    (a) Vein stripping is more likely to be needed in the patient with nonsuppurative phlebitis.
    (b) If the patient has a bacteremia and has not improved within 24 hr, despite antibiotic therapy, extremity elevation, and line removal, the vein is stripped.
    (c) If a phlebitis is identified and the patient manifests septic shock or major systems failure, the vein should be stripped immediately.

5. **Arterial line infection** Compared to intravenous catheters, arterial lines are less likely to be associated with a septic process. Arterial line infection relates to
   —The use of cutdown technique as opposed to percutaneous insertion
   —Poor technique at the time of insertion
   —Length of time the catheter has been in place
   a. **Manifestations**
      (1) Leukocytosis and/or fever
      (2) Induration, erythema
      (3) Purulence
      (4) Distal septic emboli
      (5) Pseudoaneurysm
      (6) There may be no gross evidence of infection at the catheter site.
   b. **Prophylaxis**
      (1) The arterial catheter should be removed as soon as the line is not needed.
      (2) Use aseptic technique at the time of insertion.
      (3) Provide diligent daily line care.
      (4) Minimize unnecessary manipulations of the line.
   c. **Treatment**
      (1) Remove the line.
      (2) Antibiotics are indicated if there is evidence of systemic toxicity or positive blood cultures.
      (3) If the infectious process does not clear by removing the line or using antibiotics, removal of the pseudoaneurysm, periarterial clot, and/or infected artery may be indicated.

6. **Central nervous system infection** such as brain abscess, ventriculitis, and/or meningitis may occur following
   —Open CNS injury
   —Craniotomy
   —Intraventricular catheter, which has been present for more than 72 hr
   —Cerebrospinal fluid leak
   a. **Manifestations**
      (1) Sudden decreased level of consciousness
      (2) Stiff neck ±
      (3) Fever and/or leukocytosis
      (4) Seizures
      (5) Focal neurologic deficit
   b. **Diagnosis**
      (1) Cerebrospinal fluid specimen
         (a) Decreased glucose
         (b) Increased protein
         (c) Leukocytosis (predominantly polymorphonuclear leukocytes)
         (d) Organisms seen on Gram stain
         (e) Positive culture
         (f) Increased cerebrospinal fluid pressure

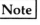 **Note** The CSF specimen should be obtained under the direction of the neurosurgeon.

  (2) CAT scan may reveal a brain and/or parameningeal abscess.
 c. **Prophylaxis**
  (1) Prophylactic antibiotics are not administered to patients with cerebrospinal fluid leaks.
  (2) Nasal tubes are not used in patients with cerebrospinal fluid rhinorrhea, to minimize colonization of the nasal cavity.
 d. **Treatment**
  (1) **Antibiotics** If central nervous system infection is likely (i.e., CSF chemistries and cell count and clinical evaluation suggest central nervous system infection) and no organisms are seen, nafcillin, chloramphenicol, ticarcillin and amikacin are administered to cover for Gram-positive and Gram-negative organisms. This antibiotic regimen has been successful in sterilizing the cerebrospinal fluid in greater than 90% of patients who subsequently prove to have a nosocomial meningitis. If Gram-positive cocci are seen on Gram stain, the patient is begun on nafcillin. If Gram-negative rods are seen on Gram stain, the patient is administered chloramphenicol, ticarcillin, and amikacin. The amikacin is initially given parenterally; however, should the organism be resistant to chloramphenicol or ticarcillin, but sensitive to amikacin, amikacin is administered into the ventricle. The patient's response to antibiotic therapy is monitored with sequential cerebrospinal fluid specimens.
  (2) If the patient has an intra- or extracerebral abscess and there is a mass effect and neurologic deterioration, drainage is indicated.
  (3) If there is localized inflammation (cerebritis) as defined by a CAT scan and a positive cerebrospinal specimen, the patient is managed with antibiotics. Serial CAT scans should be obtained to detect abscess formation. If there is mass effect from the cerebritis, surgical decompression may be necessary.

7. **Wound infections** Infections may develop in surgical or traumatic wounds. Most wound infections manifest 5–7 days after the surgery or trauma and are usually caused by staphylococci or Gram-negative rods. Streptococcal or clostridial wound infections may occur within 24 hr of contamination; therefore, all febrile patients without an obvious source of fever should have their wounds inspected, even if the classic 5–7 days have not elapsed.
 a. **Manifestations**
  (1) Fever and/or leukocytosis
  (2) Erythema, induration
  (3) Increased wound pain
  (4) Purulent discharge
  (5) Subcutaneous crepitus
  (6) Cutaneous bullae
  (7) Systemic stress response
 b. **Prophylaxis and treatment** See pp. 191 and 261.

8. **Urinary tract infections** are an uncommon cause of sepsis in our trauma patients. Indwelling Foley catheterization increases the likelihood of urinary tract infection. Enterococcus and Gram-negative rods are the most common cause of urinary tract infections in our trauma patients.

   a. **Manifestations**
      (1) Fever and/or leukocytosis
      (2) Flank tenderness
      (3) Enlarged and tender prostate with prostatitis
      (4) Enlarged and tender epididymis
      (5) Suprapubic pain

   b. **Diagnosis**
      (1) Urinalysis
         (a) Bacteria on the Gram stain of an unspun fresh urine specimen
         (b) Pyuria   10 WBC/high power field (unspun specimen)
      (2) Urine culture   Greater than 10^5 organisms/ml

   c. **Treatment**
      (1) Remove the Foley catheter, if possible.
      (2) Maintain urinary output to dilute the organisms.
      (3) Antibiotics are selected after a review of the Gram stain of the urine and sensitivity of the isolated organism.

9. **Sinusitis**   A relatively obscure but frequent source of fever and leukocytosis in our patients is paranasal sinusitis. The incidence seems to be most frequent in patients with nasal tubes (nasogastric or nasotracheal), maxillofacial fractures, and immobilization. A preponderance of the supine position is likely to cause poor sinus drainage and subsequent infection. These infections usually do not cause bacteremias.

   a. **Manifestations**
      (1) Fever and/or leukocytosis
      (2) Purulent nasal discharge may or may not be present.

   b. **Diagnosis**
      (1) Opacification of sinuses or an air-fluid level on x-ray
      (2) Sinus aspiration positive on Gram stain or culture

   c. **Treatment**
      (1) Remove nasal tubes.
      (2) Mobilization from the supine position
      (3) Antibiotics are selected on the basis of a Gram stain of the sinus aspirate. A variety of Gram-negative organisms have been isolated and specific antibiotic therapy cannot be recommended without review of the Gram stain.
      (4) Nasal decongestants
         (a) Pseudofed
         (b) Afrin
      (5) Sinus tap and irrigation as a therapeutic/diagnostic procedure in a patient who has an air-fluid level on x-ray or for failure to clear the sinusitis, medically.
      (6) Nasal-antral windows may be necessary for recalcitrant sinusitis.

10. **Pancreatitis** is uncommon in the trauma patient and may occur secondary to pancreatic trauma or an abdominal operation. This diagnosis should be entertained in any patient with fever and/or leukocytosis when there are no other sources identified.
   a. **Manifestations**
      (1) Fever and/or leukocytosis
      (2) Abdominal tenderness ±
      (3) Ileus
      (4) Pleural effusion
   b. **Diagnosis**
      (1) Elevated serum amylase
      (2) Elevated urine amylase
      (3) Elevated serum lipase
      (4) Abdominal x-rays
         (a) Ileus
         (b) Colon "cut-off sign"
   c. **Treatment**
      (1) NPO
      (2) Nasogastric suction is recommended but its efficacy is unknown.
      (3) Cardiovascular support (maintain adequate intravascular volume expansion)
      (4) Monitor for complications
         (a) Abscess
         (b) Pseudocyst
         (c) Respiratory failure
         (d) Hypocalcemia
         (e) Hemorrhage

11. **Abdominal abscess** See p. 185.

12. **Cholecystitis** The diagnosis of cholecystitis requires a high index of suspicion because the presentation is often subtle. Acalculous cholecystitis usually develops in a patient who is critically ill, has been without enteric feedings, and has usually received opiates.
   a. **Manifestations**
      (1) Fever
      (2) **Right upper quadrant tenderness**
      (3) Leukocytosis
      (4) Ileus
   b. **Diagnosis**
      (1) **Ultrasonography** may reveal a hydroptic gallbladder and stones, if present.
      (2) **Hepatobiliary imaging** If the scan visualizes the common bile duct and the duodenum, yet fails to visualize the gallbladder, this represents cystic duct obstruction. These scan findings in conjunction with right upper quadrant tenderness, fever, and leukocytosis suggest the likelihood of cholecystitis. If the gallbladder visualizes and fails to

contract after the administration of cholecystokinin, acalculous cholecystitis is presumed.

Note A bacteremia with a "biliary organism" (klebsiella, enterococcus, E. coli, enterobacter) suggests cholecystitis as a possible etiology.

c. **Treatment** Cholecystectomy is the treatment of choice.

13. **Vascular prosthesis infection** We feel that this entity is rare but should be considered in any patient with a new or old vascular prosthesis. We commonly insert short Dacron grafts for ruptured thoracic aortic injuries and usually use saphenous vein grafts for peripheral arterial injuries, which is a low-risk situation for infection.
    a. **Manifestations**
        (1) Graft leak
            (a) Hemorrhage
            (b) Hematoma (pseudoaneurysm)
        (2) Wound infection (seen if a peripheral wound)
        (3) Graft thrombosis
        (4) Septic emboli
        (5) Fever and leukocytosis
        (6) Bacteremia
        (7) Frequently, the diagnosis is one of exclusion, i.e., a bacteremia with an unidentifiable source.
    b. **Prophylaxis**
        (1) Prophylactic antibiotics are given when Dacron or Gortex grafts are inserted. Antistaphylococcal coverage with cephalothin or nafcillin is provided until invasive lines are discontinued.
        (2) Provide adequate initial debridement of nonviable tissue.
        (3) Remove invasive lines as soon as possible.
        (4) Aggressively treat foci of infection (pneumonia, sinusitis, etc.).
        (5) Delay wound closure if the wound would be closed under tension or if there is a question of adequate debridement.
        (6) Cover the suture lines at least partially with healthy soft tissue; preferably, the entire graft is covered with healthy tissue.
        (7) Use autogenous vascular structure (vein), whenever possible.
    c. **Treatment**
        (1) Remove the graft.
        (2) Proximal and distal ligation
        (3) Extra-anatomical bypass, but only if there is ischemia after the graft is removed
        (4) Antibiotics are administered based on the Gram stain and culture.
        (5) Treat the associated wound infection (see pp. 191 and 261).

14. **Bacterial endocarditis** This is a localized disease involving the endocardium of the heart chambers or valves, yet it presents clinically as a systemic disease. The organisms most commonly involved are staphylococci (coagulase-posi-

tive or -negative), less frequently streptococci (enterococcus; alpha-hemolytic streptococcus), and, rarely, Gram-negative rods. There has been an increase during the past decade in the incidence of right-sided endocarditis, probably secondary to the use of central venous lines and Swan-Ganz catheterization.

a. **Manifestations**
   (1) Fever and/or leukocytosis
   (2) Cardiac murmur ±
   (3) Embolization
       (a) Right heart—septic pulmonary emboli
       (b) Left heart
           i. Kidneys (urinalysis may reveal RBC and/or RBC casts)
           ii. Brain (decreased level of consciousness and/or onset of focal neurologic deficit)
           iii. Spleen (infarction and/or splenomegaly)
           iv. Skin (petechiae and/or septic cutaneous foci, i.e., furunculosis)

b. **Diagnosis**
   (1) If the patient is not on antibiotics, the causative organism will be cultured in the blood in 85–90% of cases.
   (2) Three to four blood cultures in 24 hr from separate puncture sites should reveal the responsible organism.
   (3) If the patient is extremely ill (acute bacterial endocarditis), three cultures should be obtained from different sites and antibiotics should be initiated.
   (4) Echocardiogram is occasionally helpful.

Perspective
The patient is usually systemically ill (toxic) and has a positive culture for staphylococcus or streptococcus; the diagnosis requires a high index of suspicion.

---

15. **Osteomyelitis** may be primary (direct implantation) or secondary (hematogenous). Usually primary osteomyelitis is secondary to
    —An open fracture
    —A penetrating wound (e.g., gunshot wound)
    —A surgical procedure (open reduction)
The organisms are variable and may be staphylococcal, streptococcal, or Gram-negative rod infections.

a. **Manifestations**
   (1) Fever and/or leukocytosis
   (2) Local bone pain may be present.
   (3) Decreased range of motion

(4) Soft tissue wound infection
  (a) Local pain
  (b) Erythema
  (c) Induration
  (d) Suppuration
(5) Positive blood culture for staphylococcus may be suggestive.

b. **Diagnosis**
  (1) Gram stain and culture of the wound may be positive and suggest an associated osteomyelitis.
  (2) X-rays reveal rarefaction (lucency) at the site of infection with surrounding subperiosteal new bone formation. These changes usually do not appear for 2–4 weeks in adults and may not appear until later if the patient has been on antibiotics. X-rays may reveal soft tissue swelling, which may be secondary to infection.

c. **Prophylaxis**
  (1) Open fractures are prophylaxed with cephalothin or nafcillin for 3–5 days post-injury.
  (2) Initial debridement and irrigation of the wound must be adequate and followed with delayed primary or secondary closure. If there is a question regarding the advisability of wound closure, quantitative tissue cultures are obtained.

d. **Treatment**
  (1) Open the wound and encourage adequate external drainage.
  (2) Debride the wound of necrotic tissue.
  (3) Remove nonviable bone.
  (4) Immobilize the limb.
  (5) Antibiotics are chosen based on the Gram stain and cultures.
  (6) Frequent dressing changes of the wound are performed.

16. **Atelectasis** See pp. 106 and 323.

17. **Drug fever** Eosinophilia may be present. The fever is often out of proportion relative to the improving clinical state of the patient. The patient's fever may improve with antipyretics or totally resolve in 2–3 days, if the offending drug is discontinued.

18. **Subarachnoid hemorrhage** No specific therapy.

19. **Large hematoma** Drain, if possible, after liquefaction (about 2–3 weeks).

IV. **Miscellaneous**

A. **Protocol for aminoglycoside levels** Aminoglycoside antibiotics remain the mainstay for the treatment of Gram-negative sepsis. The only way to monitor the effectiveness and safety of therapy is by monitoring serum aminoglycoside levels. Although many nomograms have been published for dosing these antibiotics, they are derived using averages for many patients, and it has become apparent that frequent serum levels are mandatory, especially in the unstable patient. Radioimmunoassay is reliable and quick.

1. **Subjects** are those receiving gentamicin, tobramycin, or amikacin for more than 24 hr.

2. **Dosing** Patients are dosed according to established nomograms or preferably by the use of the MIEMSS computer program. The desired serum levels are as follows:
   a. Gentamicin: peak of 6 μg/ml, trough of ≤1 μg/ml
   b. Tobramycin: peak of 6 μg/ml, trough of ≤1 μg/ml
   c. Amikacin: peak of 25 μg/ml, trough of ≤8 μg/ml
   All i.v. doses of aminoglycosides are to be run in over 30 min, unless otherwise stated.

3. **Levels** After the fourth dose of an aminoglycoside, serum levels are obtained in the following sequence: Obtain 5 ml of blood in a red stopper tube labeled with the patient's name at 15 min post-infusion and immediately prior to the next dose. On each successive day in unstable patients, one pre- and post-dose level are obtained. Levels are not obtained through the same tubing in which the drug was infused.

4. **Handling of specimens** The MIEMSS laboratory spins the sample and freezes the serum. The sample is picked up by the clinical pharmacology representative from the MIEMSS Critical Care Branch, and levels are run and recorded on the patient's chart. The levels are brought to the Team Leader's attention and subsequent doses are determined by using the patient's serum level and aminoglycoside clearance as guides.

5. **Levels at dialysis** All patients undergoing hemodialysis or peritoneal dialysis have aminoglycoside levels obtained immediately prior to and immediately following dialysis (see p. 354).

B. **Splenectomy** There is increasing evidence that adults as well as children who have undergone splenectomy for trauma have a higher than normal risk of developing fulminating bacteremias with encapsulated organisms. It has long been the custom to give splenectomized children prophylactic penicillin for some length of time, usually 2–4 years. With the recent introduction of the pneumococcal vaccine (Pneumovax), it seems appropriate that all patients who undergo splenectomy should receive immunization with this vaccine. The vaccine is given at the time of splenectomy or within the first 72 hr of hospitalization.

C. **Tetanus** is a risk associated with all traumatic wounds, yet it is a preventable disease. Tetanus toxoid is very effective, long-lasting, and relatively free of side effects. Protection can be achieved for at least 10 years following full immunization.

1. Patients with **clean minor wounds** need no tetanus prophylaxis if the patient has had a tetanus toxoid booster within 10 years.

2. Patients with **major wounds** should receive absorbed tetanus toxoid, 0.5 ml, if they have had primary vaccinations, but no booster in the last 5 years, or cannot give a history of previous immunization.

3. **Tetanus immune globulin,** 250 units, is given to all patients with uncertain or no vaccination history and to all patients with major wounds who have had fewer than three previous doses of tetanus toxoid. Patients with no history or incomplete immunization histories should have a full series of tetanus immunization consisting of three doses of adult toxoid, i.m., with the second dose 4–6 weeks after the first, and the third dose 6 months to 1 year later.

Section VII
NUTRITION

INTRODUCTION

Nutritional support is designed to provide the patient with sufficient amounts of substrate for energy production, i.e., lipids and carbohydrates. Water, electrolytes, vitamins, trace elements, and protein must be supplied to maintain cellular function. The purpose of nutritional support is to maintain or to minimize the destruction of the visceral and somatic protein pools. Examples of visceral proteins are albumin, transferrin, thyroxine-binding prealbumin, retinol-binding protein, lymphocytes, immunoglobulins, and enzymatic systems. The somatic proteins (muscle) are involved in locomotion and respiration.

Starvation, sepsis, and/or trauma (accidental or surgically induced) result in degradation of the protein pool. With degradation of the protein pool, there is impairment of physiologic systems, such as the immunologic, hormonal, and metabolic systems. Protein depletion predisposes the patient to sepsis and cellular deterioration and exacerbates existing cellular dysfunction.

27

NUTRITIONAL SUPPORT OF
THE CRITICALLY ILL PATIENT

I. **Manifestations of Inadequate Nutrition**

   A. **Depletion of parietal muscle**

   1. Etiology is inadequate caloric intake, despite an adequate protein load.

   2. The patient presents with a starved appearance that has manifested itself over a prolonged period.

   3. Measurements of the visceral protein stores are within normal limits.

   4. The clinical course of the patient shows a reasonably preserved ability to respond to short-term stress.

   B. **Visceral protein attrition**

   1. The etiology is generally inadequate nitrogen (or protein) intake, despite adequate caloric input.

   2. The patient appears well nourished. Other signs may be edema or hair that is easily pluckable.

   3. Measurements of the visceral protein stores show depressed serum albumin, diminished lymphocyte count, depressed serum transferrin levels, decreased total iron binding capacity, and inability to recall a response to common antigens such as candida, mumps, purified protein derivative (PPD), and streptokinase-streptodornase (SKSD).

   4. Along with the above laboratory findings, the patient may show depressed wound healing as well as sepsis or other complications.

   C. **Varying combinations of visceral protein attrition and parietal muscle depletion**

   1. The combination of severe stress along with depressed calorie and nitrogen intake causes this form of malnutrition to be the one most frequently suffered by trauma patients.

   2. The patient may show evidence of wasting.

   3. Laboratory findings resemble those of visceral protein attrition.

   4. The patient suffering this form of malnutrition shows signs of depressed wound healing, an incompetent immune system, and a variety of complications, including sepsis.

II. Maintenance versus Repletion Therapy

A. Maintenance nutrition provides a balanced intake of energy and structural substrate designed to maintain a neutral or slightly positive nitrogen balance.

B. Repletion of nutritional balance is designed to effect a positive nitrogen balance, i.e., an anabolic state.

III. Modes of Nutritional Support

A. **Total parenteral nutrition (TPN)** is a hyperosmolar solution given by a central route. TPN supplies the patient with the needed nutrients to maintain or replete the protein pool, i.e., a neutral or a positive nitrogen balance.

B. **Partial parenteral nutrition (PPN)** is an amino acid solution whose osmolality allows administration via a peripheral vein (less than 700 mOsm/liter), with or without concurrent administration of an emulsified, intravenous lipid preparation. PPN is designed to **minimize** negative nitrogen balance.

C. **Enteral alimentation** is the administration of food or liquid formulas for oral or tube feedings. Enteral alimentation may be total or partial nutritional support.

D. A **combination** of enteral and parenteral nutrition may be given.

IV. Components of Nutritional Support

A. **Calories** Up to a point, a linear relationship exists between the number of calories supplied and the degree of nitrogen balance attained when sufficient nitrogen is delivered concurrently. Patients need a certain amount of non-protein calories to utilize nitrogen. In trauma patients, this is approximately 120–170 non-protein calories/gm of nitrogen. By measuring the total body oxygen consumption in the multiply traumatized patient, indications are that approximately 1,800–2,500 non-protein calories are needed per day. Actual needs vary from patient to patient, depending on the degree of trauma. Administration of **carbohydrate** calories in excess of requirements increases lipogenesis (especially in the liver), with attendant changes in liver function tests. While modest increases in liver function tests can be expected during nutritional support, severe elevations in bilirubin, alkaline phosphatase, serum glutamic oxaloacetic transaminase (SGOT), serum glutamic pyruvic transaminase (SGPT), and lactate dehydrogenase (LDH) may indicate excessive carbohydrate infusion. When this happens, the course open to the clinician is to decrease carbohydrate calories and/or increase nitrogen administration.

Carbohydrate calories in excess result in increased carbon dioxide production. Excess carbohydrate calories are stored as fat; this is an energy-requiring step. Glucose calories are not efficiently utilized when glucose is administered at a rate greater than 4–5 mg/kg/min. Most Americans consume 40–50% of their daily caloric intake as **fat.** An attempt is made to approximate this proportion in the trauma patient.

B. Nitrogen The protein requirement for adults is 1.0 gm/kg/day in the normal nonstressed state. As the patient undergoes varying degrees of stress from trauma, surgery, or infection, the requirement for protein will increase to approximately 1.5–2.0 gm/kg/day. If the blood urea nitrogen (BUN) increases significantly and other causes of azotemia have been ruled out, the patient may be receiving either too much nitrogen or not enough non-protein calories. Nitrogen balance is helpful in determining nitrogenous needs.

C. Trace elements are administered beginning after 2 weeks of TPN therapy, unless signs of trace element deficiency are seen before that time. Enteral alimentation usually furnishes adequate quantities of trace elements. If a deficiency develops while enteral alimentation is administered, the trace elements are administered parenterally.

1. **Chromium chloride**
   a. Manifestations of deficiency
      (1) Weight loss
      (2) Glucose intolerance
      (3) Marginal nitrogen balance
      (4) Decreased respiratory quotient (RQ)
   b. Daily requirement is 10–15 μg/day.
   c. Excreted primarily in the urine (Use judiciously in renal failure patients.)

2. **Copper sulfate**
   a. Manifestations of deficiency
      (1) Hypochromic, normocytic anemia
      (2) Leukopenia (neutropenia)
      (3) Hypoproteinemia
   b. Daily requirement is 0.5–1.5 mg/day.
   c. Use judiciously in patients with biliary tract obstruction.

3. **Manganese chloride**
   a. Manifestations of deficiency
      (1) Weight loss
      (2) Ill defined dermatitis
   b. Daily requirement is 0.15–0.8 mg/day.
   c. Use judiciously in patients with biliary tract obstruction.

4. **Zinc chloride**
   a. Manifestations of deficiency
      (1) Diarrhea (first to occur)
      (2) Alopecia
      (3) Paranasal, periorbital, and perioral dermatitis
   b. Daily requirement is 2.5–4.0 mg/day.
   c. Urine zinc excretion increases in stress.
   d. If there are significant intestinal losses, such as fistula, diarrhea, or ileostomy losses, 9.0 mg/day is given.

5. **Iron** (as iron dextran)
   a. Manifestations of deficiency
      (1) Hypochromic, microcytic anemia

      (2) Low serum iron concentration

      (3) Increased iron-binding capacity

    b. Once per month, the total iron-binding capacity (TIBC) and serum iron are measured. If an iron deficiency is revealed, intravenous iron dextran (Imferon) is administered to replace hemoglobin and bone marrow stores.

$$\text{mg iron} = 0.3 \times \text{wt in pounds} \times \left(100 - \left(\frac{\text{patient's Hb} \times 100}{14.8}\right)\right)$$

D. Electrolytes The amount is variable and depends on serum and urine chemistries. Electrolyte needs are affected by gastrointestinal losses, chest tube losses, and open wound drainage.

1. Sodium (as chloride or acetate), 80–120 mEq/day

2. Potassium (as chloride or acetate), 80–120 mEq/day

3. Calcium (as gluconate or gluceptate), 4.5–13.5 mEq/day

4. Magnesium (as sulfate), 8–16 mEq/day

5. Phosphorus (as sodium or potassium salt), 15–40 mmol/day. Stock potassium phosphate solutions contain 3 mmol of phosphorus and 4.4 mEq of potassium/ml. Stock sodium phosphate solutions contain 3 mmol of phosphorus and 4.0 mEq of sodium/ml. Order phosphate in millimoles, not milliequivalents. Millimole calculations are constant regardless of the solution pH.

| Note | Potassium, magnesium, and phosphate are intracellular ions and are subject to great variations, depending on the degree of anabolism or catabolism and on the status of renal function. During catabolism or cellular breakdown, these electrolytes enter the serum. During anabolism, these electrolytes tend to enter the cell and frequently result in low serum levels.

E. Water

1. Approximate requirements are 35–40 ml/kg/day.

2. Major variations in water requirements are seen with
    a. Exogenous losses, i.e., urine, nasogastric, diarrhea, fistula, etc.
    b. Temperature
    c. Increased requirements with hemodynamic instability and third space losses

F. Albumin Serum albumin levels become depressed during stress (trauma, burns, or infection) and are slow to respond to adequate nutritional support (serum half-life of endogenous albumin is 20 days). If serum oncotic pressure is low due to low serum albumin (less than 2.5 gm %), albumin may be administered at doses of 12.5–25 gm/day until the serum albumin level rises.

While albumin is compatible with all TPN solutions, it must be administered separately because it may not pass through the 0.22 micron filter. Exogenous albumin has no nutritional value because it is tryptophan-deficient.

G. Vitamins Adult requirements (children 11 years of age and over)

Vitamins	RDA adult range	i.v. formulation
A	4,000–5,000 IU	3,300
D	4,000 IU	200
E	12–15 IU	10
Ascorbic acid	45 mg	100
Folacin	400 μg	400
Niacin	12–20 mg	40
Riboflavin	1.1–1.8 mg	3.6
Thiamine	1.0–1.5 mg	3.0
B$_6$ (pyridoxine)	1.6–2.0 mg	4.0
B$_{12}$ (cyanocobalamin)	3 μg	5.0
Pantothenic acid	5–10 mg	15.0
Biotin	150–300 μg	60

The following vitamins are given during TPN:

1. MVI-12   10 ml added to i.v. solution every other day; alternated with B complex solution such as Solu-B-Forte (10 ml) or Berocca-C (4 ml).

2. Vitamin K (AquaMEPHYTON)   10 mg once weekly (i.m.)

3. Folic acid   1.0 mg i.v. daily; 5 mg daily in patients with history of alcohol abuse

4. Vitamin B$_{12}$ (Cyanocobalamin)   100 μg i.m. on the first of every month

V. Parenteral Nutrition

A. Partial parenteral nutrition (also known as modified TPN and partial TPN) is not generally used for longer than 7 days. This form of nutritional support is indicated to minimize protein loss; rarely will a positive nitrogen balance be achieved. We administer PPN solutions as amino acids and Intralipid (a 10% soybean oil preparation) or as amino acids, Intralipid, and dextrose. If the patient is obese, amino acids plus 100 cc of Intralipid (to prevent essential fatty acid deficiency) are administered. If the patient is not obese, amino acids, plus dextrose in hypocaloric concentrations, plus emulsified intravenous lipid (100 cc) are administered.

1. Obese patients
   a. Amino acids 8.5% (500 ml)
   b. Sterile water (500 ml)
   c. Plus electrolytes, vitamins, and 100 cc of intravenous lipid

2. Non-obese patients
   a. Amino acids 8.5% (500 ml)
   b. D10W (500 ml)
   c. Plus electrolytes, vitamins, and 100 cc of intravenous lipid

We recommend administering 1.5 gm of protein/kg/24 hr. Partial parenteral nutrition solutions are not designed to induce positive nitrogen or caloric balance. They can "spare protein" and lessen the amount of nitrogen lost. If adequate nutritional support has not been started by day 7 by the oral route, total parenteral nutrition should be initiated.

B. Total parenteral nutrition

1. TPN is most commonly supplied as a solution of 8.5% amino acids and hypertonic dextrose (30–70%) in equal parts. TPN must be given via a central line and is designed for long-term nutritional support. Accordingly, when TPN is given through a central line, the rules under "TPN Catheter Care Protocol" (below) governing the maintenance of a central venous line hold fast. TPN is not given via a peripheral line or through a "long line," if at all possible.

2. Preferred procedure for proper and aseptic **catheter placement** (subclavian vein)

   a. Assemble equipment Large Deseret Intracath, a sterile prep tray, acetone, surgical scrub and solution, hydrogen peroxide, 3-0 nylon sutures, i.v. solution, and i.v. tubing for TPN with inline filter.

   b. It may be helpful to have the patient's shoulder hyperextended over a rolled sheet or towel placed longitudinally between the scapulae.

   c. Once the rolled sheet or towel is in place, place the patient in a Trendelenburg position (head down at 15°) to enable maximum dilation of the subclavian vein.

   d. Shave carefully (if necessary) the skin over the neck, chest, and/or axilla.

   e. Thoroughly defat the skin with acetone.

   f. Wear mask, sterile gloves, and hat.

   g. Wash the skin with an appropriate antiseptic scrub and then with solution (remove the residue from the scrub) in a manner identical to preoperative skin preparation.

   h. Remove gloves and put on new gloves and a sterile gown.

   i. Drape the field with 3 or 4 sterile towels.

   j. Infiltrate 0.5% or 1% lidocaine (Xylocaine), **without epinephrine** and **from an unopened bottle,** into the skin, subcutaneous tissue, and periosteum of the clavicle at the inferior border of the clavicle.

   k. Remove catheter (containing the wire stylet) from the needle and mount the needle on a syringe.

   l. Take the patient off the respirator briefly, to avoid inadvertent pneumothorax, until the vein is punctured and the catheter is introduced through the needle.

   m. Make the venipuncture with the needle, maintaining a slight negative pressure in the syringe.

   n. Once the vein is entered (as evidenced by a surge of blood in the syringe), advance the needle a few millimeters to ensure that the entire needle bevel is within the lumen of the vein.

   o. Immobilize the needle and carefully withdraw the syringe from the needle.

   p. While holding the needle stationary, advance the catheter through the needle.

q. Withdraw the needle point from the skin and apply the needle guard.
r. Withdraw the wire stylet from the catheter and aspirate through the catheter to ensure that blood can be withdrawn, to indicate proper placement in the vein.
s. Attach the extension tubing with an inline filter to the catheter and infuse isotonic i.v. solution (e.g., normal saline (NS) or D5W), until a chest x-ray can be taken to determine the position of the line. The extension tubing is secured to the skin, as is the catheter (see u, below) and, except for the proximal connector, is covered by sterile pads (see z, below). It is designed to absorb the traction generated when the line is manipulated and provides a Leurlok connection to the hub of the catheter.
t. Apply pressure with a sterile sponge gauze if there is bleeding from the insertion site.
u. Secure the catheter and extension tubing with sutures of 3-0 nylon around the catheter guard.
v. Remove the drape from the patient.
w. To enhance the security of the catheter connection with the extension tubing, they may be tied together.
x. Wipe blood or clot from the area with hydrogen peroxide.
y. Apply an antiseptic ointment to the puncture site and around the tubing-catheter connection.
z. Using a single layer of sterile pads, cover the entire device (2 × 2 sponge on the puncture site and a 4 × 4 sponge over the catheter), including the needle hub and distal i.v. extension tubing.
aa. Protect the nipple with a 2 × 2 sponge, if needed.
bb. Fix the sterile gauze dressing with tincture of benzoin and several 5-inch long strips of Elastoplast tape (or nonporous tape). The purpose of the tincture of benzoin is to create a sticky surface to which tape adheres well. Pressing nonporous tape firmly over the area seals the site.
cc. Reinforce the edges of Elastoplast tape with strips of adhesive tape.
dd. Mark the date of insertion on the adhesive tape and make a procedure note in the patient's chart.
ee. Order a chest x-ray.

3. **TPN catheter care protocol**
   a. No other entries will be made into the system. To achieve safe long-term central venous catheterization, avoid the following, except in an emergency situation:
   (1) Administration or withdrawal of blood
   (2) Administration of blood products
   (3) Antibiotics
   (4) Heparin (except any added in the TPN solution)
   (5) Corticosteroids
   (6) Any other medications
   (7) CVP measurement
   (8) Back flow of blood through the line
   (9) Placement of stopcock in the line

b. A central venous line, which has already been used for the above (**a, 1–9**), should not be used to deliver hyperalimentation solutions (TPN) on a long-term basis (longer than 3 days).

c. To avoid breaking the system, intravenous fat solutions will be administered via a peripheral venous line.

d. Do not break the system unless absolutely necessary. Any break in the system must be documented in the patient's chart.

e. The expiration date of the TPN solution will be determined and noted on the bottle by the pharmacy. The tubing down to the extension hub and the in-line filter will be changed every 24 hr.

f. Dressing changes are done every 48 hr by using aseptic techniques.

    (1) Assemble equipment   The same is used as listed on p. 440 for catheter insertion, except for the prep tray.

    (2) Masks must be worn by all persons involved.

    (3) Care must be taken not to move, pull out, or push in the catheter during the dressing change. The extension tubing is designed to avoid this complication.

    (4) With sterile gloves, remove the old dressing taking care not to dislodge the catheter. Remove gloves.

    (5) Observe the insertion site and surrounding skin for inflammation, erythema, drainage, etc.

    (6) With change of sterile gloves, remove old clot, crust, etc., from the pucture site, catheter, and extension tubing with hydrogen peroxide. Remove gloves. Pain at the insertion site upon examiner's finger pressure is a good indication to remove the line.

    (7) With a third set of sterile gloves, follow defatting, scrubbing, and dressing procedures previously outlined.

4. Length of time lines may be used   Since it may be necessary to leave catheters in place for up to 30 days (or longer), strict adherence to catheter care is mandatory. The result of any deviation from protocol may be sepsis.

a. For TPN, see "TPN Catheter Care Protocol."

b. PPN may be given peripherally or centrally.

    (1) PPN given peripherally causes that peripheral line to be treated like any other peripheral or long line.

    (2) If PPN is given via a central vein and the line is to be maintained as an inviolable central line, only PPN may be infused through that line. If medications, i.v. fluids, and PPN are infused through a central line, this line is **not** a long-term line and must be changed according to infectious disease guidelines relating to short-term central lines. In short, PPN can be considered as similar to any other i.v. solution, and lines through which PPN is infused can be treated like any other lines through which a variety of i.v. fluids are infused.

5. Available solutions

a. Travasol 8.5% without electrolytes

    (1) Delivers 7.15 gm of nitrogen/500 ml of solution (45 gm of protein equivalent).

(2) Travasol 8.5% is the crystalline amino acid solution of choice for patients who are hyperphosphatemic.
  b. FreAmine III 8.5%
    (1) FreAmine III 8.5% delivers 6.5 gm of nitrogen/500 ml of solution (45 gm of protein equivalent).
    (2) FreAmine III is the solution of choice in patients for whom modest increased amounts of branched chain amino acids are desired and in whom serum phosphorus levels are not a problem.

6. **Determining ingredients of the solution**
  a. Average **caloric needs** in trauma patients varies between 1,800–2,500 kcal/day or approximately 30–35 kcal/kg/day. This is only an approximation and some patients will require more (see p. 454).
  b. Determining caloric needs by the total oxygen consumption method

$$A - V\ O_2\ (\text{ml }\%) \times CO\ (\text{liter/min}) \times 72 = \text{kcal consumed/24 hr}$$

  c. A judicious number of dextrose calories should be administered; the ultimate goal is the administration of approximately 4–5 mg/kg/min of **dextrose**. It must be remembered that excess calories will result in fatty metamorphosis of the liver, a respiratory quotient approaching or exceeding 1.0, and storage of carbohydrate as fat. Accordingly, the projected dextrose load for a 70-kg patient will be 403 gm (70 kg × 4 mg/kg × 1,440 min/day = 403,200 mg or 403.2 gm of dextrose/day).

  The patient is not started out at this rate. The initial rate and concentration of the TPN solution are governed by the patient's water needs and glucose tolerance.

  Fats supplement the glucose in meeting the caloric needs. The initial goal of 4–5 mg/kg/min of dextrose is subject to clinical judgment, and if a "satisfactory response" is not seen within 7 days, the glucose concentrations may be increased by small increments. Consider increasing the glucose load if
    (1) A rising BUN suggests "inadequate utilization" of protein
    (2) The RQ is remaining near 0.7–0.8
    (3) Nitrogen balance is negative
    (4) Alkaline phosphatase, bilirubin, and hepatocellular enzymes are not markedly elevated

  Along with intravenous lipids and intravenous dextrose, approximately 1–1.5 gm of **protein** eq/kg are administered to the patient. Every ingredient is added with special consideration to the clinical picture of the patient. Each solution is tailored to the patient with emphasis on water, electrolyte, caloric, and protein needs.

7. **Intravenous lipids**
  a. Intralipid (10%)
    (1) Contains 54% linoleic acid
    (2) Provides 1.1 kcal/ml
  b. Indications for Intralipid
    (1) Essential fatty acid deficiency

(2) Protein sparing

(3) Source of calories during TPN

c. Dosage is generally one 500-ml bottle/day given intravenously over 4–6 hr. Dosage range may be up to 1,500 ml/day.

d. Six to eight hours after infusion, intravenous fat should be cleared from the serum. If the serum is turbid at this time, it is not being efficiently utilized.

e. Contraindications   Hepatic and pulmonary insufficiency are **relative** contraindications.

f. A 20% solution is available if fluid restriction is necessary.

8. Heparin may be added at a concentration of 1,000 units/liter to avoid catheter clotting and to eliminate the formation of a fibrin sheath at the catheter end. The fibrin sheath may enhance the colonization of blood-borne bacteria on the catheter tip. Five hundred units/liter is insufficient heparin and 1,000 units/liter has no effect on the partial thromboplastin time (PTT). Heparin should be avoided in selected patients with severe coagulopathies.

9. Insulin

a. Insulin should not be given to the patient until one has determined the patient's ability to tolerate a glucose load. It is better to give too little insulin than to give too much and induce hypoglycemia.

b. Hyperglycemia in the septic patient is best managed by decreasing the glucose load, since the administration of insulin in these patients may induce a fatty liver.

c. Glucose intolerance in the diabetic patient can be managed by

(1) Giving insulin intravenously as a continuous infusion by adding 50 units of regular insulin to 500 ml of ½NS, and by flushing out and discarding the first 50 ml of solution. Begin the rate at 1–2 units/hr and make adjustments according to the serum glucose. Change the rate of insulin infusion no more often than every 3 hr.

(2) Adding regular insulin to the TPN bottle beginning with 10–15 units/bottle (after you are certain of the response of the patient to the glucose load). Note that 8–12 units of insulin will adhere to the bottle and tubing.

(3) Giving subcutaneous insulin as a sliding scale based on serum glucose.

10. Complications

a. Catheter-related complications

(1) Pulmonary embolization of clots

(2) Phlebitis

(3) Perivenous extravasation

(4) Venous thrombosis

(5) Arterial puncture

(6) Catheter-related sepsis

(7) Hydrothorax

(8) Pneumothorax

(9) Catheter embolism

(10) Air embolism

b. **Septic complications**
   (1) Candida proliferates in TPN solutions.
   (2) Continuous use of in-line micropore filters (0.22 micron) is mandatory even if other solutions (for example, D10W) are used periodically.
   (3) No additives should be made to the TPN solution by nursing personnel. All additives are handled and controlled by the pharmacy.

c. **Metabolic disorders**
   (1) **Hyperglycemia** causes an osmotic diuresis. Rule out diabetes or infection.
   (2) **Hyponatremia** is secondary to GI losses, urinary losses, or water intoxication.
   (3) **Hypokalemia** is secondary to GI or urinary losses.
   (4) **Hypomagnesemia** is due to GI or renal losses. An insufficient amount is added to TPN solutions.
   (5) **Hypophosphatemia** Insufficient amounts of phosphorous given relative to glucose load administered; excessive calcium administration
   (6) **Prerenal azotemia** Dehydration; insufficient dextrose calories administered; excessive protein load
   (7) **Hyperammonemia** Hepatic dysfunction (impaired ammonia-urea cycle); excessive protein load. Rx: decrease protein load and increase arginine.
   (8) **Hyperchloremic metabolic acidosis** Excess chloride ion administration or bicarbonate loss. Rx: decrease chloride and increase acetate.
   (9) **Hypoglycemia** Abrupt cessation of TPN solution or too much insulin administered
   (10) **Hypocalcemia** Hyperphosphatemia; depressed serum albumin
   (11) **Hyperphosphatemia** Depressed renal function; hypocalcemia; administering excessive phosphate
   (12) **Hypermagnesemia** Impaired renal function
   (13) **Essential fatty acid deficiency** Lack of fat in nutrition regimen. The clinical manifestations of essential fatty acid deficiency are dry, scaly dermatitis, hair loss, and delayed wound healing. Calories (8–10%) should be furnished by Intralipid to correct the deficiency.
   (14) **Hypoalbuminemia** Acute stress, liver dysfunction, or malnutrition
   (15) **Metabolic alkalosis** Chloride depletion due to aspiration of large volumes of gastric secretions or inadequate chloride administration; or excess bicarbonate or acetate administration
   (16) **Hepatic steatosis** Too many glucose calories, too little protein, essential fatty acid deficiency, or amino acid toxicity (tryptophan)

11. **Monitoring nutritional support therapy**
   a. Daily serum (initially)
      (1) Sodium
      (2) Potassium
      (3) Osmolality
      (4) Glucose

    (5) BUN

    (6) Creatinine

b. Daily urine (initially)

    (1) Sodium

    (2) Potassium

    (3) Osmolality

    (4) Glucose

    (5) Ketones

c. Daily temperature and input/output of fluids

d. Weekly serum

    (1) Calcium

    (2) Phosphorus

    (3) Magnesium

    (4) Albumin and total protein (low level implies visceral protein deficiency)

    (5) Liver function tests: alkaline phosphatase, SGOT, SGPT, bilirubin, LDH

    (6) Ammonia

e. Total lymphocyte count ($<1,500$/mm^3 implies visceral protein deficiency.)

f. Nitrogen balance is the difference between nitrogen input and output. Input is the amount of nitrogen infused, and output is the amount of urine urea nitrogen (UUN) excreted per day plus a 4-gm factor which represents other urinary, cutaneous, and fecal nitrogenous compounds. By using these values, the daily nitrogen infused can be compared with approximate daily nitrogen excretion. For example, given the following values: daily urine volume=2,310 ml, UUN=615 mg %, N$_2$ out=14.2 gm+4 gm=18.2 gm; if N$_2$ in=15.6 gm, a negative N$_2$ balance exists (-2.6 gm). The calculated nitrogen balance carries negligible significance if the patient has large open wounds or draining cavities.

g. Daily weights are useful in selected patients, but are of questionable clinical value in patients with frequent changes in orthopedic casts or widely fluctuating volume status. Obviously, daily weights should not be attempted in the severely unstable patient. In the stable patient, weight gain or loss should be no more than 0.75 kg/day. Values in excess of this reflect expansion or contraction of total body water.

h. Delayed hypersensitivity tests for anergy Anergy or relative anergy may be caused by malnutrition or stress. Skin tests may be helpful in monitoring the adequacy of nutritional support. Failure to develop a response after nutritional support may imply inadequate nutritional support. The tests customarily used are SKSD, PPD, mumps, and candida. Anergy is defined as no response to skin tests, relative anergy as response to only one skin antigen.

i. Low transferrin (TIBC <250 μg/dl implies visceral protein depletion.)

j. The presence of ketones Monitoring for urinary and/or serum ketones is mandatory in patients who are receiving no dextrose and only amino acids plus intravenous lipid. Acetest reagent tablets are used for a semiquantitative determination of ketones. Acetest measures only the presence of acetoacetic acid and acetone, and not betahydroxybutyric acid. Ketosis may be marked only by an increased ratio of betahydroxybutyric acid to acetoacetic acid and acetone, i.e., an increase only in the former. The Acetest in this case will give a negative result. Ketosis is often equated with toxicity, but this is not always correct since ketosis occurs with the utilization of fat and is an expected physiologic response.

   k. Monitoring intravenous fat administration
      (1) Temperature may rise 3°–4°F, a consideration in a patient monitored concurrently for infection.
      (2) Serum triglycerides can be expected to increase for a few hours post-infusion. Follow the patient for lipemic serum, and obtain a serum triglyceride level if there is poor clearance.
      (3) Serum cholesterol Hypercholesterolemia may occur but resolves after the infusion of intravenous fat has stopped.

   l. Summary of nutritional assessment
      (1) Somatic or skeletal protein status is monitored using the creatinine-height index. Excreted urinary creatinine depends upon height (muscle mass) of the patient. Decreased creatinine excretion with normal renal function implies muscle wasting (somatic protein deficit).
      (2) The visceral protein status is monitored by
         (a) Delayed hypersensitivity skin testing (cell-mediated immunity)
         (b) Total lymphocyte count
         (c) Transferrin (TIBC)
         (d) Albumin
      Failure to react to skin tests and/or a low albumin, lymphocyte count and transferrin level may imply malnutrition.

12. Nutritional support in renal failure Nephramine 5.4% (essential amino acid injection) delivers 1.6 gm of nitrogen/250 ml of solution. The basic theory behind the administration of this solution is that supplying the patient with the essential amino acids plus sufficient calories will allow the patient with renal failure to manufacture nonessential amino acids by using endogenous urea nitrogen.

   The efficacy of essential amino acids for use in patients with renal failure has not been conclusively documented. In order for such a patient to "recycle" endogenous urea nitrogen, administration of hypertonic dextrose seems to be the rate-limiting step in the process.

   a. The goal in such patients is to
      (1) Administer decreased amounts of nitrogen (both essential and nonessential amino acids)
      (2) Provide the patient with a maximum dextrose load to effect a progressive fall in the BUN. The patient is begun on a solution of moderate dextrose concentration, e.g., D20W or D30W. This concentration is increased as the patient tolerates the glucose load. A positive response is seen when the BUN begins to decrease. At that time the glucose concentration is maintained and nitrogen is increased.

b. We administer crystalline amino acids (CAA) 8.5% 125 ml with D50W (or another appropriate concentration) 500 ml; e.g., 125 ml of Travasol 8.5% delivers 1.79 gm of N_2, and 125 ml of FreAmine III 8.5% delivers 1.63 gm of N_2.

c. Major consideration should be given to the presence of phosphate in the above solutions Travasol 8.5% contains no phosphorus; 125 ml of FreAmine III 8.5% contains 2.5 mEq of phosphorus. Administration of hypertonic dextrose acts to decrease serum phosphate as the dextrose is metabolized in the glycolytic pathway.

d. Monitor the renal failure patient in a pattern similar to that for a patient with normal renal function, with special emphasis on serum phosphorus, magnesium, and potassium levels. The nitrogen concentration is increased as the patient's BUN allows, and the carbohydrate concentration is increased according to calorie requirements and changes in the liver function tests.

13. **Cyclic hyperalimentation**
    a. Indications
       (1) TPN therapy longer than 6 weeks without becoming anabolic
       (2) "Fatty liver" (markedly elevated liver function tests and/or hepatomegaly)
    b. Theoretically, cyclic hyperalimentation will develop a postabsorptive state during which calories stored as fat can be mobilized as an energy source, thus requiring fewer exogenous calories.
    c. Cyclic hyperalimentation entails
       (1) 16 hr of amino acids + dextrose
       (2) 8 hr of amino acids with no dextrose calories
    d. Regimens decided by the clinicians are dependent upon the calorie and nitrogen needs as well as fluid requirements. For example, following is a regimen to deliver 3,000 ml total volume/24 hr. Bottles 1 and 2: CAA 8.5% 500 ml; hypertonic dextrose 500 ml. Rates: (bottle 1) 50 ml/hr × 1 hr, 75 ml/hr × 1 hr, 125 ml/hr × 1 hr, 150 ml/hr × 5 hr; (bottle 2) 150 ml/hr × 5 hr, 125 ml/hr × 1 hr, 75 ml/hr × 1 hr, 50 ml/hr × 1 hr; (bottle 3) CAA 4.25% 1,000 ml at a rate of 125 ml/hr × 8 hr.
    e. The most critical laboratory measurement until the patient is stabilized is the serum glucose. Hypoglycemia may occur when the dextrose-free bottle is begun. One hour after the dextrose-free bottle is hung, obtain a serum glucose.

14. **Nutritional support in hepatic insufficiency**
    a. Indications for precautions
       (1) Known liver disease
       (2) Hepatomegaly
       (3) Abnormal liver function tests

b. Precautions

    (1) Protein load Branched chain (FreAmine III) amino acids may be efficiently utilized and may decrease the propensity to develop encephalopathy. The quantity of protein will be determined by

        (a) Nitrogen balance

        (b) Ammonia level

        (c) BUN

    (2) Glucose load An excessive carbohydrate load will induce or exacerbate hepatic steatosis.

    (3) Cyclic TPN may be better tolerated than other solutions in patients with a "fatty liver."

    (4) Intralipid may be used **cautiously** as a source of calories to decrease excessive glucose administration.

VI. Enteral Nutrition

A. Indications

1. Tube feedings are indicated whenever a patient is unable to tolerate oral feedings and the GI tract functions.

2. The chemically defined or partially chemically defined diet is indicated when there are digestion and absorption problems or where an extremely minimal residue reaching the distal bowel is desired.

3. Oral liquid supplements are indicated in addition to regular meals when daily nutritional requirements are not met.

B. Types of enteral mixtures

1. **Polymeric** High molecular forms of fat, carbohydrate, and protein

    —Relatively low osmolality

    —1–2 kcal/ml

    —Requires normal proteolytic and lipolytic digestion

    —Less expensive

    a. **Balanced tube feeding** provides a complete range of nutrients in physiologic quantities and proportions.

        (1) Ensure

        (2) Ensure Plus (1.5 kcal/ml)

        (3) Isocal

        (4) Precision Moderate Nitrogen

        (5) Osmolite

        (6) Meritene

        (7) Magnacal (2 kcal/cc; 70 gm of protein/liter)

b. **Low residue**
      (1) Low fat
         —Precision LR
         —Precision High Nitrogen
         —Vital

2. **Elemental diet (monomeric)**
      —Amino acids are the protein source.
      —Oligosaccharides or monosaccharides are the carbohydrate source.
      —Hyperosmolar
      —Very small fat content
      —Minimal digestion is needed.
      —Expensive
      —1 kcal/ml
      —Low residue
   a. Vivonex
   b. Vivonex HN
   c. Travasorb HN
      (1) 1.06 kcal/ml
      (2) Contains di- and tripeptides and *l*-amino acids (direct absorption)
      (3) Low viscosity
   d. Travasorb STD
      (1) 1.06 kcal/ml
      (2) Contains di- and tripeptides and *l*-amino acids (direct absorption)
      (3) Low viscosity
   e. Travasorb MCT
      (1) 1–2 kcal/ml
      (2) Requires proteolysis
      (3) Low viscosity

3. **Caloric additives**
   a. **Carbohydrate**
      (1) Controlyte (2 kcal/ml)
      (2) Polycose (2 kcal/ml)
   b. **Fat**
      (1) Medium chain triglyceride oil (low residue) Fatty acids varying from 6–10 carbons, which pass through the intestinal epithelium as free fatty acids.

C. **Special formulations**

1. Amin-Aid
   a. 1–2 kcal/ml
   b. Essential amino acids
   c. Indicated for **renal disease**
   d. Expensive
   e. Requires supplemental vitamins and electrolytes

2. Hepatic-Aid
   a. High branched chain amino acids
   b. Relatively low aromatic amino acids
   c. Indicated for **liver disease**
   d. Not indicated for hepatic encephalopathy
   e. Expensive
   f. Requires supplemental vitamins and electrolytes
   g. Constipation may be a problem

D. **Enteral feeding content**

   1. Isocal   8 fl oz = 8.1 gm of protein; 250 kcal; 300 mOsm/liter

   2. Precision High Nitrogen   12.5 gm of protein/2.93-oz packet; 300 kcal; 557 mOsm/liter

   3. Precision Moderate Nitrogen   10.8 gm of protein/2.75-oz packet; 333 kcal

   4. Precision LR   7.5 gm of protein/3-oz packet; 300 kcal; 525 mOsm/liter

   5. Precision Isotonic   7.5 gm of protein/2.06-oz packet; 250 kcal; 300 mOsm/liter

   6. Vivonex Standard Diet   6.2 gm of protein/80-gm packet; 300 kcal; 550 mOsm/liter

   7. Vivonex High Nitrogen Diet   12.5 gm of protein/80-gm packet; 300 kcal; 844 mOsm/liter

   8. Osmolite   250 kcal/8 fl oz; 8.8 gm of protein; 300 mOsm/liter

   9. Ensure   250 kcal/8 fl oz; 8.8 gm of protein; 450 mOsm/liter

   10. Ensure Plus   355 kcal/8 fl oz; 13.0 gm of protein; 600 mOsm/liter

   11. Magnacal   2 kcal/cc; 70 gm of protein/liter; 590 mOsm/liter

   12. Amin-Aid (renal failure   80-gm packet; 5 gm of protein; 670 kcal; 900 mOsm/liter

   13. Hepatic-Aid (liver disease)   14.5 gm of protein; 560 kcal/packet; 900 mOsm/liter

E. **Routes and techniques for enteral hyperalimentation**

   1. **Small nasogastric catheters** (Keofeed or Dobb-Hoff) or pediatric feeding tubes obviate the discomfort and adverse effects of large-bore tubes.

   2. When long-term enteral feeding is required, a surgically placed **jejunostomy, esophagostomy, or gastrostomy** tube may be preferred to a nasogastric tube.

   3. The **needle catheter jejunostomy** is useful for beginning alimentation soon after admission.
      a. This is well tolerated because the small bowel appears to function following blunt trauma.

    b. Monomeric mixtures are generally infused by this route.

    c. Begin with one-fourth strength Vivonex at 50 ml/hr; increase the rate over the first 48-hr period until fluid requirements are met. If the patient is tolerant to the feedings, gradually increase the strength until calorie and protein requirements are met.

    d. Give continuous infusion to avoid diarrhea.

    e. Care must be taken that the set-up is not confused with an intravenous administration set.

F. **Physical and chemical considerations**

    1. The greater the osmolality and rate of administration, the greater the likelihood of cramping and diarrhea. Flavoring packets increase the osmolality.

    2. Bolus feeding results in more gastric retention than continuous feeding.

    3. Lactose-containing polymeric solutions are too viscous to flow through narrow catheters.

    4. Lactose-containing solutions should be avoided in protein-calorie–starved patients because their atrophic small intestine may be deficient in lactase.

    5. Supplemental infusion of a parenteral nutritional solution should be considered if a patient is unable to tolerate full enteral alimentation.

    6. Electrolyte, vitamin, and essential fatty acid needs must be assessed.

    7. Elemental diets are expensive and are hyperosmolar. They should be reserved only for patients who have alimentary tract fistulas, jejunal feedings, short bowel syndrome, or a need to reduce colonic bulk. In the absence of these indications, other solutions should be used.

    8. Check for history of diabetes; insulin may be required.

    9. Check serum albumin. If it is low, the patient may have difficulty absorbing micronutrients.

G. **Administration of tube feedings (gastric)**

    1. Initiate hyperalimentation using ½ kcal/cc.

    2. Daily water administration should be about 35 cc/kg. This is a rough estimate and each case should be individualized.

    3. Drip at a constant rate beginning with 50 cc/hr.

    4. Observe for gastric retention, glucosuria, diarrhea, and the presence of normal peristalsis.

    5. In the absence of the above complications, the rate of feeding may be sequentially advanced to 75 cc/hr, then to 100–125 cc/hr.

    6. After the patient has received ½ kcal/cc/hr for 24 hr without glucosuria or diarrhea, the caloric density can be increased to ¾ kcal/cc and subsequently to 1 kcal/cc. Do not simultaneously increase rate and concentration.

H. **Complications of enteral feedings**

1. **Occluded tube**
   a. Blenderized formulas usually do not flow well.
   b. Physically well mixed formulas with a low viscosity flow easily.
   c. Formulas using egg albumin as the protein source (Precision) will thicken and not pass through the tube if excessively shaken.

2. **Bronchial aspiration of feedings from the stomach**
   a. Verify tube placement in a patient with a depressed level of consciousness. X-ray confirmation of tube placement is strongly suggested in these patients.
   b. Continuous feeding helps to prevent accumulation of the feeding in the stomach.
   c. Keep patient's head and chest elevated at 30° or higher while instilling the feedings.
   d. Administer feedings at room temperature (warm liquids are emptied from the stomach more quickly than cold liquids).

3. **Diarrhea and/or cramping**
   a. Decrease rate of feedings.
   b. Decrease osmolality of feedings.
   c. Rule out a drug-induced cause of diarrhea, such as magnesium-containing antacids or antibiotics (especially ampicillin or clindamycin).
   d. Treat with an antidiarrheal drug, Paregoric or diphenoxylate hydrochloride (Lomotil), given orally or added to formula; or administer intramuscular codeine.
   e. Supply enough water to compensate for water losses.
   f. Bolus feedings may cause "dumping."

4. **Bloating or vomiting**
   a. Warm formula slightly, at least to room temperature.
   b. Decrease rate of administration.
   c. Decrease osmolality of formula.

5. Any **electrolyte, fluid, or metabolic abnormality** is possible with enteral nutritional support.
   a. Hyponatremia: water excess or sodium deficiency
   b. Hypernatremia: water deficiency
   c. Glycosuria: osmotic dehydration
   d. Excess protein: may cause an excessive osmotic load to the kidney and cause an increased water loss

6. **"High" residual volume after administration**
   a. Depends a great deal on the appearance of the aspirate
   b. For reference, keep in mind the following gastric secretion rates
      (1) Fasting: 74 ml/hr (0–176)
      (2) At night: 46 ml/hr (12–99)
      (3) After meals: 101 ml/hr (13–217)

    c. A residual of less than 300 ml in a patient receiving 50–100 ml/hr may be acceptable if the appearance of the aspirate is not identical with the formula infused, i.e., if there is bile and/or gastric content.

I . **Monitoring** (See p. 445.)

VII. **Practical Considerations**

  A. **Routes of nutritional support**

    1. Parenteral versus enteral, or both   If the intestinal tract is functioning, enteric feedings are preferred over parenteral feedings, since they are cheaper and as effective, and there are generally fewer metabolic and septic complications.

        If the intestinal tract is not functioning, parenteral nutrition should be used. Occasionally, the enteral and parenteral routes are used simultaneously if adequate support cannot be obtained by either route alone.

    2. If oral feedings are likely within 3–5 days, specific nutritional support is not suggested.

    3. If oral feedings are likely to be initiated by day 7, PPN is suggested during the interim.

    4. Oral feedings are frequently not tolerated within 7 days by patients
      a. With head injuries
      b. Requiring prolonged ventilatory support
      c. Requiring laparotomy for major abdominal injuries
These patients tend to have a high gastric residual volume when trying to initiate gastric tube feedings. The use of a catheter needle jejunostomy is suggested in these high-risk patients. If the above patient is identified upon admission, the catheter can be inserted at laparotomy. If laparotomy is not performed, the peritoneal lavage incision is enlarged slightly and the catheter is inserted. If a catheter jejunostomy was not inserted at the time of admission and the patient remains critically ill for 7–10 days post-admission and is not accepting gastric or duodenal tube feedings, insertion of a catheter needle jejunostomy should be considered.

    5. If enteric tube feedings are not being tolerated by 7 days post-admission, total parenteral nutrition should be instituted.

    6. The more critically ill the patient is, the greater the need for early institution of nutritional support. Enteric feedings, whenever possible, are generally preferable to parenteral nutrition.

  B. **Sources and quantity of nutritional support** From the nutritional standpoint, the trauma patient may be classified into one of three categories:
      —Nonstress state
      —Nonseptic stress state
      —Septic stress state

Following major trauma or major surgery, the patient's catecholamine and glucocorticoid levels are markedly elevated. These hormonal changes result in hypermetabolism and hypercatabolism, when compared to the nonstress state. Hypermetabolism produces an increase in energy requirements; hypercatabolism leads to an increase in protein wasting and urinary nitrogenous losses. After 2–7 days, if the patient is stabilized and the initial insult has been relatively minimal, the stress state abates and the patient enters a nonstress state. If the initial insult was associated with multiple systems trauma and/or major shock, the stress state may last significantly longer. The nonseptic stress state may eventuate into a septic stress state if there is a superimposed septic complication. The septic state leads to a number of physiologic derangements such that the patient is hypermetabolic and hypercatabolic; in addition, there is usually inefficient utilization of energy and nitrogenous substrates.

Nutritional support in each of these three states is debated. The quantity of calories and protein needed by the patient depends upon which state the patient is in and whether the goal is maintenance or repletion therapy. Maintenance therapy implies that the clinician is seeking to obtain neutral nitrogen balance; repletion therapy implies that the clinician is trying to obtain positive nitrogen balance to restore a depleted visceral protein pool. In the nonstress and nonseptic stress states, the patient seems to be able to utilize calories and protein in a relatively efficient manner. In the septic stress state, there is inefficient utilization of energy. Also, the patient appears to be more dependent upon protein, especially branched chain amino acids, as a source of energy.

The following are **approximate estimations of caloric and protein requirements:**

1. **Nonstress state**
    a. 1,500–2,000 cal and 1 gm of protein/kg/24 hr (maintenance)
    b. 2,000–2,500 cal and 1.5 gm of protein/kg/24 hr (repletion)
    The calories are supplied as approximately 40% fat and 60% carbohydrates.

2. **Nonseptic stress** 2,000–3,000 cal and 1.5 gm of protein/kg/24 hr. Calories are supplied as approximately 60% carbohydrates and 40% fat.

3. **Septic stress state** 2,500 cal and 1.5–2 gm of protein/kg/24 hr. The calories are supplied by 50–60% carbohydrates and 40–50% fats.

Due to inefficient utilization of sources of energy in the septic stress state and the apparent increased utilization of proteins as a source of energy, calories are not "pushed" upon the patient in a vigorous manner. There may be some advantage to increasing the protein load in the septic patient with an increased proportion of branched chain amino acids. For these reasons, calories are supplied in modest quantities and relatively more protein is administered, compared to nonseptic patients. A significant rise in the BUN would imply inadequate utilization of administered protein. In the septic stress patient, protein may be increased in amount if there is not a significant rise in the BUN. It is incumbent upon the physician to appropriately **control the septic process** with suitable antibiotics and adequate drainage of pyogenic foci. The latter step will change the patient to a nonseptic stress state and is the most important step in nurturing the patient in septic stress.

Each day, the clinician should assess the quantity and need of each of the following:
—Water
—Calories
—Protein (nitrogen)
—Calcium, phosphorus, magnesium
—Sodium, potassium
—Vitamins
—Trace elements

Too much or too little of these substances may harm the patient; therefore, they must be evaluated on a daily basis.

Section VIII
PRINCIPLES, TECHNIQUES, AND PROCEDURES

INTRODUCTION

The patients at MIEMSS are usually multiple trauma victims with varying degrees of instability. The following section deals with the application of invasive techniques to monitor and/or treat pathology. The primary intention of each technique is to improve the patient's state of well-being. Each technique is associated with its own complications. Prior to performing an invasive technique, the benefit versus the detriment of the technique should be scrutinized. In a given patient, the detrimental aspects of a technique may outweigh the potential benefit.

To maximize benefit and minimize detriment to the patient, appropriate technique is indicated. Since sepsis is a frequent sequela to invasive procedures, aseptic technique during and following these manipulations is absolutely mandatory.

Complications secondary to invasive techniques may be minimized by appropriate supervision. Physicians in training may have inadequate experience in the performance of invasive techniques, but feel that they can probably perform the technique if given the opportunity. Pride frequently inhibits one from saying, "I'm not sure how to do this procedure." If there is doubt regarding the ability to perform a procedure, assistance should be sought from the surgical or critical care staff. Supervision, from the educational standpoint, elicits two responses: reinforcement of a skill or information previously learned, or acquirement of knowledge or ability to perform a given skill. In rendering patient care, there is rarely a situation in which a physician will be criticized for seeking assistance; on the other hand, if the patient suffers from an inexperienced operator, the physician is appropriately subject to criticism.

The patient's best interest should be of utmost priority. Patient comfort during any procedure should be a paramount consideration.

A procedure note is entered into the chart describing the procedure performed. The procedure note should provide information regarding the indication for the procedure, the facility with which the procedure was performed, and the result of the procedure.

28

ARTERIAL CATHETERIZATION

I. **Femoral** Critically ill and injured patients often need continuous intra-arterial pressure monitoring and frequent withdrawal of blood samples to follow physiologic parameters: blood gases, hematocrit, electrolytes, etc. Femoral arterial catheterization meets these needs. Because of the danger of traumatizing a vessel involved with atherosclerosis and thereby causing vascular compromise, an alternate approach should be considered in the elderly patient. The femoral arterial catheter is larger than radial or brachial lines and, in general, lasts longer since it is less likely to occlude.

The **technique** for femoral arterial catheterization is as follows. The groin is prepped and draped. The pulse is palpated about 1–2 cm below the inguinal crease. A small area of skin and subcutaneous tissue is infiltrated with lidocaine immediately caudad to the pulse. A 1- to 2-mm puncture is made through the epidermis and dermis with a No. 11 scalpel blade. A needle is obtained from a 14-gauge Cathlon in which the plastic catheter has been removed and the hub broken from the needle. It is held at a 45° angle to the surface of the anterior thigh and advanced, with the bevel up, through the cutaneous puncture site. The needle is advanced until arterial flow is apparent; this requires only puncture of the anterior wall. The flexible-tipped guidewire is advanced into the arterial lumen. After removal of the needle, pressure is placed in this region to prevent extravasation of blood around the guidewire. The 16-gauge, 6-inch arterial catheter is placed over the guidewire and advanced into the arterial lumen. The guidewire is removed and the catheter is connected to the monitoring line and sutured in place.

A survey at MIEMSS comparing the efficacy and safety of femoral versus radial arterial line catheters showed that femoral lines lasted significantly longer than radial lines. The complication rate of the two catheters was not different. We would agree that a pseudoaneurysm of the common femoral artery is a more devastating problem than that involving the radial artery. We encourage the use of this catheter in the younger patient. We advise against recannulation after the femoral artery has once been used.

II. **Radial** The distal radial artery is one of the safest and most accessible sites for arterial cannulation. However, catheterization is not without complications. The vessel is easy to palpate and stabilize; the collateral circulation is usually adequate via the ulnar artery (about 3% of the population has absent ulnar pulses bilaterally); if periosteal puncture is avoided, the procedure is relatively pain-free.

A reliable maneuver to determine palmar arch patency is the Allen's test, which is performed as follows:

—The radial and ulnar arteries are occluded by the examiner's fingers while the patient repeatedly opens and closes the hand.

—The patient is requested to open the hand, but avoids complete extension and wide separation of fingers, which can occlude the transpalmar arch. A blanched palm and fingers are noted.

—The examiner releases the pressure from the ulnar artery and if the arch is patent, a blush over the entire palm and fingers is seen. If the blush does not appear within 5 sec, collateral circulation is inadequate and the test is positive. A 15-sec filling time has a 10% incidence of distal ischemia following radial line insertion.

The hand must be frequently observed for arterial insufficiency. If there is evidence of an ischemic hand, the catheter must be removed.

A. **Percutaneous technique**   Percutaneous radial artery cannulation should be performed with the wrist dorsiflexed over a roll, towel, or gauze sponges at a 60° angle. Then hand and forearm are fixed to an arm board. Following sterile preparation, the radial artery is palpated for a distance of 1 inch proximal to the crease of the wrist to appreciate its anatomical course. A small skin wheal is made with 1% lidocaine and a small skin incision is made with an 18-gauge needle to facilitate entrance of the catheter and minimize the likelihood of shearing or obstruction. A 20-gauge Teflon catheter should be inserted along the course of the radial artery at a 15° angle to the surface of the skin. A spurt of bright red blood indicates entry into the vessel; at this point, the needle should be held fixed and the cannula advanced into the arterial lumen. The needle is withdrawn and the cannula is connected to the pressure-monitoring tubing. The catheter is sutured with 3-0 nylon. Povidone-iodine (Betadine) ointment is applied at the cutaneous puncture site and covered with a sterile dressing.

B. **Cutdown technique**   Where the pulse is either absent or so faint that percutaneous catheterization is not feasible, cutdown technique is indicated.

The wrist is dorsiflexed and secured with a board. The skin is prepped and draped. Beginning at the radial styloid and extending in an ulnar direction, a transverse cutaneous incision is made, about 2 cm in length. The subcutaneous tissue is bluntly dissected with a hemostat parallel to the direction of the radial artery. The artery is tractioned to the skin level. A size 18 cathlon is passed through the skin about 1 cm distal to the transverse incision. The catheter is passed into the lumen of the artery and advanced proximally. The catheter is sutured to the skin with 3-0 nylon. The incision is closed with 3-0 nylon suture and dressed with Betadine ointment and a sterile gauze dressing. A suture should not be tied around the artery to secure the catheter.

III. **Pulmonary**   Right-heart catheterization is accomplished by the insertion of a flow-directed, pulmonary artery catheter. Information from the Swan-Ganz catheter contributes to the evaluation of the cardiovascular and pulmonary systems.

A. **Route**   The internal jugular, subclavian, antecubital, and femoral veins may be used as a point of entry. Percutaneous vascular access is preferable, but the cutdown technique may be required.

B. **Technique**   After the skin has been prepped and draped, the PA (yellow) and CVP (blue) ports are attached to the pressure tubing and flushed. The monitor is calibrated and the balloon is tested with 1.5 ml of air by using a 3-ml syringe. The vein is cannulated with a 16- or 18-gauge Jelco catheter. A guidewire is inserted and the catheter is withdrawn. A 3-mm skin incision is made with a No. 11 blade adjacent to the wire. The introducers (black, then white) are gradually inserted using constant pressure and rotation. The guidewire and black introducer are withdrawn and a syringe is attached to the white introducer and aspirated to confirm its intravascular position. The Swan-Ganz catheter is inserted into the introducer and advanced.

Under continuous monitor visualization of the pressure waveform and EKG, the catheter is advanced into the thorax, which is evidenced by respiratory fluctuation in the waveform. The tip will be in or near the right atrium when it has been advanced approximately 40 cm from a right or 50 cm from a left antecubital vein, 15 cm from the right or 20 cm from the left internal jugular or subclavian vein, or about 30 cm from the femoral vein. At this point, the balloon is inflated with 1 ml of air and the catheter is passed through the right atrium, right ventricle, pulmonary artery, and into the wedge position. The right ventricle is reached about 10 cm from the point that the catheter enters the thorax and the pulmonary artery wedge position is reached about 10 cm from the right ventricle. The pressure waveform aids in identifying the various vascular compartments. As the catheter advances into the right ventricle, the amplitude and mean pressure rises significantly. As the catheter enters the pulmonary artery, the mean pressure changes minimally, but the amplitude significantly decreases. As the catheter enters the wedge position, the mean pressure usually drops and the amplitude of the waveform decreases (Figure 1).

Never withdraw the catheter with the balloon inflated. If the right ventricle is not reached at the appropriate distance, deflate the balloon, withdraw the catheter, and start over. After the catheter is positioned, withdraw the white introducer, and suture the catheter to the skin and apply an antibiotic dressing.

| Note | PA lines may be a cause of arrhythmias, which usually disappear after catheter withdrawal.

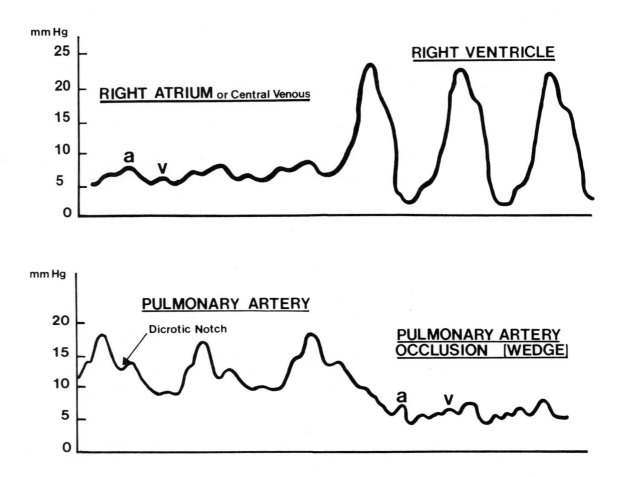

Figure 1. Swan-Ganz catheter insertion via pressure tracings. *a* wave = atrial contraction; *v* wave = passive atrial filling during atrial diastole.

29
BRONCHOSCOPY

I. **Philosophy** As most thoracic surgeons agree, bronchoscopy can be life-saving. Some say the severely traumatized patient is too ill to be bronchoscoped; actually the patient may be too ill not to be bronchoscoped.

II. **Indications** Bronchoscopy is performed for diagnostic or therapeutic reasons. Both the rigid and the fiberoptic bronchoscopes are available. The latter should be used whenever possible. We use bronchoscopy primarily to evaluate the patient for tracheobronchial injuries or evacuation of endobronchial secretions. Chest physiotherapy and postural drainage will clear most areas of atelectasis if secondary to endobronchial plugging by secretions. If an area of atelectasis fails to clear with intensive chest physiotherapy after 4–6 hr, bronchoscopy is used to remove the secretions. Delayed bronchoscopy (>12 hr) will rarely be successful in clearing an area of atelectasis. In certain instances, bronchoscopy may be life-saving by removing large mucous plugs from the tracheobronchial tree. There may be concern for "disrupting" the patient's positive end-expiratory pressure (PEEP), but in this case the patient is too sick not to be bronchoscoped.

A. **Diagnostic**

1. Bronchial or tracheal tear
   a. Large pleural air leak
   b. Mediastinal emphysema
   c. Subcutaneous emphysema
   d. Inability to expand the lung with a chest tube

2. Post-extubation respiratory distress
   a. Tracheomalacia
   b. Tracheal stenosis

3. Observe the mucous membranes and obtain secretions for culture and sensitivity.

4. Assess trauma after smoke inhalation.

5. Signs or symptoms of laryngeal trauma

B. **Therapeutic**

1. Remove a foreign body (e.g., teeth).

2. Intubate patient (e.g., a quadriplegic) in whom cords cannot be visualized.

3. Remove secretions that do not clear with chest physiotherapy.

4. Suction the tracheobronchial tree following aspiration.

III. **Rigid Bronchoscopy**   Bronchoscopy should not begin until the patient is properly positioned and all equipment is checked. The operator must carefully position the patient so that the patient's head is extended and the neck is flexed. Infusion poles or other obstacles are removed. The operator then dons cap, mask, face shield, and gloves and then checks and assembles the equipment. This procedure includes attaching the light carrier to the power source and switching the light on; attaching the suction tip to the suction tubing and wall outlet; attaching the oxygen tubing to the oxygen intake port on the bronchoscope; and preparing the Lukens tube to obtain secretions for culture, and a syringe containing sterile saline for tracheobronchial lavage.

At least one physician, in addition to the nurse, should be present to assist the surgeon. The nurse should watch the monitoring oscilloscope and notify the operator if arrhythmias develop. The inspired oxygen should be 100%.

A. The **oral route** must be used where there is no tracheostomy. Unless the patient is anesthetized, unconscious, or greatly obtunded, topical anesthesia of the hypopharynx and larynx will be necessary. In addition, premedication with diazepam (Valium), 10–20 mg i.v., should be given 5–10 min prior to the examination. The hypopharynx is sprayed with an atomizer containing 5% Cyclaine or 4% lidocaine (Xylocaine). By using a laryngeal mirror, a syringe, and a long blunt cannula, the same agent is dripped onto and through the larynx, until anesthesia is obtained. With the patient supine and the head extended and neck flexed, the bronchoscope is passed along the tongue, over the epiglottis, and into the larynx and trachea.

B. The **tracheostomy route** should be used where a tracheostomy is already present. The tracheostomy tube is removed and bronchoscopy performed. A new tracheostomy tube is inserted after bronchoscopy.

IV. **Fiberoptic Bronchoscopy**   Fiberoptic bronchoscopy is less traumatic and can easily be performed without interruption of mechanical ventilation or positive-end expiratory pressure. It is performed via a tracheostomy tube, a translaryngeal tube, or through the nostril.

The technique is as follows:
—Assemble and inspect the equipment. Test suction and light source.
—Attach the bronchoscopy swivel connecting piece between the ventilator tube and the tracheal tube.
—Place the patient on 100% oxygen.
—Instill topical anesthesia.
—Orient and then insert the bronchoscope.
—Sputum is collected for Gram stain, culture, and sensitivity.

At the completion of the procedure, the instrument is cleaned by the OR nurses. The bronchoscope should be returned immediately following use.

When a bronchoscopy is performed in an intubated and mechanically ventilated patient, there are two major ventilatory concerns: hypoxia and partial obstruction of the tracheal tube and/or tracheobronchial tree. Arrhythmias, bradycardia, hypotension, and/or bronchospasm may occur. These problems are usually avoided by increasing the FiO_2 to 1.0 before, during, and after the procedure.

An expeditious endoscopy minimizes complications. Sedatives and/or narcotics are used in those patients who are apprehensive, alert, or uncooperative. Topical lidocaine improves patient compliance.

30

CENTRAL VENIPUNCTURE

Central venipuncture is performed via the internal jugular or subclavian vein. A central venipuncture may be used at the time of admission when other venous sites are inaccessible. The central venous route is frequently used to administer maintenance fluids and intravenous drugs when other venous sites are not available. A central venipuncture is commonly used to insert a catheter into the superior vena cava to monitor right-sided cardiac filling pressures for the regulation of volume infusion. Because parenteral hyperalimentation is so hypertonic, it must be administered through a high-flow system such as a central vein to minimize venous thrombosis and phlebitis. A central venipuncture is often used to insert a Swan-Ganz catheter to assess cardiac performance. Even though central venipuncture has numerous clinical uses, it is associated with potential complications. Pneumothorax and arterial puncture are the two most common complications seen with this technique. To reduce the number of complications associated with this technique, the operator should be meticulous and skilled. As with all venous cannulation, sepsis is a complication which must be minimized to reduce patient morbidity.

I. **Jugular** The percutaneous lateral approach to the internal jugular vein is easy to perform, safe, and can be easily performed at the head of the operating table during surgery.

Internal jugular venipuncture is enhanced if the patient is placed in the Trendelenburg position, or 5–7 cm PEEP is applied. A bolster placed under the patient's scapula will accentuate extension of the neck. The head is turned contralateral to the side of entry, and the skin is prepped and draped. The point of skin puncture is along the lateral border of the sternocleidomastoid muscle just cephalad to the point where the external jugular vein crosses it. A skin wheal is made with lidocaine, and a small incision is made with an 18-gauge needle to facilitate the entrance of a No. 18 2-inch Jelco catheter. The catheter is attached to a 12-ml syringe. The catheter is advanced slowly in a plane just beneath the belly of the sternocleidomastoid muscle and directed toward the sternal notch. Within 5 cm of the cutaneous puncture, venipuncture is evidenced by free-flowing blood. If blood is not evident, the unit is slowly withdrawn while aspirating; a brisk blood flow will usually appear. The needle and syringe are securely immobilized, and the plastic catheter is advanced over the needle into the vein. A guide wire is passed through the catheter into the vein, the catheter is pulled out, and a 16-gauge catheter is introduced. The catheter is sutured to the skin and an antibiotic dressing is applied. For additional security, the tubing is looped behind and over the ear and taped.

A second and relatively easy method is to palpate the carotid artery in the mid-neck and puncture the jugular vein lateral to the carotid pulsation.

II. **Subclavian** One method of approaching the subclavian vein is by the infraclavicular technique.

The Trendelenburg position is assumed and a bolster is placed between the scapulae. The infraclavicular skin is prepped and draped. The skin puncture is performed immediately lateral to the point where the first rib is palpated to pass under the clavicle. A skin wheal with 1% lidocaine is made. The periosteum of the clavicle is infiltrated with lidocaine. A large intracatheter needle is attached to a 12-ml syringe, and the needle is initially directed into the subcutaneous tissue for about ½ cm. The inferior clavicle is touched with the needle tip to be certain of its relationship with the clavicle. The syringe is held about 15° anterior to the chest wall. The needle is slowly advanced immediately posterior to the clavicle and toward the suprasternal notch. Aspiration with advancement will yield a brisk, venous blood return when the subclavian vein is entered. The syringe is disconnected from the needle and the catheter is inserted. The needle is withdrawn and the needle guard is applied. The catheter is sutured to the skin with nylon and an antibiotic ointment and dressing are applied. If difficulty in performing the venipuncture is anticipated, the vein may be approached with a smaller catheter by using the Seldinger technique. The catheter should never be withdrawn through the needle because of the possibility of shearing the catheter into the vein.

If the subclavian artery is punctured, the blood will be arterial in color (bright red). If the artery is punctured, the needle should be withdrawn and pressure placed superiorly and inferiorly to the clavicle. After bleeding has stopped, the needle may be redirected as indicated for venipuncture.

Possible **complications** include:
—Pneumothorax
—Arterial puncture
—Brachial plexus injury
—Sepsis
See p. 444.

| Note | This procedure is not one that should be attempted by a novice without supervision. The ability to puncture the subclavian vein requires anatomical knowledge and experience.

31
CHEST TUBES

Because the multiple trauma patient frequently sustains injury to the thorax and its contents, chest tube management plays an important role in the care of the physiologic defects created by the injury.

I. **Considerations for Chest Tube Insertion**

—**Pneumothorax**   All cases receive a tube if the patient is on a ventilator, going to surgery, or must be transported. If the pneumothorax is small and the patient is not on a ventilator, clinical judgment must be used regarding chest tube insertion; serial chest x-rays should be done. Only the occasional patient should not have a tube inserted.

—**Hemothorax**   This blood is autotransfusable.

—**Hemopneumothorax**

—Patients on ventilators who develop **subcutaneous emphysema**

—**Penetrating wounds** to the chest associated with evidence of pneumothorax, hemothorax, or subcutaneous emphysema

—**Empyema**

—**Super-PEEP** (bilateral chest tubes may be indicated)

—**Chylothorax**

II. **Procedure for Chest Tube Insertion**   The procedure differs depending on whether one is inserting an apical tube for a pneumothorax or a basilar tube for a hemothorax. Both apical and basilar tubes are inserted for a hemopneumothorax.

An **apical tube** is best placed with the patient in the semi-Fowler position. A No. 28 tube should pass obliquely upward through the second intercostal space so that it is directed toward the apex of the thorax. The skin incision should be in the midclavicular line in the third intercostal space and guided upward such that the pathway of the tube moves obliquely forward to enter the pleural space through the second intercostal space.

A **basilar chest tube** should be inserted with the patient in a semi-Fowler or lateral decubitus position. The objective is placement of the tube tip into the paravertebral gutter posteriorly and immediately above the diaphragm. The skin incision is vertical and over the fifth intercostal space in the midaxillary line. The tube should enter the pleura through a subcutaneous tunnel, approximately 2–3 cm posterior to the cutaneous incision.

The **technique** for inserting the tube is similar regardless of the site of insertion:
—Prepare the skin over a wide area of the chest wall with Betadine scrub and solution.
—Drape the area with sterile towels.
—Infiltrate the skin and intercostal space with ½–1% lidocaine.
—Make the skin and subcutaneous incision about 3 cm in length.
—By using a curved hemostat, a subcutaneous tunnel is developed by blunt dissection. The intercostal muscles are bluntly dissected and a puncture is made into the pleura. The dissection should be immediately above the upper edge of the lower rib.
—Measure and mark the appropriate length of the tube that is to be inserted into the pleural space, so that the chest tube length is adequate, yet will not kink. Grasp the end of a clamped chest tube longitudinally with a curved clamp and push it into the pleural space. The last hole of the chest tube should be well inside the parietal pleura. The tube should be rapidly connected to the water seal. Then remove the chest tube clamp to establish continuity.
—Suture the tube to the skin with two sutures of No. 0 silk.
—Insert a mattress suture of No. 0 silk into the skin about 1 cm across the incision on either side of the chest tube. This suture is left untied and coiled. After removal of the chest tube, it is tied, thus closing the hole.
—If appropriate, pleural fluid should be sent for culture and chemical or hematologic analysis.
—Secure the connections.
—Apply a sterile dressing around the chest tube at the skin incision site. Secure the dressing and the chest tube with adhesive tape.
—Obtain a portable chest x-ray to check the tube position and lung expansion.

Note | An improperly placed tube may be adjusted by withdrawing the tube the necessary length. The position of a tube must **never** be adjusted by advancing it after the initial insertion. **The reinsertion of a tube must always be through a new opening in the chest wall.** Never remove the first tube before inserting the second tube. Never insert a tube so far posterior on the chest wall that a patient will lie on it.

III. **Indications and Procedure for Removing Chest Tubes**   Chest tubes can be removed when there has been no air emerging through the tube for 24 hr and when the drainage of fluid through the tube is less than 100 cc in 24 hr. The only exception to this rule exists when the tube has been inserted for a pneumothorax and the patient is on the respirator. The tube should be left in as long as the patient is on the respirator **up to a period of 5 days;** then reevaluate the situation. A tube left in the chest longer than 5 days increases the likelihood of empyema formation (see p. 420).

To assure that no air leak is present, the patient should be encouraged to cough several times before removal of the chest tube. Inform the patient that cooperation is very important. The tube should be removed quickly, at the peak of inspiration during a Valsalva maneuver. While holding pressure over the thoracostomy incision to prevent air leak, the pursestring is tied and a dressing is applied. A portable chest x-ray is obtained to exclude a pneumothorax.

IV. Standards for the Care of Chest Tubes

A. Insertion technique   A scrub suit, sterile gown, mask, cap, and gloves are necessary. A sterile gown is ideal but frequently impractical in an unstable patient at the time of admission.

B. Drainage system

1. Sterile Pleur-Evac (disposable "3 bottle" unit for underwater seal drainage of pleural cavity) is utilized for drainage of the pleural cavity.

2. Fill water seal and suction control chambers with sterile water.

3. Precautions   Do not remove rubber tubing, clamp the tubing in transit, or allow the drainage apparatus to be positioned higher than the chest.

C. Chest tube care

1. Do not change dressings until ready for removal by the physician. Petroleum jelly gauze is not required.

2. Inspect insertion site for signs of erythema, odor, purulent drainage, and security of sutures if there is evidence of sepsis; note on the chart any abnormalities.

D. Change **Pleur-Evac** only when the chambers are full.

E. Bacteriologic surveillance

1. Culture when there is concern for the presence of an empyema.

2. A specimen obtained from the rubber tubing may not be reliable. Such a specimen may represent colonization; therefore, a thoracentesis is more accurate.

3. Send samples according to the culture procedure for sterile body fluids.

V. Complications and Management

A. Lacerated intercostal artery

1. Remove the chest tube.

2. Insert a large Foley catheter, inflate the balloon, and withdraw the catheter to provide tamponade.

3. Insert a new chest tube to resolve the original problem.

4. A thoracotomy may be necessary.

B. **Nonfluctuating tube (nonfunctional) with residual pneumothorax**

1. Never clear the tube with a Fogarty catheter or a sterile suction catheter; this will contaminate the pleural space.

2. Never irrigate a tube.

3. Never insert a new tube through an old site.

C. **If the tube is fluctuating (functional) and the patient has a residual pneumothorax,** the pneumothorax may be cleared by

1. Inserting an additional chest tube

2. Partially withdrawing the tube. This may disrupt visceral and parietal pleural adhesions around the tube.

3. Increasing the suction on the chest tube

D. **Partial removal of the chest tube** by slippage with one or more holes out of the thorax, thus creating a residual pneumothorax

1. Remove the tube.

2. Insert a new tube through a new site.

E. **Chest tube traversing the mediastinum**   Withdraw the tube tip to the proper site, or remove and insert a new tube.

F. **Chest tube in the soft tissues of the neck** (outside the rib cage)   Remove the tube.

G. **Chest tube lacerating the lung.**

1. Pull tube back.

2. Possibly use a second tube to drain blood or control air leak.

3. A thoracotomy may be required.

H. **Excessive pain at insertion site**

1. Local anesthetic

2. A new tube site may be necessary.

Note   If chest tubes are not managed properly, serious complications such as bronchopleural fistulae and empyema may result. In the multiple trauma patient who is severely compromised, chest tube mismanagement can cost the patient's life. Infection and empyemas resulting from chest tube insertion are the result of poor technique.

32
ESOPHAGEAL OBTURATOR AIRWAY

I. **Authorization**   Only those individuals who have been properly trained and certified by MIEMSS are authorized to initiate intubation with the esophageal obturator airway.

II. **Principles of Design and Use**   The esophageal obturator airway is an endotracheal tube with the following modifications:
 —A soft plastic obturator tip which occludes the tube's distal end
 —Sixteen airholes located near the proximal end, at the level of the pharynx
 —The proximal end houses a 15-mm bit block which fits into a clear face mask and adapts to standard bag and resuscitator equipment fittings.

The airway is used to intubate the esophagus, rather than the trachea; consequently, no laryngoscope or special equipment is required. Its cuff, when fully inserted, lies below the carina and does not impinge upon the trachea or bronchi. The cuff, when inflated with 35 cc of air, occludes the esophagus and prevents air from passing into the stomach. It also prevents gastric contents from being regurgitated and aspirated into the lungs. Air, delivered by mouth, bag, or resuscitator, passes through the holes in the pharynx into the trachea and lungs.

III. **Clinical Benefits**   The airway's greatest advantages are its ease and speed of insertion. Passage of the esophageal obturator airway follows normal anatomical contours. Victims in respiratory or cardiac arrest can be intubated with the esophageal obturator airway in seconds; CPR can be continued without interruption. Other special resuscitative measures, such as defibrillation, can be initiated rapidly. The prevention of aspiration is important.

IV. **Clinical Limitations**   The esophageal obturator airway is intended primarily for emergency use and should be inserted in patients who
 —Are **not** breathing
 —Are unconscious, and without a gag reflex
 —Are over 5 feet tall
 —Have not ingested any corrosive fluids
 —Have no known esophageal disease

V. Intubation Procedure

—Begin artificial ventilation first, by using mouth-to-mouth, mouth-to-nose, or bag-valve-mask ventilation. Initiate CPR if cardiac arrest has occurred.

—Prepare to insert the esophageal airway during the interval between two respirations.

| Note | The tube may be lubricated with K-Y or lidocaine jelly.

Grasp the patient's jaw between thumb and index finger and lift the jaw straight upward.

—Hold the esophageal airway in the other hand (approximately at the middle of the tube) and insert the tip into the mouth. Passage is easiest along the side of the tongue or in the midline.

—Advance the esophageal airway ensuring that its curvature is in the same direction as the curvature of the pharynx. Continue to advance, gently "bouncing" (feeding) the airway into the esophagus until the mask is seated firmly over the mouth and nose.

—Hold the mask firmly on the face with both hands; take a deep breath and blow into the red adaptor. If the chest rises, the airway is properly positioned in the esophagus. This occurs in most instances. If the chest does not rise, the airway has probably passed into the trachea and has blocked it. In this case, remove the airway and continue mouth-to-mouth, mouth-to-nose, or bag-valve-mask ventilation, and prepare for a second attempt to insert the esophageal airway. Proper positioning and ventilation are checked by listening for breath sounds with the stethoscope.

—When assured that the airway is properly placed in the esophagus, prepare to inflate the cuff during the interval between two respirations.

—Fill the 35-ml syringe with air and attach the syringe to the one-way valve.

—Inject the 35 ml of air into the cuff and remove the syringe immediately. The one-way valve effectively seals itself and prevents deflation of the cuff.

—Maintain a seal at the face and continue airway ventilation until effective spontaneous ventilation returns, or until an endotracheal tube has been placed for long-term ventilation.

VI. Considerations for Hospital Personnel

A. **Translaryngeal intubation**   If ventilatory support or airway control is necessary, an endotracheal tube is passed while the esophageal airway is in place. First, place both hands on the mask with fingers grasping each side and with the thumbs located on the red adaptor. Exert upward pressure on the mask and remove it. Position the airway to one side. At this point, a laryngoscope blade is positioned and an endotracheal tube is passed. The airway is not removed until the cuff of the translaryngeal tube is inflated and suction is available to clear the pharynx of regurgitation. Removal of the airway is frequently associated with regurgitation.

Do not cut the one-way valve or tubing to relieve the pressure from the distal 35-cc cuff.

B. **Esophageal damage** Esophageal rupture occasionally occurs; pneumomediastinum or a hydrothorax may be manifestations.

33
MILITARY ANTI-SHOCK TROUSERS

The following protocol describes the employment of Military Anti-Shock Trousers (MAST) within MIEMSS. The trousers "mobilize" blood from the lower extremities and abdomen to autotransfuse 750–1,000 cc of blood to the heart-brain-lung circulation.

I. **Criteria for Utilization**

    A. **Indications**

        1. Systolic pressure below 80 mm Hg

        2. Systolic pressure below 100 mm Hg, if associated with manifestations of shock

        3. Pelvic fractures

        4. Fractures of the lower extremities

    B. **Contraindication**   Acute respiratory distress

II. **Application of the Trousers**

    —The left leg is applied first, then the right leg and abdominal component. The abdominal segment is inflated after the legs.

    —MAST should be placed immediately below the patient's costal margins.

    —Proper inflation is achieved when air pressure is increased to the point that the velcro fasteners begin to loosen and safety valves begin to vent (which corresponds to an inflation pressure of approximately 105 mm Hg) or the systolic blood pressure reaches 100 mm Hg.

    —The trousers may remain inflated up to 48 hr if the pressure does not exceed 40–50 mm Hg.

> **Note**   A compartment syndrome may develop if the MAST are used for a prolonged time in patients with tibial fractures.

III. **Removal of the Trousers**

    —The greatest danger associated with utilization of the trousers is the rapid removal by persons unaccustomed to their use. The proper sequence of deflation begins with the abdominal segment followed by deflation of the individual leg segments.

—Before the trouser is deflated, a large bore i.v. catheter should be inserted and fluid administered.
—Each segment should be slowly deflated with frequent checks of the vital signs. Any drop of more than 5 mm Hg in systolic blood pressure should signal the need for reinflation of the trousers, followed by additional fluid support.
—Premature removal of the trousers may result in profound shock or cardiac arrest.

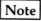 Military Anti-Shock Trousers are expensive and should not be cut from the patient, but should be removed by separating the velcro fasteners.

34

TRACHEAL INTUBATION

I. Tracheostomy

A. Elective

1. **Considerations for tracheostomy**
   a. Prolonged ventilatory support
   b. Tracheobronchial access (hygiene)
      (1) Removal of secretions
      (2) Bicarbonate instillation
      (3) Hyperinflation of lungs
   c. Upper airway obstruction (e.g., laryngeal fracture)
   d. Inability to pass a translaryngeal tube
   e. Airway protection in head-injured patients
   f. Tracheal injuries

2. **Technique** The soft tissue incision is horizontally made. Under the advice of the ENT service, the tracheal incision is vertically made and includes the second and third rings, and the upper portion of the fourth tracheal ring. No tracheal cartilage should be removed. Two tracheal stay sutures should be placed lateral to the tracheal incision for the first 5 days until a well developed tract has formed. The transtracheal tube should be secured at the flange to the skin for the first 5 days to prevent expulsion. Use of 3-0 prolene suture is recommended.
   Tracheostomy tubes recommended are
   —Adult male: Shiley No. 8–10; Portex No. 36–39
   —Adult female: Shiley No. 6; Portex No. 33

   There is a controversy regarding the length of time a translaryngeal tracheal tube may safely remain in place. To answer this question, we recently performed a tracheal intubation study. Patients were randomized into an early versus a late tracheostomy category. The early tracheostomy group received transtracheal intubation 3–4 days after translaryngeal intubation, and the late tracheostomy group received transtracheal intubation 14 days after translaryngeal intubation.

   The study revealed no difference between early and late tracheostomy in regard to laryngotracheal pathology. The rigid head-injured patient (decorticate/decerebrate) had a 40% complication rate; an early tracheostomy (3–4 days) did not "protect" these patients. These patients should be laryngoscoped prior to extubation. There was no difference in the incidence of respiratory infection between the early and the late group.

3. **Anesthetic considerations** Preanesthetic sedation should be individualized according to the patient's neurologic status and/or antecedent pain. Any preoperative regimen of sedatives, narcotics, and/or muscle relaxants should be continued throughout the procedure.

Prior to transportation to the operating room, the mouth, oropharynx, endotracheal tube, and nasogastric tube (NGT) should be suctioned until clear.

During the transportation of patients with pulmonary failure, a Mapleson system with 100% oxygen and high flow is used. Positive end-expiratory pressure (PEEP) is maintained by controlling the pop-off valve. Hyperventilation should be maintained in head trauma cases. A portable EKG is used for monitoring during transportation.

Patients with unstable lower extremity injuries, hip fractures, or high intracranial pressure (ICP) should be maintained in their preoperative position during the procedure.

Once in the operating room, the patient is placed on intermittent positive pressure ventilation (IPPV) with the Engstrom ventilator, and pretransportation ventilator settings are used. Initially, the patient is placed on 100% oxygen. If the initial vital signs are stable, the FiO_2 is reduced to the pretransportation level. Preoperative inotropics, vasopressors, hyperalimentation, and i.v. medications should be continued. Therapy for elevated ICP is continued. No anesthetic is needed if the patient is in barbiturate coma.

Before the patient is draped, the mouth, pharynx, endotracheal tube, and NGT are suctioned until clear. Before the trachea is incised, 100% O_2 is administered and the tube is untaped. If appropriate, the Trendelenburg position is recommended to avoid aspiration of secretions that lie above the cuff and/or the surgeon should suction these secretions through the tracheal incision. The cuff is deflated and the translaryngeal tube is withdrawn until it disappears from the stoma. Following insertion of the tracheostomy tube, the cuff is inflated until a seal is obtained. Chest motion and breath sounds are evaluated for bilateral equality. One hundred percent O_2 is administered for 3 min, then appropriately decreased.

Under direct laryngoscopy, the translaryngeal tube is removed and the epiglottis and vocal cords are evaluated. A note is written in the chart describing the appearance of the cords, the tube used, its size, the level of tracheostomy, and the amount of air injected into the cuff.

B. **Emergency** The majority of patients with airway obstruction or inadequate ventilation may be managed by one of several options. Most airways are readily cleared and the patient may be ventilated with an Ambu bag. When a skilled nurse or physician becomes available, an endotracheal tube may be passed to secure the airway and ventilate the patient. There are certain patients in whom a patent airway cannot be obtained; therefore, these patients cannot be ventilated. The majority of such patients can be handled by immediate insertion of a translaryngeal tracheal tube. On the other hand, there is a **small** but significant number of patients in whom a translaryngeal tube either cannot be passed or is potentially detrimental to the patient:

—Anatomical variation (e.g., short, fat neck)
—Massive facial swelling secondary to fractures
—Intraoral hemorrhage
—Cervical spine fracture
—Laryngeal fracture

Under these circumstances a cricothyroidotomy is the preferred route for expeditious tracheal intubation. The cricothyroid membrane is readily located and easily entered surgically.

The **technique** for emergency cricothyroidotomy is as follows. The neck is rapidly prepped. The thyroid notch is palpated with the index finger. The finger moves caudally until the prominence of the cricoid ring is palpated. A 3-cm transverse incision through the skin and subcutaneous tissue is made immediately above the cricoid ring. The cricothyroid membrane is punctured transversely with a No. 11 scalpel blade. A hemostat is inserted into the puncture site and spread transversely. A second hemostat is inserted in a perpendicular fashion and spread vertically. The hemostats are removed and the tracheostomy tube is inserted. In emergency tracheostomies, a tube one size smaller than usual should be used:

—Adult male: Shiley No. 8; Portex No. 33
—Adult female: Shiley No. 6; Portex No. 30

The tube is secured as described on p. 481. The decision regarding relocation at the second or third tracheal ring is at the discretion of the surgeon, but is encouraged if prolonged intubation on a ventilator is required.

Emergency cricothyroidotomy may be associated with major complications in the hands of an inexperienced operator. The anatomy must be well known, and the indication must be a patient who has an insecure airway which cannot be stabilized with another technique.

This technique is reserved for emergency use only.

II. **Endotracheal intubation** Successful intubation requires familiarity with the equipment and its location, rapid anatomical evaluation of the airway, correct position of the patient's head, and atraumatic manipulation of the laryngoscope. Ineptness at intubation is fraught with hazard. Under emergency conditions, the safest way to secure an artificial airway is usually by the placement of a transoral endotracheal tube.

A. **Indications** Intubation may be indicated for patients unable to maintain an airway, patients who need ventilator support or hyperventilation, patients with respiratory insufficiency, and patients in shock who need rapid cellular resuscitation. Specific indications are as follows:

1. Many patients are admitted with an esophageal obturator in place. After the face mask is removed from the esophageal tube, translaryngeal intubation is performed. When it is certain that the endotracheal tube is in proper position

and the cuff is inflated, the esophageal cuff is deflated and the tube is removed. Removal of the esophageal obturator is usually accompanied by regurgitation of gastric contents into the mouth; hence, the previously placed cuffed endotracheal tube helps to prevent aspiration.

2. Upper airway obstruction in an unstable patient

3. Unconsciousness (unprotected airway)

4. Head trauma (to induce hyperventilation)

5. $PaO_2 \leq 60$ torr on room air or 80 torr on supplemental O_2, or $PaCO_2 \geq 55$ torr

6. Persistent respiratory rate greater than 35

7. Systolic pressure at admission less than 80

8. If surgery is anticipated, intubation and sedation facilitate the resuscitation and diagnostic evaluation.

B. **Technique**

1. **Precautions against full stomach** All patients entering MIEMSS are considered to have a full stomach, since many were eating or drinking prior to injury. The physiologic response to trauma and pain is to delay gastric emptying, thus compounding the full stomach problem. Sellick's maneuver is to apply external pressure to the cricoid cartilage by placing the thumb and first two fingers over the anterior neck at the level of the cricoid cartilage and forcing the cricoid cartilage posteriorly into the esophagus. This maneuver can provide a pressure of up to 100 cm H_2O to seal the upper esophagus and prevent gastric contents from entering the mouth. Active vomiting against well applied cricoid pressure can rupture the distal esophagus. Anesthetized, paralyzed patients cannot vomit. Passive regurgitation of gastric contents is easily controlled in an anesthetized, paralyzed patient with cricoid pressure. Although the head-up position increases the gastric pressure that is required for regurgitation, this position enhances pulmonary aspiration of any material in the mouth. The Trendelenburg position, which forces gastric contents or blood in the mouth to run out of the nose and not into the trachea, is the safest position to prevent aspiration.

2. **Intubation** Upon admission, measurements of arterial blood gases (ABG) are obtained on room air, after which oxygen is administered at 10–15 liters/min with a nonrebreathing face mask if the patient is breathing. If the cervical spine x-ray is normal, the head is placed in the "sniffing" position, which is obtained by slightly flexing the neck and extending the head, thus forming a straight line between the open mouth and the glottis. Not uncommonly, the patient requires emergency intubation before a C-spine x-ray has been obtained to rule out a fracture or dislocation in which case the neck is held neutral.

Hypoventilating patients require bag and mask ventilation while the physician is preparing for endotracheal intubation. These patients should be placed in the Trendelenburg position with cricoid pressure applied by an assistant until intubated. Bagging the patient without cricoid pressure tends to insufflate the stomach and predispose to vomiting.

To facilitate intubation, the patient is induced with a bolus of thiopental sodium followed by succinylcholine. Constant cricoid pressure is applied. Gently insert the laryngoscope on the right side of the mouth and advance it until the base of the epiglottis is visualized. At this point, the blade is moved to the midline; this maneuver pushes the tongue toward the left. As the laryngoscope is lifted at a 45° angle, the glottis is visualized. An 8.0-mm tube is recommended for the adult female, and a 9.0-mm tube for the adult male. The cuff should be lubricated with a water-soluble lubricant to minimize trauma to the vocal cords. The endotracheal tube is advanced under direct visualization until the cuff has passed the vocal cords. The cuff is inflated with the amount of air necessary to minimize or prevent air leak. The lungs are checked for symmetrical expansion. Cricoid pressure is released after the cuff is inflated. The patient is placed on IPPV and 100% O_2 for 5 min, after which O_2 is decreased to 50%. ABG levels are checked while the patient is on 50% oxygen. An oral airway is inserted to prevent the patient from biting the endotracheal tube. The face is cleaned and the skin is sprayed with benzoin. The tube is secured with adhesive tape. Umbilical ties may be used if adhesive tape will not adhere to the face. An 18F Salem sump tube is passed into the stomach via the mouth and placed on low suction. While the patient is on 100% O_2, the endotracheal tube is suctioned for material that might have been aspirated following injury.

C. **Variations**

1. **Unconscious and unresponsive patients** may be intubated without medication.

2. If the patient is **hemodynamically unstable,** only succinylcholine is given.

3. If a **cervical collar** is in place, the anterior portion is removed to facilitate cricoid pressure and jaw mobilization. Remove the collar after the patient is quiet from thiopental.

4. Neither barbiturates nor neuromuscular blockers should be used if there is **partial airway obstruction** or a question of **severe intraoral trauma.** In the awake patient, nasotracheal intubation may be attempted with a topical anesthetic, if there is no mid-face fracture. If performed **prior to aggressive fluid replacement,** oral intubation is usually not a problem in patients with oral fractures. A patient with severe masseter muscle spasm will need muscle relaxation to open the mouth.

5. **Laryngeal trauma** is a relative contraindication to translaryngeal intubation.

6. Patients with clinical evidence of **cervical spine injury** who need mechanical ventilatory support should be managed with nasotracheal intubation, if awake, or tracheostomy. Use of the fiberoptic laryngoscope permits intubation without neck manipulation. If oral fiberoptic intubation is used, an oral airway or bite blocks should first be placed in the mouth to prevent damage to the laryngoscope.

7. Use a bolus of pancuronium bromide, **not succinylcholine,** in the patient with a severe burn, crushed muscle, or eye injury.

8. If emergency intubation is required and the cords cannot be visualized, jet needle ventilation or cricothyroidotomy may be needed (see pp. 45 and 482).

III. **Suctioning the Airway** A patient with an artificial airway is unable to produce an effective cough to clear tracheal secretions. Mobilization of secretions is facilitated by chest physiotherapy and airway suctioning.

We use a 22-inch, soft, sterile plastic catheter with a two-eye whistle tip. There is a proximal vent which is larger than the internal diameter of the catheter and a plastic sleeve which maintains catheter sterility. The external diameter should be no larger than one-half the internal diameter of the tube suctioned.

A. **Technique** The patient is administered 100% oxygen and hand-ventilated with at least five deep breaths. The catheter is inserted without vacuum until the carina is approached or until the left or right main stem bronchus is entered. The catheter is withdrawn with intermittent suction and rotational movement. Suctioning is done for about 10 sec and no longer than 20 sec. The ventilator system is closed for 1 min and suction repeated, if needed. The patient is hand-ventilated with at least five deep breaths and the oropharynx and nose are suctioned. If there are any complications, the patient is mechanically ventilated with an FiO_2 of 1.0 and evaluated.

B. **Complications** Atrial and ventricular arrhythmias, cardiac arrest, hypotension, hypoxia, and atelectasis can occur and are most likely the result of improper technique. In these critically ill patients, the above method is associated with the fewest number of complications.

Section IX
MONITORING

INTRODUCTION

Monitoring is the process of observing, regulating, or controlling a system relative to volume, intensity, quality, or quantity. This process is accomplished through visual, auditory, or printed techniques and can be simple or complex. At MIEMSS, physiologic, biochemical, and bacterial monitoring provides continuous information which is valuable for the management of critically ill patients. Conventional transducer and electronic monitoring equipment is used with digital readouts, trend recorders, and visual/auditory centralized and bedside alarms incorporating computer recall. The degree a patient is monitored will vary with the severity of the injury or illness, the degree of biochemical and physiologic derangement, and the detrimental factors associated with the monitoring process.

Critical injury implies that the patient's life is in peril and gross physiologic dysfunction is usually present. Many patients develop single or multiple system dysfunction following shock, trauma, sepsis, or other major systemic insults, with central nervous system, cardiovascular, and pulmonary dysfunction posing the most severe and immediate threat to life. The gastrointestinal tract and its accessory organs, the kidneys, and other peripheral tissues are also vital for survival and depend on appropriate function of the cardiovascular and pulmonary systems.

The ideal approach to the victim of major trauma or critical illness is total body monitoring to provide maximum information and early warning signs of impending complications and system failure. We monitor the following body systems: coagulation, respiratory, hematologic, cardiac, renal, central nervous, metabolic, gastrointestinal, peripheral sensory/motor, and bacteriologic. Monitoring commences immediately upon admission, first clinically, then followed as rapidly as possible with electronic monitoring. On admission, treatment begins with assessment and aggressive resuscitation. Once adequate ventilation and appropriate volume infusion have commenced, blood pressure recordings, pulse rate, central venous pressures, EKG, and urinary output monitoring are begun. An arterial and venous sample of blood is obtained soon after admission to evaluate blood gas, biochemical, and hematologic parameters. This information is obtained within minutes following admission and relayed to the Admitting Area by computer technology.

Since invasive monitoring can be associated with septic, vascular, and miscellaneous complications, it must be evaluated on a daily basis to ascertain the risk/benefit ratio. As potential and actual risk approaches or exceeds the level of benefit, the monitoring device should be discontinued.

Intensive monitoring is indicated in the critically ill patient in order that deterioration of physiologic systems is detected early. If organ-system dysfunction is diagnosed early, it is more likely that this system may be adequately supported until resolution can occur. As the patient moves out of the critical phase, the simpler forms of monitoring are sufficient.

35
METABOLIC AND
PHYSIOLOGIC MONITORING

There are physiologic and metabolic parameters that should be monitored to optimally evaluate the total patient. The older the patient, the more systems that are dysfunctional, and the greater the degree of injury in a given organ, the greater the intensity of the monitoring that is required. The following indices are important in monitoring the critically ill patient.

I. **Cardiovascular System**   Routine evaluation by **physical examination** and by monitoring the **heart rate** and **blood pressure** is performed in all patients to assess cardiovascular function. A baseline **EKG** is obtained in all patients to substantiate the presence or absence of abnormal electrical cardiac function. Continuous **cardiac monitoring** of the heart rate is important to assess acute changes in stress and/or the development of arrhythmias. The **central venous pressure** is helpful in providing objective information regarding fluid infusion and cardiovascular function. If the patient has obvious cardiovascular insufficiency or is likely to have cardiac insufficiency, but its presence is uncertain, a Swan-Ganz catheter must be inserted. The Swan-Ganz catheter will provide information regarding the **cardiac output, systemic vascular resistance, wedge pressure, central venous pressure,** and **arterial-venous oxygen content difference.** These parameters will provide objective information such that the appropriate component may be manipulated to improve perfusion (optimal oxygen consumption). All **medications** that possess a cardiovascular effect must be scrutinized to make certain that their benefit outweighs the risk or detriment associated with this drug. See p. 335.

II. **Respiratory System**   Physical examination, **chest x-ray,** and **arterial blood gases** are important in all trauma patients. With physical examination, the clinician should note the presence of an effective cough, chest wall splinting, respiratory rate, rhonchi, rales, wheezes, and symmetrical quality of the breath sounds. If a **chest tube** is in place, the quantity of fluid drainage, the presence of an air leak, and functional assessment of the tube is noted. If the patient is on a ventilator, the PaO_2/FiO_2, **level of PEEP, minute ventilation volume, ventilator rate, patient respiratory rate, $PaCO_2$, pH,** and **bicarbonate** are assessed. Prior to the removal of ventilatory support, the PaO_2/FiO_2 **(shunt), vital capacity, maximal inspiratory force, compliance,** and **dead space** must be acceptable. **End-expiratory gases** are followed in the critically ill patient by a mass spectrometer and fed into a computer to analyze pulmonary and cellular function (respiratory exchange ratio, CO_2 production, oxygen consumption, dead space, etc.). See p. 313.

III. **Central Nervous System**   **Physical examination** is helpful in assessing patients with head and spinal cord injuries. The level of consciousness, brain stem function, and extremity response to command or pain should be closely noted and followed. Any deterioration of central nervous system function warrants a prompt investigation for structural and metabolic abnormalities. The **CAT scan** is indicated for head-injured patients, to provide diagnostic information at the time of admission, and is repeated, as necessary, during the hospital course to assess intracranial pathology. **Intracranial pressure monitoring** allows the clinician to detect the presence of intracranial hypertension early in order that edema may be treated at the earliest possible moment; otherwise, intracranial hypertension may not be apparent until later when an obvious change occurs on physical examination. See pp. 215, 228, and 309.

IV. **Gastrointestinal System**   **Physical examination** is important in assessing normal or abnormal gastrointestinal function. A flat, soft abdomen in which normal bowel sounds can be auscultated implies normal peristalsis. If the patient is passing flatus and/or stools of normal consistency, functional peristalsis is present. If a gastric tube is in place and the **gastric drainage** is less than 1,000 cc/24 hr, it is likely that peristalsis is intact. The **gastric pH** should be followed and controlled in the critically ill patient to prevent stress gastric and duodenal ulceration. The quality and quantity of any abdominal drainage should be monitored to assess intra-abdominal pathology. An elevated **bilirubin, hepatocellular enzymes,** or **amylase** level usually indicates abnormal biliary or pancreatic function. **Peritoneal lavage** generally provides more information about the presence of abdominal injury than physical examination.

V. **Renal Function**   The **quantity of urine/hr** reflects, to some degree, renal function. A urinary output less than 30 cc/hr implies decreased renal blood flow, renal parenchymal dysfunction, or urinary obstruction. A **creatinine clearance** should be routinely performed daily in the critically ill patient to follow glomerular function. The **free water clearance, urine osmolality, urine specific gravity,** and **urinary sodium** reflect renal tubular function. A rise in the **BUN** usually represents hypermetabolism, catabolism, or renal insufficiency. The **urinalysis** usually helps to confirm the state of renal function and presence or absence of urinary sepsis. The presence of **hemoglobinuria** or **myoglobinuria** should prompt careful monitoring of renal function. See p. 349.

VI. **Musculoskeletal System**   Extremity function is primarily assessed by **physical examination.** Color, capillary refill, palpation of the pulses, and inspection of the extremities for edema are useful to assess vascular function. Soft tissue wounds are inspected for the presence of necrosis and sepsis. Sensory and motor function of the extremity is assessed to detect central or peripheral neural pathology. Skeletal abnormalities are usually detected by the presence of deformity, abnormal motion, pain, and ecchymosis. **X-rays** assist the clinician in detecting skeletal pathology. See p. 241.

VII. **Hematologic System** The **hematocrit/hemoglobin** provides the clinician with information regarding the presence of red blood cell loss, red blood cell production, red blood cell destruction, and/or dilution. The hematocrit and hemoglobin should be serially monitored in the critically ill patient until the patient is stable. In the extremes, the **white blood cell count** may reflect the presence of sepsis. In this instance, potential sources of sepsis must be thoroughly investigated. A **platelet count** may reveal the presence of thrombocytopenia which may be secondary to dilution, disseminated intravascular coagulopathy (DIC), sepsis, decreased platelet production, and/or increased platelet destruction. Each entity must be investigated as soon as thrombocytopenia presents.

VIII. **Coagulation** Abnormalities of coagulation must be assessed quantitatively and qualitatively. It is important to note on **physical examination** in a patient who has a numerical coagulation abnormality whether there is cutaneous petechia or bleeding from wounds, vascular lines, urinary tract, gastrointestinal tract, etc. The absence or presence of obvious bleeding will often dictate whether a coagulation abnormality should be treated. **Thrombocytopenia, hypofibrinogenemia,** or a prolonged **prothrombin time (PT)** or **partial thromboplastin time (PTT)** may be secondary to dilution and/or DIC. Elevated **fibrin split products** and **thrombin time** usually indicate the presence of DIC. The bleeding time may be increased if there is a qualitative or quantitative platelet defect. Evaluation of **clot formation** and **dissolution** may assist in the detection of a coagulation factor abnormality, platelet dysfunction, or increased fibrinolysis. These factors should be closely followed in the patient with major quantities of blood loss or lesser hemorrhage in which vital structures are injured, e.g., brain contusions/hematomas. Coagulation abnormalities may be secondary to malnutrition or sepsis. See pp. 37 and 414.

IX. **Metabolism**

A. Since there is a propensity toward glucose intolerance during stress, the serum **glucose** should be followed in the critically ill patient. Hyperglycemia usually causes a major extracellular fluid shift and causes excessive water loss by an osmotic diuresis, both of which lead to intracellular dehydration. Impairment in glucose metabolism is likely if steroids are administered or the patient is starved, septic, or diabetic.

B. The **osmolality** usually reflects the state of hydration of the critically ill patient. Hypertonicity usually implies cellular dehydration, and hypotonicity usually implies cellular swelling. The osmolality may be elevated if the patient is azotemic or hyperglycemic or if there is a circulating osmolar active agent, e.g., mannitol or ethanol. Extremes of osmolality usually cause abnormal cellular function.

C. **Fluid input and output** data provide the clinician with an approximation of the patient's total body water content. These figures in conjunction with an assessment of insensible water losses, physical examination, and chemical information such as the serum osmolality, sodium, BUN, etc., are useful in determining appropriate fluid and electrolyte requirements. The greater the degree of stress and hemodynamic instability, the more frequently the input and output figures and fluid and electrolyte needs must be assessed.

D. The **electrolytes**, such as sodium, potassium, calcium, magnesium, and phosphorus, should be followed frequently, until the patient is stable. Abnormalities of electrolytes create cellular dysfunction and disruption of homeostasis.

E. Daily **weights** are helpful in determining changes in total body water and lean body mass if the patient is hemodynamically stable and third space loss is minimal. A weight change of greater than ½ pound/day usually implies water gain or loss. The unstable and critically ill patient tends to sequester fluid in the extravascular space; total body water usually increases, since excessive fluid is necessary to maintain normal intravascular volume to provide normal organ perfusion.

F. **Nitrogen balance** is helpful in determining the patient's state of metabolism. If nitrogen output is greater than nitrogen input, the patient is catabolic. If nitrogen input is greater than nitrogen output, the patient is anabolic. The goal of metabolic support is to maintain neutral nitrogen balance or anabolism to prevent or minimize destruction of the protein pool. Nitrogen balance should be followed during the period of stress and after its abatement until protein depletion is restored.

G. The daily **caloric intake** should be compared to the caloric expenditure. The greater the caloric expenditure and the longer the caloric output is greater than the caloric intake, the greater the protein depletion and the likelihood that cellular dysfunction will follow. It is suggested that calorie demands as estimated by oxygen consumption be met as soon as clinically feasible.

H. The serum **albumin** reflects to some degree the patient's stores of protein. A low albumin implies inadequate nutritional support or liver dysfunction. The sequel to hypoalbuminemia is usually a net increase in water flux from the intravascular to the interstitial compartment, i.e., edema. An albumin level should be obtained each week to follow the nutritional state of the critically ill patient.

I. The **pH** is affected by respiratory and metabolic function. If the pH is not maintained in a relatively narrow range, cellular dysfunction will follow. The more critically ill the patient, the more frequently the pH should be monitored, as well as the specific respiratory and metabolic functions which affect it.

J. The **bicarbonate level** reflects the acid-base balance of the blood. A deficit of bicarbonate represents a metabolic acidosis either as a primary problem or compensatory to a respiratory alkalosis. An excess of bicarbonate represents a metabolic alkalosis, either as a primary event or to compensate for a respiratory acidosis. The bicarbonate level should be followed frequently in the critically ill patient to detect metabolic and respiratory dysfunction.

K. There will be an increase in **lactate** formation if the cell enters anaerobic metabolism secondary to an impairment of cellular perfusion (shock). In general, the greater the impairment of perfusion, the greater the lactate level. As perfusion is restored and the oxygen debt is repaid, lactate will normalize.

L. Shock and hypoxia commonly cause ischemic changes in the liver. The **SGOT, SGPT, LDH,** or **bilirubin** may rise following necrosis/ischemia of the liver. Jaundice, which develops secondary to liver ischemia, usually peaks approximately 5–8 days after injury and becomes normal by the 10th–14th day. Persistent jaundice at this time usually implies an additional insult such as sepsis and a poorer prognosis. See p. 436.

M. The **respiratory exchange ratio** (RER) estimates the actual respiratory quotient (RQ) and is the ratio of carbon dioxide production to oxygen consumption. The RER provides information regarding the type of substrate being utilized: 0.7 for fat, 1.0 for carbohydrates, and 0.8 for protein. If all three of these substrates are being metabolized the RER is usually about 0.85. The clinician can ascertain what substrates are being metabolized if the RER is obtained. If exogenous substrate is administered to the patient, the RER should reflect whether this substrate can be utilized or not.

N. **Oxygen consumption** is obtained to assess overall cellular function. Oxygen consumption may be low secondary to inadequate cellular perfusion or decreased oxygen demand. A low oxygen consumption (less than 150 cc of oxygen/min) is associated with a poor prognosis and a normal or increased oxygen consumption is generally associated with a good prognosis during shock resuscitation. It is important to optimize oxygen consumption in the critically ill patient as a useful end point to follow during manipulation of cardiorespiratory therapy.

O. It may be beneficial to know the **carbon dioxide production** to better understand the patient's metabolism. Increased carbon dioxide production may be a manifestation of excessive carbohydrate calorie administration or increased metabolic rate. This may be clinically important in a patient with increased dead space, who is being weaned from a ventilator.

X. **Infection Monitoring** is an important aspect of managing critically ill patients, since sepsis is a common cause of morbidity and mortality. Frequent **white blood cell count** and **temperature determinations** are necessary to detect the presence of sepsis. Routine **surveillance cultures** are useful in critically ill patients, since bacteremias and sepsis frequently stem from organisms which have colonized the patient during the initial hospital course. Routine cultures are taken from the urine, sputum, wounds, and drains. Wounds and catheter sites should be routinely inspected for evidence of inflammation. If the patient develops fever, leukocytosis or **physiologic systems instability,** all potential sources of sepsis should be aggressively investigated by **radiologic techniques, sampling body fluids,** and **physical examination.** The length of time prophylactic and therapeutic **antibiotics** are used should be monitored regarding their risk/benefit ratio.

Perspective

Various physiologic and biochemical parameters were recorded in 300 shock patients at MIEMSS and evaluated relative to survivors and nonsurvivors. A critical analysis of the physiologic and biochemical data indicates a major disturbance of metabolic functions at the tissue and cellular levels. These metabolic disturbances are frequently present despite the presence of "normal" physiologic parameters that are commonly monitored, such as blood pressure, electrolytes, and blood gases. Oxygen and glucose utilization appear to be decreased as evidenced by increased anaerobic metabolism, with elevated lactate and pyruvate levels and increased blood glucose levels in nonsurvivors. The coagulation mechanism is frequently abnormal in nonsurvivors. Hypoxia of the liver apparently accounts for many of the biochemical abnormalities identified. Oxygen consumption and cardiac outputs were statistically greater in survivors than nonsurvivors; however, the difference in blood pressure between the two groups was not significant. High lactate levels are usually associated with a markedly elevated mortality rate. A critical assessment of the metabolic sequelae of shock/trauma may offer further insight into these physiologic derangements. We plan to continue evaluating physiologic and biochemical data to better understand the parameters which most affect survival. If these factors can be identified and favorably altered, we may further improve patient survival.

We have found the computer to be valuable in providing "automatic" computations from physiologic and metabolic information entered into this system. The computer has the capability of providing on-line recall and trend analysis of various parameters. We feel that the ability to follow trend analyses provides practical clinical information regarding the presence of stability or deterioration, which in turn will dictate the necessity to continue or alter current therapy.

In summary, the mortality rate of critically ill and injured patients will only be reduced when clinicians realize that in-depth monitoring and analysis are necessary.

Section X
HYPERBARIC MEDICINE

INTRODUCTION

Hyperbaric oxygenation is the use of oxygen under increased atmospheric pressure, resulting in an increased amount of oxygen physically dissolved in the blood.

Provided the temperature remains constant, the volume of the gas is decreased under pressure. The decrease in volume is directly proportional to the increase in pressure. For each 33 feet below sea level, the pressure of a given volume of gas is increased by 1 atmosphere absolute (ATA). At 2 ATA pressure, the volume of the gas is decreased by one-half. Since liquids are not compressible, body fluids and tissues are not directly altered by atmospheric pressure changes.

The therapeutic value of the hyperbaric chamber is due to a combination of pressure and oxygen, resulting in an increase in the partial pressure of oxygen. At 3 ATA with the patient breathing 100% oxygen, approximately 6.4 vol % oxygen is physically dissolved in the plasma, enough to support life even with no hemoglobin. If exposure to 100% oxygen under pressure exceeds safe time limits, it can cause oxygen toxicity to the lungs and central nervous system (CNS). Continuous treatment with 100% oxygen at 3 ATA (66 feet salt water) for more than 90 min produces oxygen toxicity.

36
CLINICAL PROBLEMS AMENABLE TO HYPERBARIC THERAPY

I. **Conditions Treated**

Condition		Category
Gas gangrene	I	Emergency
Smoke inhalation	I	Emergency
Carbon monoxide poisoning		
Cyanide		
Decompression sickness (bends)	I	Emergency
Air embolism	I	Emergency
Spinal cord injuries (research)	II	Emergency
Compromised skin grafts	I	Semi-emergency
Anaerobic infections	I	Semi-emergency
Radionecrosis (bone and soft tissue)	II	Non-emergency
Chronic osteomyelitis	II	Non-emergency
Bone graft	II	Non-emergency
Wound healing enhancement	I and II	Semi-emergency
Other		

II. **Terminology**   The atmosphere (air) has a weight (pressure) which is equal at sea level to a column of water 1 inch in diameter and 33 feet high (10.4 m) or 760 mm Hg or 14.7 pounds per square inch (psi). Engineers express pressure in psi and scientists express this pressure in mm Hg. A further method of expressing hyperbaric pressure is by depth equivalent in feet of salt water which is zero at sea level. Pressure in "feet of salt water" is common U.S. Navy parlance.

Feet salt water (FSW)	Atmosphere absolute	psi	mm Hg	Volume of gas (%)
0 (sea level)	1	14.7	760	100
33	2	29.4	1,520	50
66	3	44.1	2,280	33⅓
99	4	58.8	3,040	25

The chamber pressure gauge is set to read zero at sea level (1 ATA); thus, all readings on the gauge below 14.7 psi reflect negative atmospheric pressure.

III. **Personnel Qualifications** Chamber operators should be graduates of the Naval Diving School with a minimum of 6 years experience with high pressure environment. MIEMSS operators are retired Navy divers and are responsible for all chamber operations and functions.

All medical and nursing staff who participate in hyperbaric medicine treatment must have a chest x-ray and EKG to exclude pulmonary and cardiac disease. Those with a history of chronic sinusitis or ear problems must be approved by an ENT surgeon. Obese people are excluded from daily diving because of problems related to nitrogen retention and release; however, an occasional dive is acceptable, after a chest x-ray and EKG are shown to be within normal limits. Each person must take a qualification dive which consists of pressurizing with a bounce dive to 112 feet and a return to 60 feet while breathing 100% oxygen for 30 min. This exposure is to test for oxygen tolerance.

IV. **Supplies and Equipment in the Chamber** The MIEMSS chamber complex consists of two large chambers, the surgery chamber and the therapy chamber. The two chambers are connected by a third smaller chamber, an entry lock. The surgery and therapy chambers have small medical locks for passing materials, laboratory specimens, etc., in and out.

Two volume ventilators for controlled ventilation and anesthesia are present in the surgery chamber. In addition, there is wall suction, oxygen and air outlets, and a K-thermia blanket for hypo- and hyperthermia. A junction box with the capability of monitoring heart rate, blood pressure, pulmonary artery pressure, central venous pressure, intracranial pressure, and temperature in two patients is available. The scopes and modules are outside the chamber and can be easily seen through the portholes. An emergency and cardiac arrest drug box is available. There is a defibrillator available for use in the chamber.

A two-way intercom and telephone is available for communication. Each chamber is monitored by a closed circuit television camera.

V. **Prohibited Materials** As a general rule, nothing which could produce static electricity or a spark is allowed in the hyperbaric chamber. Toxic materials such as paints, insulation, adhesives, mercury, and equipment containing oils, or components that would burn or give off toxic fumes at operation temperature should not be installed or used in a manned hyperbaric chamber.

Prohibited material include the following:
—Alcohol or alcohol-based solutions
—Cigarettes
—Matches and lighters
—Aerosols of any kind
—Flash cameras
—Flammable anesthetics
—Toxic gases
—Volatile flammable liquids
—Mercury or components containing this metal

—Beryllium or components containing this metal
—Magnesium or alloys containing magnesium
—Synthetic clothing—nylons, dacrons, double knits, garters, girdles, synthetic slips, shoes with exposed metal bottoms (taps)
—Nondiving watches
—Fountain pens
—Radios
—Motors of any kind

Note Patient and medical staff must wear scrubs and/or cover gowns during treatment in the hyperbaric chamber under normal conditions. If the oxygen concentration in the chamber exceeds 22%, ventilation of the chamber air must be undertaken. If venting is not possible, the dive must be aborted. Patients will always be accompanied by at least one doctor and/or nurse. On dives to 3 ATA, it may be necessary to have two people accompany the patient. This will be determined by the physician in charge of hyperbaric medicine.

Personnel must be observed for at least 1 hr following any dive requiring decompression. There must be no flying for 12 hr after a dive.

VI. **Order of Command** The chamber operator is in charge of operating the chamber for dives and emergencies. Standard diving tables including speed of compression and decompression are used. Treating decompression sickness (bends) is the responsibility of the chamber operator with the physician serving as a consultant. The physician is in charge of patient management and may abort the dive only if a life-threatening complication has occurred in the chamber.

All abnormal reactions of the patient or diving staff must be reported to the operator, who must then consider continuing or aborting the dive.

The nursing staff is in charge of the care of the patient. The inside nurse and chamber operator work together to make certain that the patient receives maximum benefit from the treatment.

VII. **Routine Patient Management**

A. **Routine care of the acute critically ill, unstable, or unconscious patient**

1. Chest x-ray
   a. Prior to first dive
   b. After first dive
   c. After each dive if a chest tube is present

2. Bilateral myringotomies prior to first dive

3. Sedation to prevent breath holding or struggling. Dosages: Valium, 5–10 mg i.v. before dive; phenobarbital, 100 mg i.v. before dive

4. Gastric decompression with a nasogastric (NG) tube

5. Endotracheal tube cuff is filled with water, **not air.**

6. Exclude air bubbles in i.v. lines.

7. Administer i.v. fluids in plastic bags. If a glass bottle is used, it must be vented.

8. Patient is placed on the ventilator and 100% oxygen is used at whatever volume is prescribed by the anesthesiologist.

9. Be aware of the signs and symptoms of oxygen toxicity.

10. Chest tubes must be patent at all times, **never clamped.**

11. Pneumothorax and pulmonary edema are excluded by frequent auscultation. Meticulous tracheobronchial toilet is necessary to avoid mucous plugs and air trapping.

12. Drugs are available in the chamber for cardiopulmonary arrest.

13. Technical procedures which require skill should not be attempted at 2.8 ATA (60 feet) or more, unless directed by personnel outside the chamber. Any such procedure must first be cleared by the physician in charge of hyperbaric medicine.

14. Dressing changes, debridement, and fasciotomy may be done.

15. Record vital signs as per routine. Record the patient's tolerance to the dive and the appearance of the affected area.

B. **Routine medications and medical problems** The full complement of drugs designed for use in the intensive care environment should be available in the hyperbaric chamber. These drugs do not have known major complicating problems when used under hyperbaric pressure.

1. **Seizures** The drug of choice for the treatment of seizures is diazepam (Valium, 10 mg) given intravenously. There are no major interactions or complications with the use of this drug in the hyperbaric environment.

    Dilantin and barbiturates can be considered for seizure treatment, but concern for barbiturate toxicity under hyperbaric oxygen conditions has not yet been resolved.

2. **Cardiac arrhythmias** Often, the seriously ill patient requiring hyperbaric oxygen has a cardiac arrhythmia. Many such arrhythmias are relatively benign and do not require treatment. Those requiring treatment should be treated in the normal manner with the use of agents such as Digoxin, Quinidine, Procainamide, and other antiarrhythmic drugs. Electric cardioversion can be used in the chamber. Where cardioversion is undertaken, precautions must be taken to prevent sparks or open archs during the use of electrical defibrillation.

3. **Shock** Standard medications should be utilized in the treatment of septic shock. Improving cardiac performance during shock with medications, blood and fluid replacement, and treatment of infection is carried out as usual. Large doses of steroids have been used in the prevention of endotoxic shock.

4. **Allergic reactions and anaphylaxis** Anaphylactic shock may occur in the chamber. Treatment using epinephrine, large doses of steroids, and antihistaminics should be undertaken. It is essential to treat anaphylactic reactions rapidly with all the appropriate medications. The use of these drugs should not be compromised because of a concern for their use under hyperbaric conditions.

5. **Anxiety and pain** Analgesics such as morphine, pentazocine (Talwin), and meperidene (Demerol), and tranquilizers given under pressure are used with the same precautions for respiratory depression as under normal pressure. Valium is usually the best tranquilizer to administer. It is important not to alter the neurologic status of the patient since evaluation of the mental status is often an important part of the treatment.

6. **Heart failure** Acute or chronic congestive heart failure may require a variety of medications, including digitalis, diuretics, morphine, or xanthine derivatives such as aminophylline. Since there are no known detrimental interactions between these drugs and the hyperbaric environment, they should not be withheld from the patient.

7. **Respiratory failure** may occur secondary to numerous mechanisms including heart failure, drowning, smoke inhalation, severe oxygen toxicity, or shock lung. Provided oxygen toxicity is not the cause of pulmonary insufficiency, the high partial pressures of hyperbaric oxygen may be advantageous to the patient. However, this advantage is for short periods only. The rapid onset of pulmonary toxicity can occur with prolonged oxygen exposure.

8. **Hypertensive crises** There is little known about potential complications of antihypertensive agents under hyperbaric conditions. Reserpine, which enhances cerebral oxygen toxicity, should be avoided in the hyperbaric environment.

9. **Anticoagulation** has been advocated as part of the treatment of severe decompression sickness. Patients on anticoagulants should be protected from minor or major trauma in the chamber to prevent excessive bleeding. If excessive bleeding occurs under hyperbaric environment, reversal of the anticoagulant should be instituted immediately.

   Note | In the hyperbaric situation, there should be no hesitation in providing the full battery of intensive care medications or diagnostic and therapeutic procedures equivalent to that needed in the care of the patient in a normobaric environment.

10. **Emergencies** Bleeding wounds or dehiscences can be treated within the chamber as can dressing changes, fasciotomies, or debridement. A pneumothorax must be treated immediately with a chest tube or a needle. Cardiac arrest not requiring defibrillation can be handled in the chamber. If defibrillation is indicated, the patient can be defibrillated in the chamber at

depth or brought out by decompression. On dives requiring a decompression stop, an emergency team is sent into the entry lock to bring the patient out while the tenders needing decompression will go into the entry lock for decompression.

C. **Routine care of the acute conscious and cooperative patient**

1. Ear examination   Large wax buildup will need to be removed.

2. Attempt dive **without** myringotomies. If the patient fails to clear the ears, perform bilateral myringotomies.

3. Chest x-ray
   a. Prior to first dive
   b. After each dive, if a chest tube is present or chest symptoms or signs are present

4. Valium (i.v.) for sedation before dive, as needed.

5. NG tube is not necessary.

6. Oxygenation via face mask, endotracheal tube, tracheostomy tube, or head tent

7. Exclude air bubbles in i.v. lines.

8. Fluids are administered intravenously in plastic bags. If a glass bottle is used, it must be vented.

9. Be aware of the signs and symptoms of oxygen toxicity. Keep the patient as relaxed as possible.

10. If a chest tube is present, it must be patent at all times, i.e., never clamped.

11. Pneumothorax and pulmonary edema are excluded by frequent auscultation. Meticulous tracheobronchial toilet is necessary to avoid mucous plugs and air trapping.

12. Drugs are available in the chamber for cardiopulmonary arrest.

13. Skilled technical procedures should not be attempted at 2.8 ATA (60 feet) or more, unless directed by personnel outside the chamber. Any such procedure must be cleared by the physician in charge of hyperbaric medicine.

14. Record vital signs as per routine. Record the patient's tolerance to the dive and the appearance of the affected area.

D. **Routine care of the nonacute patient**

1. History and physical examination before first dive

2. Chest x-ray, EKG, CBC with differential, electrolytes, sedimentation rate, and fasting blood sugar prior to beginning series of dives

3. Cultures of lesions

4. Vital signs before dive, and when necessary

5. Record tolerance to dive and complications.

6. Be aware of oxygen toxicity signs and symptoms. Strive to keep patients as quiet as possible.

7. Ophthalmologic consultation for long-term patients

8. Photograph of lesion on admission and each 2 weeks thereafter

E. **Myringotomized patients**

1. Pressure-equalizing (PE) tubes can be retained for up to 3 months.

2. Initial care consists of Cortisporin drops (prevents clotting), three times/day × 48 hr.

3. Water must not be allowed into ears; no hair washing or submersion of head under water, while PE tubes are in place.

VIII. **Oxygen toxicity**   The two systems primarily affected by oxygen toxicity are the central nervous system and the pulmonary system. Oxygen toxicity depends upon the oxygen concentration, atmospheric pressure, and length of exposure.

A. **Central nervous system**   Symptoms and signs of oxygen toxicity of the CNS include facial pallor, sweating, bradycardia, choking sensation, sleepiness, euphoria, apprehension, fidgeting, disinterest, clumsiness, loss of visual acuity, constriction of visual fields, and tinnitus. There may be unpleasant olfactory or gustatory sensations, panting, grunting, or hiccuping. Severe symptoms include nausea, vomiting, twitching of the lips and cheek, syncope, or convulsions.

A convulsion which presents while under pressure is managed by:
—Discontinuing the oxygen by removal of the mask or, if an endotracheal tube is used, changing to compressed air
—Preventing injury
—Administering i.v. Valium
—Waiting 10 min and resuming therapy if the patient is stable

B. **Pulmonary system**   The first pulmonary symptom is a tickling sensation which occurs with deep inspiration after breathing oxygen for 3–6 hr on 100% oxygen at 3 ATA. A dry cough may develop. Following 8–10 hr of oxygen breathing, a constant burning sensation of the chest develops and may be followed by uncontrollable coughing and dyspnea at rest. Pulmonary function tests reveal a decreased vital capacity, inspiratory capacity, inspiratory flow rate, carbon monoxide diffusing capacity, pulmonary capillary blood volume, and lung compliance.

The symptoms of tracheobronchitis usually begin to diminish as soon as oxygen breathing stops; however, progressive impairment of pulmonary function may continue over the next 2–4 hr. Lung volumes return to preexposure values in 1–3 days.

All of the acute effects of hyperoxia are completely reversible if their progression has been arrested in time. Once this time frame (8–10 hr) has been exceeded, progressive pulmonary destruction results in death. The primary method to prevent oxygen toxicity is to use air breaks during the hyperoxic periods, i.e., alternation of 20 min of hyperoxia (100% oxygen) with a 5-min normoxic exposure on chamber air. Vitamin E has been used in large doses (1,200 units daily), but no controlled trials are available to prove its effectiveness.

IX. **Smoke Inhalation: Carbon Monoxide and/or Cyanide Poisoning** Carbon monoxide (CO) and cyanide poisoning are prime indications for treatment with hyperbaric oxygen. Because polyvinylchloride, wools, foam, and other synthetic materials are often used in furniture, clothing, etc., cyanide poisoning, in addition to carbon monoxide, is not unusual in smoke inhalation. A person exposed to smoke and exhibiting neurologic symptoms which cannot be attributed to trauma should be treated with hyperbaric oxygen, if possible. It is not possible to quickly make a differential diagnosis of carbon monoxide and cyanide poisoning, but both conditions are being treated by the administration of hyperbaric oxygen. Patients showing any CNS symptoms or a carboxyhemoglobin (COHb) level over 25% will be submitted for treatment with hyperbaric oxygen. Carbon monoxide and cyanide block mitochondrial enzyme function thus impairing oxygen utilization. See p. 379.

A. **Signs and symptoms correlations with COHb level***

Signs and symptoms	Serum COHb level (%)
None	0–10
Tightness across forehead, possibly slight headache, dilatation of cutaneous blood vessels	10–20
Headache, throbbing in temples	20–30
Severe headache, weakness, dizziness, dimness of vision, nausea and vomiting, collapse	30–40
Same as previous item but with greater possibility of collapse or syncope, increased respiration and pulse	40–50
Syncope, increased respiration and pulse, coma with intermittent convulsions, Cheyne-Stokes respiration	50–60
Coma with intermittent convulsions, depressed heart action and respiration, possibly death	60–70
Weak pulse, slowed respiration, respiratory failure and death	70–80

*Adapted from Roughton, F. J. W., and Darling, R. C., 1944. The effect of CO on oxyhemoglobin dissociation curve. *Am. J. Physiol.* 141:171.

Because of the variance of clinical signs and symptoms compared to the COHb level, we have undertaken a trial using psychometric testing to help diagnose diffuse brain involvement of carbon monoxide poisoning, which may occur at lower levels than the currently accepted levels that are listed above. We feel that gross neurologic methods of evaluation are not accurate or detailed enough to determine minor mental changes which enter into personality, cognitive thought, deductive reasoning, etc. For this reason, psychometric testing has been incorporated into our routine workup of carbon monoxide-smoke inhalation victims. Where the COHb level is lower than 25% and the patient shows psychometric testing abnormalities, the patient is considered a candidate for hyperbaric oxygen therapy.

The aim of therapy in carbon monoxide poisoning is the rapid elimination of carbon monoxide from the blood and tissues. Initial treatment includes removal of the patient from the contaminated atmosphere and allowing the patient to breathe room air. The addition of supplemental oxygen may be provided by either nasal catheters, a tight-fitting mask with an O_2 reservoir, endotracheal intubation, or hyperbaric oxygen.

Average half-life of COHb
—In air: 320 min
—In 100% oxygen: 80 min
—In 100% oxygen at 3 ATA: 23 min

The treatment objective is to reduce the COHb level as rapidly as possible.

B. **Admission protocol** (with the exception of disasters, all cases are brought to the Admitting Area)

1. **Fire victims** SYSCOM notifies the chamber staff (operator and nurse on call) of any unconscious patient and the staff comes in immediately. If a patient has been exposed to smoke and is not unconscious and is cooperative, but is being admitted for assessment, the chamber staff is not notified until it is decided that the patient should dive.

2. **Burns** Cases referred from regional centers with severe CO poisoning plus burns can be treated with hyperbaric oxygen, then transferred to the City Hospital Burn Unit. These patients are admitted to the Admitting Area or directly to the chamber at the Team Leader's discretion.

3. **Disasters** If two patients with smoke inhalation are involved, they will go to the Admitting Area for stabilization. If there are more than two patients, they will be admitted directly to the chamber area for assessment and two teams must be notified. The medical teams will report to the chamber area.

C. **Resuscitation** Five cubic centimeters of venous blood is obtained at the scene and placed in a purple top tube for CO analysis and marked with the date and time of sampling.

1. On admission, draw arterial blood gases (ABG) and obtain a COHb.

2. Ensure airway If patient is unconscious, intubate and ventilate with 100% oxygen; if conscious but confused, use tight-fitting mask with 100% oxygen.

3. One central i.v. line

4. Chest x-ray before dive

5. 12 lead EKG where possible

6. Bilateral myringotomies if patient is unconscious (PE tubes not necessary)

7. NG tube and Foley catheter if patient is unconscious

8. Alveolar air analysis (to be done by chamber personnel)

9. Routine bloods as per stat lab protocol

10. Psychometric testing in awake patients

D. **Treatment protocol for CO poisoning**

1. **Diagnosis**
   a. History of exposure/clinical signs and symptoms, and
   b. Alveolar CO testing and blood COHb should be taken before O_2 is administered.

2. **Treatment**
   a. If symptoms of headache, nausea, dizziness, etc., with neither a loss of consciousness nor a change in mental status, and a COHb level of 10–17% are present, 100% O_2 via tight-fitting mask is administered for 3 hr. Watch for an additional hour and return to work next day.
   b. COHb level 18–25% and no alteration in level of consciousness, 100% O_2 by tight-fitting mask for 3½ hr. Watch for a further 2–3 hr for recurrence of symptoms. Home for a 24-hr rest period and observation.
   c. Hyperbaric oxygen is administered when there is a COHb level 26% or above, or COHb level less than 2%, but
      (1) History of unconsciousness and no head trauma
      (2) Unconscious on examination
      (3) Drowsy, unable to answer questions coherently or only able to give yes/no responses
      (4) **a** or **b** with no improvement clinically on 100% oxygen
   d. Repeated CO exposures   Treat more aggressively for lower COHb levels. There is no cumulative effect of CO on lungs; however, there is more damage to neural tissue. The home or work environment should be checked for CO leakage. Information should be obtained whether or not the patient is using a protective mask, etc.
   e. Patients with known heart disease, hypertension, angina, or infarction must be treated more aggressively at lower levels because of the toxic effect of CO on the myocardium.

E. **Hyperbaric oxygen treatment protocol** (dive protocol)
   —Sixty feet (2.8 ATA) × 46 min on 100% oxygen via tight-fitting mask
   —Unconscious patients or those not rapidly improving will undergo a second dive 4–6 hr after the first, at the same depth and time schedules

Since there is no dire emergency to dive the conscious CO patient, a complete workup should be performed:

—Alveolar CO samples; MINICO Tester
—Blood samples for COHb from scene, Admitting Area, and hourly
—Psychometric testing battery: pre- and post-treatment
—Exhaled CO sample during dive
—COHb post-dive and every hour until there are two consecutive levels under 10%

The chamber nurse on call sees that the above workup is done. After hyperbaric oxygen, the patient is transferred to an appropriate unit bed for observation or further treatment.

X. **Radiation Necrosis (Bone and Soft Tissue)** Following radiation therapy, there is a progressive obliterative vasculitis which may result in nonhealing wounds. Hyperbaric oxygen causes neovascularization and stimulates collagen formation and fibroblast proliferation, thus promoting healing.

Treatment protocol Referrals are from physicians only. It must be clearly understood by both the patient and the referring physician that hyperbaric oxygen is an adjunctive therapy with whatever treatment is deemed necessary by the referring physician, i.e., antibiotics, surgery, etc.

Once the patient is accepted for hyperbaric oxygen treatment, routine patient care is performed. Treatment is hyperbaric oxygen at 48 feet for 90 min on 100% oxygen. Treatment is daily, excluding weekends, for up to 60 treatments. After 40–60 treatments, the patient is given a 30-day break and then reevaluated for further treatment. In some cases, as many as 100 treatments may be indicated.

XI. **Chronic Osteomyelitis** In chronic refractory osteomyelitis, hyperbaric oxygen has been found to be effective in promoting neovascularization and osteogenesis. There is a chronic anoxic state in the bone and thus a lack of fibroblast and osteoblast proliferation. The increased O_2 levels consequent to hyperbaric oxygenation stimulate these tissues to heal.

Treatment procedure Referrals are only accepted from physicians. Hyperbaric oxygen is an adjunctive therapy with antibiotics and surgery, as indicated. Once a patient is accepted for treatment, routine patient care is continued. Surgery for the removal of necrotic tissue and bone sequestra is essential for healing to occur.

Treatment is hyperbaric oxygen at 48 feet for 90 min on 100% oxygen. Treatment is daily, excluding weekends, for up to 60 treatments. The patient is given a 30-day break and then reevaluated for further treatment. As many as 100 treatments may be necessary.

XII. **Compromised Skin Grafts** Controlled studies indicate that hyperbaric oxygen therapy is beneficial for the take of skin grafts when circulation is tenuous. The increased O_2 transport to the graft increases the chances of take.

Treatment procedure The referring physician should notify the chamber personnel regarding the date and time of surgery so arrangements can be made to receive the patient directly from the recovery room.

Treatment schedule is: q6h × 24 hr; q8h × 24 hr; q12h × 48 hr. Each treatment is at 48 feet for 90 min on 100% oxygen. Appropriate patient care is provided.

XIII. **Decompression Sickness (Bends)** People breathing air with its high nitrogen content under compression conditions have a massive uptake of nitrogen into the tissues as a result of the greatly increased partial pressure of the nitrogen. If the rate of decompression is such that the speed of release of bubbles is too great, these bubbles coalesce to form larger bubbles of nitrogen in the blood vessels and skin.

As the bubbles diffuse through the skin, they produce a skin rash, itch, and marbling (skin bends), or if the bubbles reach a size significant enough to cause occlusion of blood vessels, depending where the embolism lodges, signs and symptoms will develop. For example, if the embolism is in the brain, hemiplegia may result, and if it is in the spinal cord, paraplegia may manifest. There may be local pain in the joints of the arms and legs, itching, and, in more severe cases, dizziness, blurring of vision, dyspnea, fatigue, collapse, and coma. The pulmonary effects of the bubbles released may result in disruption of pulmonary vessels, which causes mediastinal air, pneumothorax, or soft tissue emphysema, in the midline structures. Decompression sickness may occur during surfacing and up to 6 hr post-dive.

The treatment is immediate recompression which reduces bubble size. The addition of 100% oxygen therapy allows for more rapid bubble reabsorption and resolution. Rapid recompression in a hyperbaric chamber helps eliminate intravascular bubbles by reducing their size and by replacing the nitrogen with oxygen. In addition, the high oxygen concentration establishes a steep inert gas gradient across the bubble tissue-fluid interphase, which helps eliminate the inert gas and prevents new bubbles from forming when the chamber pressure is reduced. Recompression also reduces the secondary phenomenon of cerebral edema from disrupted microcirculatory flow and increased intracranial pressure.

The recommended treatment protocol established by the U.S. Navy is 100% oxygen at 2.8 ATA, 60 feet of seawater. Sessions can be extended with intermittent air and oxygen treatments, e.g., 25 min on oxygen and 5 min on air for as long as deemed necessary. Recurrence of symptoms or nonresponse to treatment necessitates a deeper dive on air at 165 feet of seawater, 6 ATA, followed by decompression according to the schedules and clinical picture. The true incidence of decompression sickness is not known because the method of reporting casualties is poor, and experience with this problem is sparse except in the coastal regions around Florida and California where warm water encourages scuba diving.

XIV. **Scuba Diving Accidents** Any diving accident victim is admitted directly to MIEMSS; the chamber staff is immediately notified. The patient is admitted directly to the chamber if the chamber personnel are present; otherwise, the patient is taken to the Admitting Area. **Only** a neurologic examination and vital signs are performed. If time is available, a chest x-ray is taken. No sedation or i.v. lines are initiated, unless the patient is in shock.

In transporting the patient to a hyperbaric unit, further decompression in an unpressurized plane cabin is very dangerous. Thus, for short distances, transportation on ground or a low flying helicopter is advisable. Long distance plane transportation should be done in a pressurized cabin. The patient should be fully recumbent at all times with the head slightly down.

In the absence of a physician with experience in decompression sickness, the hyperbaric chamber operator is primarily responsible for treatment decisions in decompression sickness and scuba diving accidents.

XV. **Air Embolism—Arterial or Venous Gas Embolism**   Diving with compressed gas while breath-holding or local air trapping on ascent can result in "pulmonary overpressure." Pulmonary overpressure is the result of alveolar-capillary septal disruption secondary to barotrauma, which causes air to enter the intravascular compartment. The possible effects of overpressure are pneumothorax, pneumomediastinum, and systemic arterial gas embolism. Iatrogenic gas embolism of the vessels is not always recognized and treated. The iatrogenic causes of vascular gas embolism include open heart perfusion during heart surgery; intravenous lines, especially with pressure infusion; placement or disconnection of central venous catheter; neurosurgery involving the base of the brain or skull involving sinuses in the upright position; diagnostic or surgical procedures involving the lung; surgery on the aorta or carotid arteries; hemodialysis; arterial catheterization; abdominal, retroperitoneal, or uterine insufflation with gas; and mechanical ventilation. Cerebral gas embolism requires treatment in the hyperbaric chamber as soon as possible. The outcome usually depends on the time required to transport the patient to a treatment center. There have been reports of patients recovering full function even when treatment was delayed as long as 24 hr.

The initial treatment of anyone suspected of having gas embolism is to lie the patient on the left side with the head down and the feet up; then pass a central venous line and aspirate air from the right atrium and ventricle. Oxygen (100%) by a tight-fitting mask is given. A large single dose of intravenous steroids, non-dextrose containing crystalloid, and dextran are administered to establish an adequate circulatory volume. Intravenous aspirin is given because of its antagonistic action on platelets.

When gas embolism occurs during open heart surgery, vigorous efforts should be made to clear all gross bubbles from the heart and aorta. The patient should be cooled to hypothermic levels and given 100% oxygen and a single bolus of steroids. The surgery should be completed and the patient taken to the hyperbaric unit.

XVI. **Closed Spinal Cord Injuries**   All cases which do not require surgical intervention are treated in the hyperbaric chamber. All patients are given 100% oxygen and randomized into one of two groups. Half the patients are taken to a 33-foot depth; the other half are taken to an insignificant depth (1 foot) to simulate a dive.

A. The same team assesses all cases using the same format, including daily neurologic examination, BID blood gases, and a blood gas 30 min post-dive.

B. Routine spinal cord treatment in **all** cases

   1. Resuscitation in the Admitting Area

   2. Assessment by the Team Leader and neurosurgeon

   3. i.v. steroids

   4. Cervical spine immobilization

   5. Patients requiring neurosurgery or general surgery are not eligible for inclusion in the study.

   6. Once diagnosis is made of spinal cord injury and nothing further can be done for the patient, the patient is admitted into the study.

   7. It is important to dive the patient as soon as possible after the injury, preferably within 6 hr.

   8. All incomplete lesions are eligible for hyperbaric treatment up to 24 hr post-injury.

   9. Blunt chest trauma   If contusion, fractured ribs, or a hemopneumothorax is present, the patient must be intubated and mechanically ventilated. If **only** neck trauma is present, a mask can be used without a ventilator.

      Note The fact that the patient is to undergo hyperbaric oxygen therapy must not alter any other form of normal treatment of the patient. A dive in the hyperbaric chamber is no reason by itself for tracheal intubation and ventilation.

C. After routine treatment, notify the physician in charge of hyperbaric medicine to initiate hyperbaric oxygen therapy according to the study protocol. This includes: informed consent, myringotomy in intubated and uncooperative cases, and determining a diving schedule.

D. **Protocol**   On admission, the patient is rapidly resuscitated and assessed.

   1. Halo skeletal traction is applied immediately while the patient is being resuscitated and worked up.

   2. The weights are applied as soon as possible to stabilize the lesion.

   3. A CVP, peripheral, and arterial line are inserted.

   4. The patient who is conscious, cooperative, and able to tolerate mask breathing should not be intubated. When the patient cannot breathe adequately nor maintain adequate blood gases, the patient should be intubated.

5. If intubated, the patient should have bilateral myringotomies. Since the ears may close within 12 hr, PE tubes should be inserted after the first dive, but before the third dive.

6. Hyperbaric oxygen therapy   As soon as all investigative procedures, except myelogram, are complete, the patient enters the chamber for a first dive for 90 min. Spinal reduction is performed during the initial dive. An x-ray machine has been developed for use in the hyperbaric chamber up to 2.8 ATA, primarily for cervical vertebral x-ray. The patient is admitted to the chamber on a Stryker frame, where an x-ray of the neck is taken for standardization. Weights are added to the traction and x-rays are taken to determine the point of reduction and realignment. The weights are then reduced to prevent overdistraction. The reduction takes place in the chamber while the patient is on hyperbaric oxygen.

7. Myelogram   After the first dive, the patient is returned to the Admitting Area for the myelogram. Thereafter, the decision is made whether to intervene operatively. If no operation is indicated, the patient returns to the chamber for a second dive 2 hr after the first.

8. Further hyperbaric therapy   Two additional dives with 2-hr surface intervals between them will follow. Then, the patient undergoes four more dives with 6-hr surface intervals. At the end of eight dives, the patient is reevaluated. If the patient has a complete lesion, hyperbaric oxygen therapy is stopped. If the patient has a recovering lesion, hyperbaric oxygen therapy is continued BID for 5 days. The complete diving schedule will therefore be: q2h × 4 dives; then q6h × 4 dives; then reevaluate. Each dive will be at 2 ATA for 90 min. Treatment will be discontinued only by order of the chief of hyperbaric medicine or the neurosurgical attending physician.

9. If the patient requires sedation, particularly for claustrophobia, use Valium and/or morphine.

XVII.   **Gas Gangrene**   See p. 297.

XVIII.   **Synergistic Soft Tissue Infections**   See p. 299.

Section XI
DEATH AND DYING

INTRODUCTION

Although all energies in a trauma setting are geared toward sustaining an individual's life, at times the inevitable fact of dealing with death and the dying patient as well as the patient's family must be addressed.

In attempting to reckon with the issues involved in the provision of care to these individuals, the tools of our profession seem to fail us. There are no brief guidelines available that will provide us with the "right words" to make dying more bearable. There is an anxiety-producing problem at the time of death; the vision of ourselves as "healers" comes crashing to the ground. In panic, at the exposure of our vulnerable selves, we swiftly rise to the moment with all the logic and intellectual defense we can mobilize, desperately trying to ignore our feelings of impotence. The gnawing sense of failure penetrates these defenses. We experience the limitations of being humans with finite powers.

There are not many words to help the family, the patient, and health providers at this point. The suggestions presented in the following chapter are offered to provide support to the health provider, the patient, and family when facing the issues of severe trauma and death.

37

PROBLEMS RELATED TO
THE DYING PATIENT

I. **Support for the Medical Staff** The staff rapidly learns to build defenses against the "horrors" they encounter daily. Chronically working with people who suffer mutilating injuries leads one to remain distant from the object of stress, the patient and the family. We do this by talking about patients only in terms of their injuries or sometimes by not learning their names. We find ourselves interacting minimally with the patient and family and have contact with them only when necessity demands. Our avoidance patterns often lead to poor communication with our peers and other health professionals. Ultimately the emotional/physical care becomes fragmented. When the stress of working with these patients and their families is not acknowledged and verbalized, and when collegial support systems are nonexistent, anger and hostility become chronic interactive patterns. No one can survive an environment like this for long. Suggestions to the health provider:

—Recognize your vulnerability to this stress—this is the first step in initiating preventive mental hygiene.
—Have a life outside of trauma; spend time in pursuing and developing your interests.
—Develop a routine of physical exercise.
—Listen to what you are feeling.
—Share your thoughts and feelings—peer support and recognition are of.utmost importance.
—Empathetically recognize and verbalize your awareness of others' needs and concerns.
—Eat and sleep in accordance with what you would recommend to someone you care about.
—Take a break when you know you need it.
—"Punch out of the unit"—work and home need to be separated as much as possible.

The following are suggestions that might be helpful in telling a family about the death or dying process of their loved ones:

—If possible, approach the family with a supportive colleague.
—When you enter the room, introduce yourself, your role, and your colleague.
—Maintain eye contact with the people in the room.
—Ask the family to introduce themselves—you need to know the names of the key people to whom your message is being addressed.

—Sit down and take your time.

—Look at the key people—call them by name—and their loved one by name: "Mr. and Mrs. S., Johnny was flown here about two hours ago. When he got here... we did this and that [describe the procedures briefly]. Though we did everything that was possible for Johnny, Mr. and Mrs. S., we were not able to keep him alive. It's very difficult for me to tell you that Johnny died five minutes ago."

—Expect the family to react intensely (crying, screaming, pounding on walls or furniture) and accept their behavior as a way of expressing the intensity of the feeling they are experiencing.

—Stay with the family through this initial response.

—Offer physical support if you feel comfortable doing so: an arm around someone's shoulder, touching their hand while they're crying. Should they reject this and pull away, that is acceptable.

—Provide the family with information about what you attempted to do for their loved one. They need to know that all that was possible was done for their loved one.

—Remember that your presence indicates human concern and caring.

—Listen to the family should they want to tell you about their loved one or show you pictures.

—Direct them to people who can answer their questions as to what next: the funeral director, Medical Examiner, etc.

—For yourself, afterwards:

  Go somewhere quiet.

  Listen to what you are feeling.

  Seek out another colleague and validate thoughts and feelings about the experience.

Perspective

In our interactions following discharge with patients and families we are repeatedly told that the most helpful thing to them in adapting to their loss is that the doctor and nurse cared about them, by taking time to talk with them. They are thankful for the clinical expertise that their doctor and nurse provided, but many speak briefly about this issue. What stands out by far is the fact that the doctor cared and that in some way, even when death was to be the natural progression of events, they were never stripped entirely of their hope. The continued presence of the physician and nurse is symbolically reassuring.

Trauma patients and families "clutch" the words spoken by the doctor and nurse; their words are the only link to their loved one. It is difficult and frustrating to spend time with people who seem as if they do not hear the words that you bring them; the key is to persevere and empathize in addition to providing professional information. It is this empathy that makes the major difference in terms of the family's future perspective on life.

II. **Support of the Awake-and-Dying Patient** There is little information available that addresses the problems associated with the individual who, following a sudden traumatic injury, is awake and dying. The common assumption is that the trauma patient does not have the time nor the cognitive abilities to work through his or her death. The following are offered as guidelines to provide, when possible, both physical comfort and emotional support to these patients.

Even though the attempts at salvaging a patient's life involve many personnel, "lots of action and noise," it is important to talk firmly and directly to the patient, using the patient's name if you know it, providing the patient with basic facts: "You're in the hospital. There are doctors working on your injuries." Do this repeatedly, to keep the patient informed.

—Monitor your own anxieties. Often we verbalize our fears out loud—"He's bleeding out" and the like.

—Touch reassures the patient. The patient is able to differentiate between painful procedures and the gentle hand of someone who considers him or her a person.

—Provide physical comfort. Appropriately medicate the patient for pain; allow the patient to express himself or herself before inducing coma.

—Provide emotional support. Your presence relays your offer of strength and courage.

—Be honest with the patient. If the patient talks about death, remember that while the patient is alive, there is always hope, even though the injuries are very severe.

—Attempt to meet the patient's requests. Special visiting, and giving someone a message from the patient is helpful. Sometimes you must ask the patient if there is anything that you can do for him or her.

—Sometimes our own need is to run from the last moments of another's life. As the heartbeat and blood pressure drop, the tendency is to leave the cubicle or talk intellectually about the patient's injuries. The suggestion is to stay quietly with the patient, perhaps talking and letting the patient know that you are present; continue to stay.

—When possible, encourage the family to spend time with the dying patient—suggest that they talk to him, touch him and say their goodbyes.

Although the passage from life to death is one each individual makes totally alone, the presence of another, familiar or not, appears to provide patience, strength, and often peace not only to the person dying, but to the person who stays beside the patient.

III. **Interaction with the Family** The impact of trauma extends beyond the trauma victim alone. Trauma produces shock waves that have immediate, sudden, and severe impact on those closest to the victim. The family experiences a state of acute crisis when one member (or perhaps several) is critically and physically debilitated as the result of multiple injuries. The family members are faced with overwhelming adaptive tasks that they have had no time to anticipate. During the initial treatment phase, when the patient is the object of intense life-saving efforts, they must deal with the anxiety and helplessness of facing the unknown. In successive phases they may be confronted with the realities of death, permanent impairment, or the loss or disruption of a role-performance vital to the family, such as breadwinner or child care provider. Families traveling through the area, separated from their usual sources of support, and those with histories of intrafamily conflict or poor social functioning present additional problems.

Family members faced with the loss or threatened loss of a significant person experience symptoms of physiologic and psychologic disturbance. Psychologic symptoms include denial, isolation of affect, repression, and overwhelming, intense affective states. Expressions of sorrow, guilt, and anger are common. Many of these symptoms are transient and abate as the threat diminishes or the family unit is able to adapt and cope with the posttraumatic outcome. However, there are families that experience overtaxation of their adaptive, coping mechanisms and who are not able to marshal resources within the family or in the immediate social network to be able to cope with the trauma and its disruption.

Timely intervention with families of trauma victims can enhance the families' attempts to cope with the stress they are experiencing and can also help develop a problem-solving ability to cope with future life stresses. Nurse/physician intervention can enable the family to achieve a correct perception of the situation; manage affect through awareness of feelings and appropriate ventilation, which leads to tension discharge. This intervention leads to the development of patterns which enable the family to deal with others who may provide additional help. (See Lydia Rapoport in Parad, H. J., ed., *Crisis Intervention: Selected Readings*, New York, Family Service Association of America, 1965). Such intervention further increases the likelihood that the family will be able to develop these patterns of responses for more effective coping.

In a system designed to treat trauma and its sequelae, provision must be made to treat those other victims, i.e., the family, who suffer as the result of trauma. The physical and emotional care of the patient is the primary focus of the medical and nursing staff. In some instances, routine contact with the physician and nurse is sufficient to enable the family to negotiate the stress. When the family's reaction is intense, which is a sign of family decompensation under stress, or when family structure and functioning appear to be devastated as the result of a traumatic event, difficult management problems present. A trauma unit's ability to meet the psychosocial needs of the victim and family represents a holistic and progressive approach and recognizes that the patient is not an isolated entity, but is a person with attachments to a family and a wider social network. Medical and nursing staff cannot compromise patient care to divert their attention to severe family problems. The need exists for family treatment specialists.

An orientation toward the adequate care of families of trauma victims must be an integral part of a comprehensive trauma unit's program. Family treatment specialists are instrumental in providing direct service to families and in helping the MIEMSS program be more responsive to the psychosocial needs of both the patient and the family.

There are times when a family member (or members) will become emotionally out of control after the patient has arrived at MIEMSS. The range of distress can vary from anxiety to grief to overt psychosis. In most cases Family Services can deal with the situation.

There may arise unusual situations or problems necessitating aggressive management. In general, sedation is not useful in grief reactions. Mourning is necessary and should not be blunted. Let the family members ventilate and talk out their feelings. This should be done by Family Services or, in their absence, a physician or nurse. If this is unsuccessful, other family members should be encouraged to take the disturbed member to their family doctor, or to the Emergency Room. If a family member becomes violent or is threatening the staff, hospital security should be called to escort that person out of the building.

Section XII
PROTOCOLS

INTRODUCTION

Management of the critically ill and severely injured patient is one of the most complex problems that the physician must confront. Not only must the hospital care be efficient, but prompt and meticulous prehospital treatment and transportation are mandatory. Since time is crucial in the management of these critical and complex situations, there is little room for diagnostic and therapeutic errors. To ensure appropriate management, protocols or guidelines are necessary to maximize proper care. Protocols are established by experienced individuals to provide assistance to those with less tenure so that the patient receives the best possible care. Since there is no way to put in writing a protocol that will be successful for each and every clinical situation, flexibility must be maintained and clinical judgment must prevail. Prehospital and hospital protocols are an evolutionary process, since therapeutic and diagnostic procedures may change as newer techniques become available and investigations confirm or disprove old concepts. There must be continuous scrutiny of each protocol to make certain that it provides maximal care for the desperately ill patient. The protocols have been established by seasoned clinicians; therefore, deviation from these guidelines should take place only after sound reasoning.

38

PREHOSPITAL PROTOCOLS

An integral part of the management of the trauma patient involves the prehospital phase. Many areas of the United States have basic life support programs performed by emergency medical technicians. Other areas have advanced beyond this to a level of advanced life support with paramedics performing invasive medical techniques, particularly in metropolitan areas. These prehospital personnel provide immediate patient care and can perform different therapeutic modalities either according to protocol or on radio supervision by a physician located at a resource center. These personnel are trained in the immediate management of the multiple trauma patient, since medical intervention in the first hour prior to arrival at the trauma center has an impact on patient survival.

Prehospital medical protocols can be instituted by the field personnel before consultation with a physician. In addition, they may triage certain categories of injuries; for example, burns may be sent directly from the scene to the burn center, or the multiply traumatized patient to the trauma center, or the neurosurgical patient with a Glasgow Coma Scale of less than 10 may be triaged to a neurosurgical receiving facility. Appropriate triage protocols must be developed when facility designation is made to ensure that appropriate patients are fed into the appropriate facility. Protocols should be developed in regions that possess a designated trauma center capable of administering advanced life support, to include the following:

—Routine patient care protocol
—Protocol for unconscious persons
—Protocol for multiple or severe trauma
—Protocol for burns
—Protocol for pediatric emergencies
—Protocol for patients with respiratory distress
—Protocol for patients in shock
—Protocol for spinal cord injuries

The routine patient care protocol should include a routine system of initial patient assessment with triage which includes the mandatory use of a communications system. There should be protocols for endotracheal intubation, use of the esophageal obturator airway, and use of the MAST in both the adult and child. The system should also include a mechanism for assessing protocol efficacy.

A system of case review should be instituted, preferably by the physicians managing the trauma case at the receiving facilities. This should be an ongoing review, for example on a monthly basis, to allow the prehospital personnel to improve their techniques and their knowledge of the management of these critical patients. Evaluation is simplified if one has an automated data collection system such as a trauma registry or else computerized ambulance runsheets for immediate feedback and analysis.

The following is an example of triage criteria for the traumatized patient:

The patient should be mobilized to a trauma center if any of the following criteria are met:

—Systolic blood pressure less than 80

—MAST required to maintain a systolic blood pressure between 90 and 100

—Head-injured patient with a Glasgow Coma Scale of 10 or less

—Spinal injury as demonstrated by paralysis or loss of sensation

—Gunshot wound to the chest

—Extrication time greater than 30 minutes

—Accidents in which other members involved in the automobile are dead at the scene

—Multiple injuries (chest, abdomen, and extremities)

—Respiratory distress

If a patient is taken to a hospital without a trauma center designation because of its proximity, or if a facility is unable to care for the patient, then the patient is transferred to a trauma center with the appropriate capabilities. The hospital will request consultation from the nearest areawide trauma center, and ambulance or helicopter transportation is arranged.

See pp. 215, 228, 475, and 479.

39

HOSPITAL PROTOCOLS

I. **Clinical Laboratory** The Clinical Laboratory is an integral part of the team at MIEMSS in supporting critically ill patients. The Clinical Laboratory is staffed around the clock, services only those patients admitted to MIEMSS, and offers most tests needed for immediate patient care. The laboratory does an average of 18,000–20,000 tests a month, or about 700 tests per day.

To ensure efficiency of laboratory services and optimum data collection, a protocol has been developed and is automatically followed for each patient. The purpose of the protocol is to monitor the critically ill and unstable patient.

A. **Protocol studies** (Tables 1 and 2)

1. **Admission**
   a. **Trauma patients** A complete battery of tests is done. Results are sent via computer to the Admitting Area within 5 to 20 min as the procedures are finished. Admission laboratory work includes arterial blood gas, Hgb, Hct, WBC, platelet count, Na^+, K^+, osmolality, H_2O content, total solids, glucose, BUN, creatinine, lactate, urine electrolytes, and urine creatinine. Prothrombin time (PT), partial thromboplastin time (PTT), and fibrinogen are conditional tests. The laboratory will perform these automatically if admission platelets are below $200,000/mm^3$ or when specifically requested. Lactate is not considered a stat procedure. These samples are batched and run usually within 48 hr. Results are transmitted via the computer, with laboratory forms as a backup method. Stats and abnormals are also placed on the computer and the clerk is notified.
   b. **Carbon monoxide patients** A sample of anticoagulated blood is usually sent from the scene and is used to determine the initial CO level. Admission workup includes CO level, Hgb, Hct, osmolality, and BUN. After the hyperbaric dive, CO levels are received every hour until the patient is stable. Results are sent to the chamber area via telephone.

2. **Operating room** Blood studies are sent to the laboratory as needed. Typical studies include Hgb, Hct, Na^+, K^+, and blood gases. Often coagulation studies are requested. These results are transmitted via computer.

3. **Critical Care Recovery Unit (CCRU)** A patient entering the unit is initially placed in the unstable category. The patient receives blood work twice a day: a complete study at 7 a.m. and an abbreviated study at 7 p.m. As the patient progresses, he or she is moved to the stable category. The doctor determines on a daily basis the appropriate category.

Table 1. MIEMSS Clinical Laboratory protocol

Test	Admission	Operating room	CCRU Unstable 7 p.m.	7 a.m.	Stable 7 a.m.	ICU and IMCU
Blood gas	X	As needed	X	X	X	As needed
Hemoglobin	X			X	X	
Hematocrit	X		X	X	X	
WBC	X			X	X	
Platelet count	X			X	X	
Sodium	X		X	X	X	
Potassium	X		X	X	X	
Serum H_2O	X			X	X	
Total solids	X			X	X	
Osmolality	X			X	X	
Glucose	X			X	X	
BUN	X			X	X	
Creatinine	X			X	X	
Lactate	X					
Urine sodium	X			X		
Urine potassium	X			X		
Urine creatinine	X			X		
PT[a]						
PTT[a]						
Carbon monoxide	X					

Stat orders are noted as such and analyzed immediately.

[a]Coagulation studies are specifically requested, batched, and run at specified intervals unless ordered as stat.

4. **Intensive and Intermediate Care Units** Patients in the Intensive Care Unit (ICU) and the Intermediate Care Unit (IMCU) are generally not placed on the laboratory protocol. Tests are requested according to patient need. Daily blood studies are ordered by the team leader the evening prior to sampling. Specimens are sent to the laboratory before 8 a.m. and are processed. Results are usually at the patient's bedside by 11 a.m.

Table 2. Main Laboratory protocol: MIEMSS patients

Test	Admission	CCRU Unstable (M, W, F)	Stable (W)	ICU and IMCU
Hepatitis-associated antigen	X			As needed
Calcium	X	X	X	
Phosphorus	X	X	X	
Bilirubin	X	X	X	
Total protein	X	X	X	
Albumin	X	X	X	
Uric acid	X	X	X	
Amylase	X			
Ethyl alcohol	X			
Liver enzymes[a]				

[a]Admission serum stored in the MIEMSS laboratory for 7 days.

If bloods cannot be drawn by 8 a.m., it is more efficient and less costly to send samples at 7 p.m. or 7 a.m. than at other times. Emergency requests are handled at any time.

B. **Special topics**

1. **Routine studies**   At 6:30 a.m. a cart is placed in the main unit with the necessary tubes and syringes. For each patient in the CCRU, there will be a red and a lavender tube, and a heparinized syringe. These tubes are filled with the patient's blood, properly labeled (hospital plate label), and returned to the cart by 7 a.m. Blood gas samples must be placed in ice. The nurse must also complete a MIEMSS requisition, which is attached to the sample. At 7 a.m. the laboratory technologist will take the cart to the laboratory. Because the workload in the morning can be extremely pressured and heavy, late samples are discouraged.

   At 6:30 p.m. the procedure is repeated. The cart is put in the unit and each unstable patient is given a heparinized syringe and red and lavender tubes.

2. **Stat testing**   Stat tests can be performed at any time. Turnabout time for most procedures is 15 min (exceptions are coagulation studies, i.e., PT and PTT, which require 30 min).

   Every stat sample entering the MIEMSS Clinical Laboratory is done as soon as possible. Stat samples are never batched. The laboratory staff treats all stat samples with immediate attention and priority. Results are sent via computer.

3. **Urine studies**   A 2-hr urine sample is collected between 5 and 7 a.m. Urine studies are done routinely on CCRU patients and on others as requested. Between 7 and 7:30 a.m., a sample (50 cc is plenty) is placed on the laboratory cart in the CCRU.

   Routine urine tests include osmolality, urine electrolytes (Na^+ and K^+), and urine creatinine. Free water and creatinine clearance are calculated by the computer.

4. **Coagulation**   Coagulation studies (PT, PTT, fibrinogen) are not included in either profile. Although platelets would logically fall into the coagulation classification, platelet testing is done from a lavender tube and PT, PTT, and fibrinogen are done from a blue tube. Patients needing PTT studies on a regular basis should follow the protocol times if possible. A patient needing a PTT every day ideally would have blood drawn at 7 a.m. Coagulation studies may be drawn from venous or arterial lines; if so, they should be labeled as such. An order for a coagulation study includes PT, PTT, and platelets. Fibrinogen and fibrin split products must be specifically ordered.

5. **Labeling**   Joint Commission on Accreditation of Hospitals (JCAH) regulations make it mandatory that all samples entering the laboratory be labeled with the patient's name, time, and test required. Samples sent on ice should be labeled on the sample tube itself rather than on the container of ice. Blood gas syringes should be labeled on the syringe's body rather than on the plunger.

Tubes should have the label affixed vertically rather than around the circumference, as this allows the technician to separate serum or plasma from spun blood without removing the label.

6. **Postdialysis** Postdialysis blood studies are sent 2 hr after completion of dialysis. The study consists of Na^+, K^+, BUN, creatinine, osmolality, Hgb, Hct, and PTT.

II. **Death Protocol** Most cases at MIEMSS involve trauma-induced death and are under the jurisdiction of the Medical Examiner. When death occurs or is imminent, the Medical Examiner's office is notified. The Medical Examiner has the option to perform an autopsy if desired, but, as a rule, does not perform an autopsy.

If a patient is brain-dead, there is virtually a 100% likelihood that the Medical Examiner will release the body for an immediate autopsy. In this case, the Immediate Autopsy Service and MIEMSS staff receive clinical and research information. If a patient is brain-dead or is likely to be pronounced brain-dead, the Mortuary Service is called to notify them of an immediate autopsy candidate. These patients are also candidates for the Organ Procurement Service; this service should be contacted. The Medical Examiner's office should be made aware of the presence of a brain-dead patient so that they may cooperate with the Immediate Autopsy and Organ Procurement Services.

Cardiopulmonary arrest may be imminent in a patient without the patient being brain-dead. In this situation, the patient is a less than ideal candidate for organ procurement or immediate autopsy. Nevertheless, the two services should be notified. The situation has frequently arisen in which a complicated and interesting patient dies and an autopsy cannot be obtained. The following are options used to obtain an autopsy:
—The Medical Examiner will perform the autopsy.
—The Immediate Autopsy Service will perform the autopsy (if not brain-dead, chances decrease).
—Ask the Medical Examiner to release the body to the Mortuary Service and they will perform the autopsy. Permission must in such a case be granted by the family (the likelihood of obtaining family permission is variable).

Nontrauma patients are not under the Medical Examiner's jurisdiction, but an autopsy is frequently desired. In this case, a permit must be obtained from the patient's family.

A. **The dead-on-arrival patient** If a patient arrives in a helicopter and is pronounced dead on arrival (DOA) or expires on the heliport roof, the patient must be brought to the MIEMSS Admitting Area and formally admitted. The following procedures are to be followed:

1. The clerk on duty will make up a chart with a face sheet, obtain the patient's name and other pertinent information, and relay this to the admitting office as usual.

2. The Team Leader should:
   a. Obtain a history of relevant events.
   b. Examine the patient to assess the injuries and findings that confirm death. For legal reasons, do not strip off the patient's clothing.

   c. Document the information obtained from the history and physical examination and the time of pronouncement on the progress sheet.

   d. Call the Medical Examiner's office and ask for the Medical Examiner on duty.

   e. Contact the family spokesperson immediately after the patient's death:

      (1) In the case of a DOA or Admitting Area death, the next of kin, as reported by the State Police to the clerk or SYSCOM, are to be notified as soon as possible.

      (2) If it is a nonnatural death, inform the family member that the body, by law, will be taken to the Medical Examiner's office.

      (3) Give the family member the time and cause of death.

      (4) Inform the family member that the family's funeral director will arrange with the Medical Examiner for release of the body.

      (5) Inform the family that grief counseling is available to family members through the Family Services Division.

   f. Dictate a discharge summary.

B. **Immediate autopsy** The immediate autopsy is a useful research tool at MIEMSS. Knowledge gained by this technique can lead to better patient care for subsequent trauma victims. Immediate autopsy requires the immediate and thorough cooperation of the Medical Examiner, the Department of Pathology, and MIEMSS.

Immediate autopsy is defined as an autopsy performed within minutes (less than 2 min) after the clinical death (cessation of cardiorespiratory function) of the patient. After routine autopsies (usually done 3–6 hr after the patient's death), the tissues by light microscopy may appear quite normal; however, ultrastructurally the cells and organelles are completely shattered and show evidence of cell death. Therefore, in order to perform satisfactory diagnostic ultrastructure study or conduct research utilizing human tissue, it is imperative that tissues be obtained within minutes (if not seconds) after the patient's death.

Candidates for immediate autopsy are:

—**Group 1** The driver in an automobile accident, victims of industrial accidents, and street injuries under questionable circumstances (usually autopsied).

—**Group 2** Passengers, pedestrians, and assaults in questionable circumstances (possibly autopsied).

—**Group 3** Definite homicides and suicides (usually autopsied).

It is the responsibility of the Team Leader to notify Mortuary Services in the following situations:

—When death is inevitable in a patient

—In the case of brain death (notify Mortuary Services immediately on declaration).

Mortuary Services personnel will state whether an autopsy is required under Medical Examiner's law (see **1.** below). If not, an attempt should be made to get a regular permit or Anatomical Gift Act permit (see **2.** below).

1. **When an immediate autopsy is authorized by the Medical Examiner's office,** inform Mortuary Services of situation, notify the organ procurement team, and notify the family of the patient's impending death and have them visit the patient. While they are there, explain to them that the case is a Medical Examiner's case and an autopsy has to be performed.

a. In the case of **brain death:**
  (1) Notify the neurosurgical chief resident, who with the neurosurgical staff determines brain death.
  (2) Notify Mortuary Services of the result.
  (3) Maintain cardiorespiratory status as near normal as possible. Try not to use vasopressors, but keep the respirator going.
  (4) After brain death is declared, notify the family and call Mortuary Services.
  (5) Get terminal blood sometime in the hour before death for total study including SMA-12.
  (6) If kidneys are to be obtained, the patient is declared brain-dead and taken to the operating room. It is important that the autopsy team be available before the patient is to be released from the operating room.
  (7) After declaration of brain death, the immediate autopsy team and/or organ procurement team assumes cadaveric responsibility.
  (8) No further progress notes should be added to the patient's chart after the declaration of death.
  (9) A discharge summary should be dictated.

b. In the case of **cardiorespiratory death:**
  (1) Call Mortuary Services immediately when cardiorespiratory death is anticipated.
  (2) Notify the organ procurement team.
  (3) Maintain cardiorespiratory and renal status as near normal as possible. Try not to use vasopressors, but keep the respirator going.
  (4) Get terminal blood sometime in the hour before death for total study including SMA-12.

2. **Autopsy by permission under the Anatomical Gift Act**
  a. Mortuary Services personnel will state whether an autopsy is permissible without a permit. If not, an attempt should be made to get a regular permit or an Anatomical Gift Act permit.
  b. Notify the organ procurement team.
  c. Notify the family of the patient's impending death and have them visit the patient. While they are there:
    (1) Ask for permission to do an autopsy.
    (2) The family should be told that the autopsy is a valuable method to obtain additional knowledge of the particular type of illness and that such knowledge may benefit other patients.
    (3) Call Mortuary Services about the results of the consultation.
  d. Maintain the patient's cardiorespiratory and renal status as near normal as possible. Try not to use vasopressors, but keep the respirator going.
  e. If kidneys are to be obtained, the patient is declared brain-dead and taken to the operating room. It is important that the autopsy team be available before the patient is to be released from the operating room.

f. After declaration of brain death or cardiopulmonary arrest, the immediate autopsy team and/or organ procurement team assumes cadaveric responsibility.

g. No further progress notes should be added to the patient's chart after the declaration of death.

h. A discharge summary is dictated.

C. Organ procurement

1. The potential donor

a. A potential donor is a patient who has a disease or injury from which recovery is very unlikely, but which may leave transplantable tissue with normal function. Transplantable tissues include kidneys, heart, corneas, cartilage, and bone.

b. Certain disease entities and injuries are incompatible with tissue donation for transplantation. This decision will be made by the organ procurement service. Patients arriving DOA are unacceptable for kidney donation, but may fit the criteria for bone and corneal harvest.

2. The role of the attending physician

a. The responsibility of a physician attending a potential donor is to inform the next of kin regarding the seriousness of the injury or disease.

b. The attending physician should notify the Greater Baltimore Organ Procurement and Perfusion Center of a potential donor. The attending physician will then direct efforts toward the continued resuscitation of the patient. It is the responsibility of the organ procurement team to obtain procurement permission. The trauma team will assist in measures to support the patient for organ procurement. If the trauma team is unable to support the potential donor due to other patient care commitments, the organ procurement team must assume the responsibility. The feasibility of providing manpower to support the potential donor is at the discretion of the attending staff and team leader.

c. The treatment of the patient should be as unencumbered as possible from the considerations of transplantation. Thus, decisions regarding major therapeutic procedures such as diagnostic arteriograms and/or surgery will be made entirely on the basis of the potential benefit to the sick and dying patient. It is recognized that some decisions cannot be made free of considerations regarding the function of the transplantable organ. For example, it may be necessary to maintain respiratory support in order to provide the time needed to discuss matters with the family and go through the procedures necessary to ascertain brain death. When decisions of this type exist, it is appropriate to consult the transplantation team.

d. The pronouncement of death will be performed at an appropriate time and with adequate documentation. Certain guidelines have been established, but all considerations to date necessitate the use of medical judgment in the application of objective tests of cerebral function.

The pronouncement of death has been and will remain based upon physiological reasoning and not upon total cellular death of an organism.

In traditional practice, when cardiac function ceased, the patient was declared dead in spite of the fact that the epidermis, the erythrocytes, and many other tissues remained viable for days. The pronouncement was valid because it is inconceivable that any part of that person could continue functioning in the absence of circulation. The declaration of brain death is no different in principle. The inference is made that without brain function other organs will certainly fail. The diagnosis of brain death, however, is more complicated than the determination of absence of circulation.

The brain may be judged functionless if the following **criteria for brain death** are met:

(1) The patient is normothermic (95–102°F).
(2) Subcoma levels of narcotics, hypnotics, and/or alcohol, or a definite, negative history of ingestion of drugs is obtained.
(3) The patient is normotensive.
(4) Pupils are fixed and dilated bilaterally.
(5) There is total absence of pontine function as evidenced by:
    (a) no corneal reflexes
    (b) no oculocephalic reflexes (doll's eyes)
    (c) no oculovestibular reflexes (calorics)
    (d) flaccid extremities.
(6) The patient must be apneic in the presence of hypercarbia. To make this determination, an oxygen catheter is inserted into the trachea and oxygen is insufflated at 15 liters/min for 5–8 min. An arterial blood gas is obtained, which should reveal a normal PaO_2 and hypercarbia. The presence or absence of apnea is noted at this time.
(7) No evidence is present of motor response in the extremities to deep pain with the exception of minimal residual decerebrate posturing when all other criteria for brain death are met.

The routine for inhouse and stable patients will be two such examinations 6 hr apart. However, in the presence of rapidly failing vital signs and inability to stabilize the patient a single determination shall suffice.

When doubt exists, the State's Attorney's office may be approached for clarification.

An electroencephalogram may be indicated to confirm the absence of cortical function. If the EEG is isoelectric at double the standard gain for 15 min at intervals of 6 or more hr, irreversible brain death is established. It should be recognized that other tests may also be useful. For example, in cases of suspected subarachnoid hemorrhage, the arteriogram may be indicated as a diagnostic procedure to determine whether a remedial lesion is present. If this test demonstrates no filling of the internal carotid artery because of massive intracranial pressure, the diagnosis of total cerebral infarction and death is supported.

To make the clinical diagnosis of brain death, it is not necessary to have corroboration by EEG or arteriography except when the findings of the neurological examination are equivocal.

e. For medicolegal purposes, the pronouncement itself of brain death should be made with the aid and advice of at least two consultants, one of whom is specially skilled in neurological diseases. Certification of death will be made on the state death certificate. The two consultants should record pronouncement of brain death in the progress notes.

f. The final responsibility of the attending physician is to seek autopsy permission. Although this is the responsibility of the attending physician, the transplantation team should also mention to the family the desirability of performing an autopsy to exclude with greater certainty the possibility of diseases that could be transmitted to the recipient.

3. **Responsibilities of the organ procurement team**

a. The primary function of the organ procurement team is to provide tissue for transplantation.

b. The organ procurement team has established 24-hr-a-day coverage in order to respond immediately to a call from an attending physician regarding a potential donor. As soon as the family has consented to donation, the donor's red hospital plate is removed and the kidney team red charge plate will be utilized for charges.

c. The organ procurement team will manage the donor after the consent is obtained and the donor is pronounced dead.

d. The organ procurement team will coordinate harvest of all potential transplant tissue (kidneys, bone, cartilage, corneas, etc.).

III. **Automatic Stop Orders for Narcotics and Sedatives**   All orders for narcotics and sedatives will have an automatic expiration time of 8:00 a.m. on Mondays and Thursdays. Orders for these drugs must be renewed at these times.

If someone other than a member of the primary team caring for the patient writes such an order, the order must be reevaluated the next day by a member of the patient's team.

Sedatives covered by this protocol include benzodiazepines and barbiturates as well as narcotics used for sedation and analgesia. Use of barbiturates for seizure disorders or for neurosurgical use in elevated intracranial pressure will not be included under this policy.

APPENDIX

ADMINISTRATION

This section presents an overview of the clinical component (the Shock Trauma Center) of the Maryland Institute for Emergency Medical Services Systems, and discusses in general terms some of the major administrative issues and problems in the organization and operation of trauma centers. Not all factors discussed herein are relevant to the operations of other trauma centers. However, the unique mix of functions within MIEMSS has created a learning environment. This has permitted a systems approach to management of specific complex interrelationships within a trauma systems operation, some of which will have application in various trauma systems center operations throughout the country.

I. **Capsule View of MIEMSS Clinical Operations** The Maryland Institute for Emergency Medical Services Systems is a two-function program: a major clinical facility (the Shock Trauma Center) and the statewide Emergency Medical Services (EMS) program. The management of MIEMSS is integrated into both functions, with the costs of management allocated to each specific function. This section deals principally with the Shock Trauma Center.

The MIEMSS Shock Trauma Center encompasses 47,000 square feet. Facilities include 73 beds, 6 receiving bays in the admitting area, 3 operating rooms immediately adjacent to the admitting area, a clinical stat laboratory, and a hyperbaric oxygen unit. Distribution of the total bed complement is as follows: intermediate care unit, 22; critical care recovery unit, 12; intensive care unit, 20; neurotrauma, 19 (12 for intensive care and 7 for intermediate care).

The clinical staff is comprised of approximately 550 full time equivalent positions: 40 physicians, 250 nurses, and 260 support personnel. Support personnel include respiratory, physical, and hyperbaric oxygen therapists; clinical laboratory and research personnel; and administrative support personnel. Other services are provided by the University of Maryland Hospital on a contractual basis.

The physician staff consists of 25 attending physicians and 15 fellows as shown in Table 1.

Subspecialty services such as plastic surgery and urology are provided on a contractual basis from the University of Maryland Hospital and the Johns Hopkins Hospital.

Nearly two-thirds of the salary distribution (61%) is allocated to nursing; 16% is allocated to administration, 12% to physicians, and 11% for other services (i.e., clinical stat laboratory, respiratory therapy, physical therapy, hyperbaric oxygen therapy, and research).

During 1981, MIEMSS experienced 1,324 admissions amounting to 15,934 patient days, with an average length of stay of 13.3 days. The ratio of male to female admissions was 3:1. Eighty percent of the patients were white; 19% were black.

MIEMSS had 1,034 live patients discharged in fiscal year 1980. Thirty-seven percent of these patients required interhospital transfers; 20.8% went to the University of

Table 1. MIEMSS physician staff

	Attending	Fellow
Surgeons	10	6
Critical care/anesthesia	8	6
Orthopedics	2	1
Neurosurgery	3	1
Infectious disease	1	1
Director	1	0
	25	15

Maryland Hospital, whereas 16% went to other hospitals. An additional 6.3% of patients were transferred to rehabilitation facilities or nursing homes. A substantial portion of those returning home required assistance in planning for convalescence and continuing care.

More than two-thirds of the patients were between the ages of 16 and 35. More than half (51.7%) were single, with an additional 16.6% being separated, divorced, or widowed. More than half of the patients (56.5%) fell into four occupational categories in descending order of frequency: skilled laborer, student, unskilled laborer, and unemployed. The most prevalent cause of trauma was motor vehicle accidents.

The average revenue per admission was approximately $14,500. Eighty-one percent of the funds were derived from direct patient billings, with the remaining 19% provided by direct state support.

II. **The Trauma Center Designation Process**   The process of obtaining designation as a trauma center and maintaining postdesignation operations requires a knowledge of the designator/evaluator and a continued involvement with the designating agency, whether it is the Health Systems Agency, the State Health Planning Agency, or an Emergency Medical Services Authority. Designation must be performed by an agency that is empowered to grant licenses. Self-designation generally presents extremely difficult problems (with the possible exception of rural situations). Without an associated trauma delivery system, the hospital may incur significant costs without a commensurate patient load. This will precipitate cost inefficiencies and the remaining risk of rate problems for the facility. Further, designation by an agency without authority has led occasionally to legal challenges. Therefore, it is imperative to know the authority of the designators.

The hospital administrator must maintain involvement throughout the designation process and must address the following:
   —Are the designation criteria appropriate?
   —Are the projected caseload and catchment area correct?
   —Is the designation process objective (e.g., is the site survey team unbiased?)?
   —Is there integrity within the postdesignation system with regard to protocols, evaluation, reimbursement, monitoring and oversight, and legal sufficiency?

Without an understanding of these factors an effective designation process cannot and will not occur, and the trauma care system ultimately may be compromised after significant effort (and expense) has been made.

With the allocation of substantial resources, the trauma facility has a vested interest in assuring the continuing viability of the EMS designating authority and its evaluation efforts. It is this authority which provides, in effect, the "marketing effort" for the designated center.

III. **Planning for the Provision of Trauma Service**   Some insight into understanding the overall trauma system and its ultimate impact on any one facility is needed in planning for a trauma service. The planning process must begin with an assessment of the total need for trauma care and the potential for converting the need to demand for the hospital services.

The minimum data base for performing a needs assessment consists of a knowledge of the total population by age, sex, and geographic and temporal distribution from the proposed facility. The causal factors of trauma, with sufficient trend data to document their variability over time, also must be known. These combined factors determine the required facilities, equipment, and specialty personnel to provide adequate services. Special characteristics or unique criteria also must be taken into account. For example, a trauma facility at or near the intersection of major highways can be expected to serve a substantial proportion of motor vehicle accident victims. A facility located in a heavily industrialized area requires the capacity to care for victims of occupationally related injuries which may range from blunt trauma to penetrating injuries to burns. Inner city hospitals, especially those in low income areas, usually require the capability to manage increased numbers of injuries resulting from gunshot wounds, stabbings, and other assaults. The opposite situation usually exists in retirement areas. The incidence of acute trauma there can be expected to be lower, but the demand for other emergency medical services (e.g., coronary and stroke care) will be greater.

Once the demographic and etiologic factors of the patient population have been assessed, yielding the total universe of properly identified trauma, it is necessary to examine the manner in which trauma will be distributed and the impact on each facility. Where state or regional EMS coordinating agencies exist, the process of equating supply of quality trauma services with demand for those services and ensuring access to care can more readily be accomplished. Specialty services also can be distributed in an appropriate manner.

The case mix and volume determine the structure of the total trauma program. The required personnel, facility design (renovation requirement), and equipment needs must be addressed for the entire spectrum of services, including specialty services such as burns, limb reimplantation, neurological trauma, pediatric trauma, and eye trauma. The provision of rehabilitative services is extremely important. To provide service in these areas, interhospital transfer agreements may be necessary.

Services and facilities specific to each hospital must be organized to meet anticipated demands. The impact of the caseload on the trauma and emergency services as well as on general and ancillary services of the hospital must be assessed and adequate capacity provided.

IV. **Dedicated vs. Duplicated Resources**   The care of seriously injured patients requires both personal and institutional commitments. Highly trained personnel must be immediately available 24 hr a day throughout the year. Trauma patients require immediate access to sophisticated diagnostic laboratory and radiologic services, including CAT scanners, as well as operating rooms and critical care beds. Despite the expense of duplication, some of these resources must be dedicated exclusively to the care of trauma patients.

The American College of Surgeons has recommended that there be three levels of trauma care. Level I hospitals should be those which serve as regional referral centers and have the capability to treat approximately 1,000 patients per year. This volume is required for the professional team to maintain technique and performance standards as well as to justify the enormous expense of personnel and equipment.

Level II institutions usually are large hospitals that receive significant volumes of serious trauma but lack the full spectrum of available medical and surgical specialties. Although it is desirable that these hospitals have their own specifically allocated trauma beds and separately organized trauma services, trauma patients probably will be admitted into surgical or surgical subspecialty beds. Level II hospitals should have back-up and transfer arrangements with level I facilities for the immediate transfer of those patients requiring specialty coverage unavailable in the level II facility. The need for a neurosurgeon is the most frequent example of this kind of situation.

Hospitals that have only one or two neurosurgeons on staff (with those surgeons engaged primarily in private practice) may not be able to provide appropriate coverage for patients with head and spinal cord injuries on a 24-hr basis. The transfer of those patients, as soon as they have been stabilized, best serves the interests of these patients, the level II hospital, and the neurosurgeon.

Level III hospitals generally are small facilities (200 beds or less) that have commitments to the resuscitation and stabilization of trauma patients and the capability to manage certain cases. These hospitals do not, however, have the resources required for adequate treatment of the more critically injured patients or those requiring specialty care (central nervous system injury, burns, etc.). Transfer agreements and protocols in some specialty areas are essential.

These standards are designed to limit duplication of effort throughout the system and to focus caseload on one or more facilities as may be required. Therefore, a hospital must make a decision as to what level of resources can be committed and at what level, if any, it can participate as a trauma service within the trauma system. Clearly, this depends upon the factors outlined above as well as the case mix of the trauma service, and the organizational interrelationship between the trauma service and the supporting hospital. A level I and possibly a level II trauma service treating a large proportion of neurological patients usually requires its own designated CAT scanner, with recognition, however, of the need at times to utilize that scanner for purposes other than trauma. This specific example demonstrates the critical balance between the need for the resources that must be immediately available for the trauma admission and the costs of equipment and its utilization in the contemporary economic climate. The administration and the physician staff are central in achieving this appropriate balance in view of the economic climate specific to the area.

V. **Organization of the Trauma Service**   The optimal functioning of a trauma service requires strong commitments from the hospital's board of directors, medical staff, and chief executive officer. This commitment should result in the trauma service being appropriately placed within the hospital's organizational structure to permit effective staff interaction among the disciplines and services affected. In the ideal situation the trauma service would have departmental status, making its clinical chief a peer with other department chairmen.

The trauma service must be immediately responsive to patient care demands and maintain an ability to modify protocols, policies, and procedures as appropriate to ensure optimal quality of patient care. The following individuals ensure this responsiveness.

The strength of the Trauma Service Director is the central factor in determining the trauma service's effectiveness within the institution as well as in influencing and coordinating the dynamics of the medical staff. The selection of the director, therefore, is crucial and must be made through a careful credentialling and review process. The director must have clinical expertise specifically in the area of trauma, as well as proven experience in medical administrative affairs.

The Trauma Service Administrator, working directly with the Trauma Service Director, must be positioned at an organizational level in the overall hospital administrative structure to be able to address the numerous problems involved in the operation of a highly intense program experiencing considerable variability in volume. The Trauma Service Administrator must have the necessary authority to effect change as needed.

In rural community hospitals, the administrative functions of trauma services should be assumed by the hospital administrator. In larger suburban facilities, an assistant should have the responsibility for the trauma program and for as many as possible of those areas on which the trauma program will have major impact (e.g., emergency department, radiology, operating room, clinical laboratory).

Larger urban hospitals (those with organized trauma services with significant patient volume) require a program administrator with dedicated responsibility for the service. The program administrator should report directly to the assistant administrator in charge of the trauma service and coordinate directly with the Trauma Service Director.

Well organized trauma services must be holistic in their approach to patient management. Consequently, they will impact extensively on many services of the hospital, each of which is competing for resources. It is essential that the Trauma Service Administrator fully understand the systems approach to management and have the ability to communicate with personnel at all levels within the organization. The interrelationships must function smoothly at all times, although coordination may be difficult with other problems consuming the administrator's time. The administrator must determine the most applicable management techniques and use those techniques to solve problems. Trauma patients cannot wait for the services they need; they require priority throughout the institution. A Trauma Service Administrator should function as a peer with the Trauma Service Director and the Trauma Nurse Coordinator/Director in the design, implementation, execution, evaluation, and modification of policy for the trauma service and its interrelationships with other hospital services and departments. This collaborative effort should result in a matrix organization that encourages creativity, professionalism, and a team approach to patient care in which motivational levels remain high.

Finally, the Trauma Service Administrator, either directly or through superiors in the organizational hierarchy, must be able to promote the trauma service in the community at large and with federal, state, and local agencies as appropriate.

Other important individuals in the trauma service include the Physician Coordinators for anesthesia, surgery, and critical/intensive care and the Nursing Unit Coordinators for the emergency room, operating room, intensive care unit, medical-surgical areas, and rehabilitation. It is essential that the trauma team provide continuous care for the patient throughout the course of illness, convalescence, and rehabilitation, regardless of the patient's location within the hospital. The coordination point for all this is the Trauma Service Director, with the Nursing, Administrative, and Physician Coordinators as support personnel.

VI. **Financial Issues** A trauma service, assuming appropriate activity levels, should be established as a cost center to delineate specific costs and revenues and consider subsidies, if required, to cover these costs. The operating budget should be based upon projected utilization of the center. Demand projection is not an easy task and is very sensitive to uncontrollable changes. This sensitivity must be understood and analyzed before significant resource commitments are made to the trauma service.

Charges must be established that, assuming effective resource utilization, will generate revenues adequate to cover operating expenses. Trauma care by its nature is expensive and is perceived as a "loss leader." Nonetheless, with the proper approach the service can generate significant revenues in excess of expenses. Primary considerations in the establishment of charges are the financial case mix of the patient population (i.e., the proportions of various patients by payor categories and the rates at which they reimburse hospitals), any constraints that may be imposed by state regulatory agencies (e.g., restrictions on cross-subsidization), and any general or special state or other outside revenue appropriations that may aid in the payment for services to trauma patients.

Active collection efforts are necessary because of the size and nature of patient bills. At MIEMSS, 11.4% of the patients generated 51.5% of the total billings for a 1-year period; all of these bills were in excess of $25,000, nearly double the average bill.

Collection efforts for the trauma service must be well organized. Accounts receivable must be closely monitored, and written policies should exist concerning payment for services by the uninsured and underinsured, abatement of bills for those who are unable to pay them, and the pursuit of collections. Because many trauma cases (especially motor vehicle accidents) result in litigation, the hospital's chief financial officer must develop effective follow-up procedures on these cases, especially in instances where patients have no assignable health insurance.

Stand-by costs are a concern. All nursing units must be fully staffed around the clock and throughout the year. Surgeons and anesthesiologists must be available in anticipation of an admission. They cannot perform elective surgery or provide other services while they are on call for the trauma service. Resource commitments for personnel may exceed the potential for reimbursement unless there are adjustments in rates. This must be carefully considered, as in some areas stand-by costs are not reimbursable. This may result in the need to develop alternative funding sources.

Physician reimbursement presents some unique problems. Third party payors frequently do not understand the complexities of the procedures performed on trauma patients. Further, they may pay only one fee for multiple procedures. Although trauma patients usually require extraordinarily lengthy and frequent follow-up care, this often is assumed in the basic fee. Therefore, physicians may not be adequately compensated through the existing fee structure.

There are several excellent approaches to resolving this particular dilemma, most of which have potential implications for hospital costs and rates. Approaches should be cautiously addressed. One approach is for the trauma service to be a hospital-based service and place all costs in the hospital's rate base. An alternative is to form a professional corporation, either hospital-based or physician-based, to bring together all of the billings including those generated by house staff, fellows, and physician extenders as well as the physicians themselves and present a consolidated bill to third party payors. Unified billing yields significant results. It should be emphasized that in many cases physicians do not view the reimbursement issue as a problem and it should not be made a problem.

Most of the revenue generated by trauma patients occurs in the first 5–7 days following admission. It is essential to have an effective disposition process so that high intensity, high cost resources can be most effectively utilized.

VII. **Discharge Planning/Disposition Coordination**   There are few if any places in a hospital where early initiation of effective discharge planning is more needed than in the trauma service. The primary reason for such planning is to ensure appropriate placement of the trauma patients with their complex medical and psychosocial problems. However, the unpredictable inflow of patients requires an ongoing ability to transfer patients rapidly to other units or discharge them altogether in order to be prepared for new admissions. Resources must also be properly utilized to yield necessary revenues.

At MIEMSS three discharge coordinators are employed full time. These coordinators are graduates of a baccalaureate community health education program. Their role is one dedicated to the disposition process, unlike nurses and social workers whose professional aspirations generally conflict with the need for the intense disposition efforts. The process of discharge planning begins as soon as the patient's condition has been stabilized and a treatment plan developed. The disposition coordinators make daily rounds on all patients, continuously communicating with physicians, nurses, and other members of the care team to ensure that planning is ongoing and consistent with the patient's needs.

The key element in successful discharge planning is a series of established working relationships and/or formal contractual arrangements with other services in the hospital, other hospitals (where necessary), rehabilitation facilities, nursing homes, and other community resources.

The point should be made that during peak admission periods, disposition in trauma services becomes an active triage process. Frequently, patients are not ready for transfer or discharge; however, unless they are moved from the trauma service, there is an inability to admit new severely injured patients. On the other hand, it is generally difficult to predict admissions precisely. A patient should not be transferred or discharged because of anticipated admissions that never arrive. Therefore, there is a need for a mechanism to ensure the effective use of resources by having the ability to expedite transfers or discharges when absolutely required. This makes good fiscal as well as medical sense. The effectiveness of the disposition process is measured through the utilization review portion of the quality assurance program.

VIII. **Quality Assurance**   All hospitals are familiar with the Joint Commission on Accreditation of Hospitals' requirements for quality assurance programs. The guidelines within which these requirements are framed are designed with sufficient flexibility to allow individual departments or services to develop their programs within the context of unique, individualized needs. It is essential that the trauma service's quality assurance program meet certain standards and serve specific needs while simultaneously fitting within the hospital's broad plan.

The quality assurance program, which must be based upon a written plan, serves at least three major functions:

—Evaluation of the clinical care process
—Utilization review
—Risk management/liability control.

The high intensity of patient services delivered in a trauma unit demands that a strong system for the continuous monitoring of patient care be established and implemented. This system should be predicated upon written standards of care or protocols that are established and approved by a multidisciplinary committee chaired by the Trauma Service Director and comprised of representatives from the relevant surgical subspecialties, anesthesia/critical care medicine, other relevant medical specialties, nursing, and medical records and administration. Written protocols, with their obvious advantage of providing baseline data for evaluation of program progress, are essential to trauma service programs. A trauma registry and utilization program using standard trauma definitions and norms, but tailored as well to the unique requirements of each trauma center, should serve as the data base upon which to establish priorities for a quality assurance program. There exist manual and computer programs to complete this task.

Medical care evaluations should include special audits for trauma deaths, morbidity and mortality reviews, nursing audits, appropriateness of care reviews, tissue reviews, and continuous reviews of the content and adequacy as well as the timeliness of completion of medical records. In addition to assessing the quality of care on a systematic, objective basis, chart audits can serve as powerful educational tools for the correction of deficiencies identified throughout the care process. Routine and systematic audits of basic care processes can lead to the identification of areas requiring further in-depth study.

As a management tool, the quality assurance program serves two important purposes. The first of these is utilization review, to ensure that the appropriate level and mix of services is being provided to patients and that they are given in a timely manner. This relates to the comments pertaining to disposition. Cost containment objectives can be achieved without compromising quality. With good planning and management these are parallel objectives leading toward the same goal: the best possible outcome for the patient. Planning for and operation of programs that allow for the achievement of multiple objectives is one of the advantages of collaborative practice.

Effective utilization review ensures that resources are utilized according to standard. For example, it ascertains that patients requiring critical care or intensive care are moved along the continuum to more appropriate levels. Simultaneously it ensures that these scarce and costly resources are not misutilized for financial reasons. Further, it ensures that disposition (discharge) planning begins as soon as the patient is stabilized and a prognosis can be established, and that this process continues in an orderly and timely manner.

Finally, an effective quality assurance program serves a major function in risk management and liability control. Malpractice is of heightened concern today, and the trauma service is a high malpractice area. An incident monitoring system that is rationally designed and employed in a timely manner is an essential component of any quality assurance program in a trauma service because it will permit corrective actions and avoid malpractice difficulties if managed properly.

IX. **Public Relations**   The public relations function of a trauma center is an evolving part of the operation. First, the public relations plan has to be related to the designation process. After designation, good public relations is essential to the survival of the service. The trauma center must promote its public service role both to its potential patients and funding sources. In addition, it has a public education mission to perform. This should include programs on injury prevention in the home, in industry, and on the highways and athletic fields; first aid and CPR training for the public as well as medical and paramedical professionals; and continuing education programs for community-based physicians and other health professionals on the state of the art of trauma care.

Good media relations are very important. They help the trauma service to capitalize on the success of the many complex problems with which it deals.

Maintenance of good will within the health care provider sector is an essential public relations function of the trauma center. It is important to provide feedback to ambulance personnel, referring physicians, and hospitals, to make them part of the team.

X. **Conclusions**   Trauma centers in 1982 are not what they will be a decade from now; their future potential seems almost unlimited. Advances in the treatment of critically injured patients can be expected to continue, and as more and more lives are saved, technologic innovations will continue to be diffused throughout the medical care community.

The emergency health services system in general and the trauma care system specifically will continue to evolve, with each echelon increasing its capability to care for more seriously injured patients than previously. Research and training should remain the rightful purview of academic health centers. However, a system must evolve in which communication and the sharing of personnel become refined throughout a region.

Planners, rate regulators, state legislators, federal policy makers, and others concerned with trauma service delivery must clearly understand the continuing evolution of the trauma care system. Without their cooperation and active participation in the pursuit of the common goal of a better trauma system, it will be impossible to balance resource requirements with the need for services.

COMPUTERS

In most medical environments, computers are typically used for functions of administration, i.e., payroll, accounting, supplies, and billing, but the computer system at MIEMSS is used primarily to store and retrieve patient data. Clinical data are presented in formats suitable for computing indices of physiologic systems, computer-assisted therapy including drug dosage, and other similar applications.

MIEMSS is equipped with a PDP 11/70 computer, manufactured by the Digital Equipment Corporation. Other hardware and/or peripherals include patient monitors (which interface with the computer), cathode ray tube (CRT) terminals, color graphic terminals, and printers. A clinical software system developed by Quantitative Medicine, Inc. (QMI), provides real-time, continuous information. The system is operational and physicians at MIEMSS have come to depend upon it in daily care of the critically injured patient.

The system was designed with the following goals in mind:
—Efficient storage of patient data
—Automatic or semiautomatic computations
—Computer-assisted individualization of therapy, such as drug dosage
—Automatic collection of measurements in critically ill patients
—Archival storage
—Administration of treatments under computer control
—Notification to staff of the occurrence of significant events
—Assistance in organization of drug and other treatment programs
—Collection and processing of statistics on past experience
—Recommendation to staff of accepted protocols
—Generation of statistics to describe overall system operations

Most of these goals are realizable now; it is hoped the remaining few will be realizable in the near future.

The system provides entry devices at locations convenient to the sources of the data. Any terminal can request data on any patient at any time. The system is modular so that it can be changed readily or expanded as needed. It can accept data from automatic collection devices. It is transportable to different computers.

Each piece of data in the system is called an ITEM. Each ITEM has associated with it an ITEM NUMBER and a PRINT NAME (or PROPER NAME). It may or may not have SYNONYMS.

Any items can be logically grouped together to form any number of CHARTS (each of which is also an ITEM). By requesting the Main Lab chart, the user receives all the laboratory data at once.

To participate, a user consults a command menu for data input, several forms of data output, or various bookkeeping functions. The user selects the command and specifies the ITEM, usually a chart (available from a suggested menu if the ITEM number is not known).

If desired, the user can choose different ways to format data. Time may be across the top of the chart (with items down the side) or down the side (with items across the top), or one can obtain the latest values of each item, together with the times they were obtained, thus giving a capsule summary of what is known. Items and even charts can be graphed over time on a graphics terminal. Any chart or graph seen on a CRT also can be obtained on a graphics printer in the patient area.

The computer maintains a complete ward roster displaying the availability of beds and patient locations. A request to list the roster is usually followed by a command to SET the terminal to a particular patient for the purpose of recording or retrieving data about that patient.

Data stored for a patient are used to obtain indices of cardiovascular, pulmonary, and renal function. The results are stored in the data base and are available just like any other data, for output on charts or graphs.

Another important aspect of the clinical computing system is the ability to record and review accurate injury diagnosis. Diagnoses are entered by the clinical staff by stepping through menus that successively define an injury diagnosis. The coding scheme used is an extension of the ICD.9.CM. (International Classification of Diseases, Ninth Revision, Clinical Modification). Using a standard classification scheme as a basis keeps the MIEMSS data consistent with the various hospital information reporting requirements, yet allows an accurate record of diagnosis for research and later review.

Various off-line programs collect and organize the coded injuries and allow interactive queries of this data base. This system will become a statewide trauma registry.

COST EFFECTIVENESS AND UTILIZATION REVIEW

There is a growing awareness within the medical community that hospital roles are frequently inefficient. Hospitals can no longer, except in unusual circumstances, provide all the various types of primary patient care that are demanded by contemporary diseases. Hospitals are tending to specialize; for example, one hospital in a region may be the burn center while other hospitals are the spinal cord, open heart, neonatal, or pediatric centers. With the advent of specialized areas of critical care and trauma, trauma centers are developing. This concept has evolved on the premise that increased specialization produces greater expertise, and that if patients can be triaged either from the scene or from a local emergency room into these specialized referral centers, they will obtain better care.

The burn center is an excellent example of a specialty center. Not all hospitals can afford the necessary equipment of a burn unit, including specialized nurses, rehabilitation, plastic surgeons, Hubbard baths, and so forth. Therefore, patients with severe burns are best triaged by protocol into such a referral center. In Maryland, any burn of greater than 30% of the body surface area, or any burn involving the face, hands, or perineum, is triaged directly from the scene, thus providing effective utilization of these expensive facilities. Another example of specialization is reimplantation surgery, since very few centers have the necessary expertise in anastomosing digital arteries, veins, and nerves to obtain a functional hand after traumatic finger or hand amputation. Such a concentration of patients undoubtedly leads to better experience and expertise. The Union Memorial Hospital Hand Center in Baltimore now manages patients from Maryland and elsewhere. This center treats approximately 150 patients per month and manages its own hand rehabilitation center. Several trained reimplantation teams are a part of the system. Statistics for patient survival and cost effectiveness for multiple trauma are emerging at the present time and show that the survival rate for trauma victims is better when the patient is managed at a trauma center. Improved efficiency in specialty centers has been demonstrated for open heart operations and is applicable here. The mortality and utilization rate of centers performing more than 150 open heart bypasses per year is better than those performing fewer than this number.

For a designated trauma facility, it has been estimated that a center needs approximately 400 patients per year to provide a reasonable cost-benefit ratio for the cost of immediate availability of surgeons, operating rooms, and associated ancillary support. This is by no means a hard figure and can be modified by the local environment. For example, there may be a need within a geographical area for a trauma unit with fewer patients, but in order to substantiate such a center other general surgical emergencies could be included to form an emergency surgical center. Almost by necessity, trauma units are usually allied with a larger hospital so that effective utilization of ancillary support such as angiography, nuclear scanning, CAT scanning, and specialty medical support are available. It is mandatory that these ancillary support services give top priority to these critical patients.

Cost effectiveness at a trauma center can best be assessed and manipulated by performing a utilization review using a systematic trauma registry. Only in this way can an assessment be made to ensure that appropriate patients are being admitted and treated efficiently in the trauma facility. At the same time, patient flow to other institutions and home should be expeditious. Therefore, appropriate length-of-stay audits and regulations regarding patient transfer are necessary.

TRAUMA/EMERGENCY MEDICAL SERVICES SYSTEMS

The modern era of Emergency Medical Services (EMS) and the civilian systems approach to improving trauma care were initiated in 1966 by the now classic white paper, "Accidental Death and Disability: The Neglected Disease of Modern Society," prepared by the National Academy of Sciences/National Research Council Committees on Shock and Trauma. In this document some 24 recommendations were made and have become the basis of the essential EMS systems components for establishing comprehensive and effective trauma care programs. The real impact of these components has not been their individual importance, but rather their overall conceptualization, appropriate integration, and rational implementation with regard to the unique geographic characteristics of each locale and region.

There has been a maturation of thought in regard to the emergent critically ill or injured victim over the last 20 years. Not so long ago, death by serious injury was an "acceptable death." The improvements in resuscitation and surgical management of the critically injured in military and inner city trauma units in the 1960s stimulated some initial academic interest in trauma care in terms of biomedical research, clinical studies, and postgraduate surgical trauma training programs. In the early 1970s, as an outgrowth of our military experience, several pioneer regional programs showed the way for better planning, organization, and resource deployment for trauma systems in the civilian community. The experience of the mid- and late 1970s has brought an even wider implementation and modeling of trauma/EMS systems, with identification of specific patient problems, designation of trauma centers, and development of care protocols and professional teams on a regionwide basis. The acceptance of regionalized systems of care for trauma patients now makes trauma a potentially manageable disease.

I. **Management of Trauma Patients within a Regional EMS System** Trauma is a clinically demanding disease. For other conditions that have less severity, multiplicity, and fewer limitations of time and geography, protocols of care can be developed on a nonregional, nonsystem, and noninterdependent basis. For the critically injured, this is not a practical option.

Death will eventually prevail in all severe cases if definitive care is not provided within time constraints. A standard mortality curve (Figure 1) shows an emergency with eventual death in time if therapy is withheld. Each medical emergency has its own constraints and requires specific and appropriate medical care.

In trauma, the lethal event may be forestalled by early and sustained resuscitation and stabilization. The time of death is different according to the magnitude and variety of trauma pathology. With EMS response, communications and transportation, and initial basic field care, time will be saved and death prevented (Figure 2).

Trauma incidence and patient distribution within an EMS regional system show that 85% of patients can be managed at the local level, 10% need further care in standard

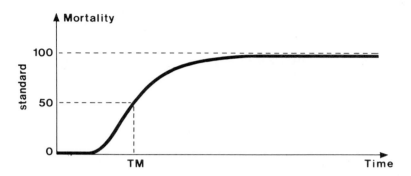

Figure 1. A standard mortality curve. *TM*, time of 50% mortality.

and intensive care settings, and 5% need special care that is available only at designated trauma centers. These figures might be reversed for spinal cord and burn injuries, with 85% requiring immediate special and total care in specialized centers.

In the past, civilian trauma centers have developed only in large metropolitan hospitals, where extensive medical and surgical resources are available. The vast rural areas in this country have infrequent accidents relative to their population and geographic area, but collectively account for over 80% of highway-related deaths. Therefore, regional EMS systems with less sophisticated trauma centers should be upgraded. The Maryland EMS system has proven that many vehicular trauma deaths can be prevented if adequate resuscitation, stabilization, and proper definitive care are performed at the regional trauma service centers.

Trauma care systems are necessary in all EMS regions across the country. Such systems would consist of immediate care for all patients at the scene, safe and efficient transportation to designated trauma centers for appropriate definitive surgery, critical care management, and rehabilitation.

The pioneering experience and lessons learned in the organization and operation of trauma units in civilian programs have been invaluable in subsequent organizational and

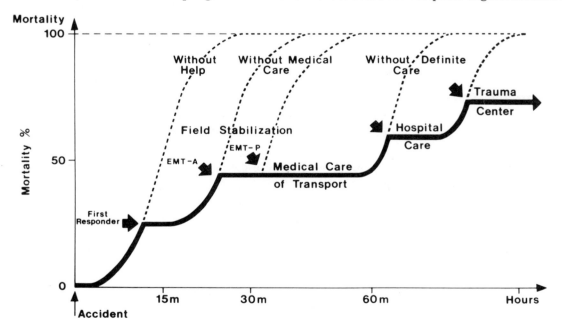

Figure 2. Effect on mortality of an organized emergency medical system.

therapeutic endeavors across the country. Of paramount importance throughout has been the concept of the "trauma team" approach in patient care, teaching, and research that evolved at MIEMSS.

The most important principles in operating a trauma center are:
—Immediate identification and transportation of the critically injured to the trauma center
—Triage of all trauma victims in a single location by a team of experienced surgeons
—Resuscitation and evaluation in a designated, fully staffed and equipped area
—A team approach used for patient care, with the general surgeon as team coordinator
—The trauma team coordinator should be a senior experienced surgeon, working closely with the anesthesiologist and emergency room physicians
—A designated intensive care area, dedicated to the needs of the critically injured patient
—Specially trained nurses and other health professionals would staff the unit
—Related hospital resources consolidated in this location
—Laboratory services available in the unit itself
—Trauma patients are given high priority at any time of the day or night in the hospital's operating rooms, x-ray department, blood bank, and elsewhere.

Effective response to a trauma emergency requires a system, preplanned at the regional level, that rapidly deploys properly trained and equipped personnel. In major trauma, only the sophisticated definitive care provided by paramedic, medical, and surgical personnel with the necessary knowledge, skills, and equipment will positively affect final outcome. This indispensible, sophisticated, intensive care capability is available only in a system of trauma care.

A trauma/EMS system is a complex arrangement of essential personnel and facilities, the coordination and management of which require an EMS lead agency to provide the necessary focus and central direction of trauma/EMS system planning, implementation, operations, monitoring, and evaluation. This EMS lead agency must represent the interests of all trauma patients and providers and assume the responsibility for all trauma patients in both the public and private sectors within the region. Uniform programs, guidelines, and protocols for patient care for the region must be identified. The lead agency's traumatologist, working with colleagues at various levels within the system, identifies problems, develops practical solutions, and deploys operational protocols for prehospital, interhospital, and trauma center care, as well as for rehabilitation from the initial planning to implementation and evaluation of the system.

Critical trauma patient care, therefore, demands a protocol approach for many of the systems operations, and for treatment given to patients as they progress through various providers and phases of care. These same protocols should be utilized during both training and daily operations, form the basis for evaluation, and provide a legal standard of care.

A regional trauma/EMS system is a first attempt at conceptualizing and implementing an operational model for a regional management entity within the health care delivery system. The system is constructed and operated by individuals who collaborate within an interrelating communication network.

This interrelated, interdependent communication and management network of a regional trauma/EMS system uses a team approach and must maintain a team-building effort on a wide geographic basis. This approach is now being utilized in industry, but has heretofore not been implemented within the health care system. It is now being used in the early stages of the development of regional trauma/EMS systems. The basic transfer agreements between rural physicians and trauma center surgeons, the development of areawide triage and treatment protocols, and regional evaluation studies are the first true examples of interdependent team interaction on a wide geographic basis. This team approach is essential to ensure integrity and competency, as well as to maintain interdependency and the quality of service that must be coordinated throughout a regionwide trauma/EMS system. These interactions are necessary for acute and demanding environmental circumstances and ensure that trauma patients will receive level-of-the-art care within the region rather than capricious, ineffective, and fragmented care.

The skills of trauma team personnel must be deployed within an overall organized regional trauma/EMS system according to protocols. What the initial EMT provider does in the field seriously affects what subsequent care providers do at later treatment stations. An overdose of a sedative, changing the neurological signs early on during resuscitation in the prehospital and/or early hospital phases, can seriously hamper later evaluations. The early Vietnam experience showed what effect vigorous shock resuscitation with crystalloid solutions had on the intraoperative and postoperative management of patients developing shock lung. The Vietnam experience was due, in part, to overresuscitation by providers early in the care process, when the patient was not under the direct medical control of the definitive care surgeons.

The many protocols essential for diagnostic, operative, and intensive care management must be initiated and reviewed periodically to assure proper care. These protocols should be uniform and rational in terms of the patient's treatment environment at specific times and places, and of sequence of care. Doing an extensive diagnostic workup on a trauma patient in a referring hospital and/or emergency department when the trauma surgical team is not available can be hazardous. The trauma surgeon should be there to observe the often subtle diagnostic information that many times is of a fleeting nature and subject to varying interpretations. Time delays caused by inappropriate diagnosis before operative care are many times crucial to subsequent management of major trauma and can result in mortality and considerable morbidity.

The "golden hour" (first 60 min after insult) should not be utilized inappropriately by persons who are not on the operative trauma team. Sometimes this time loss is inevitable by reason of geography within a regional trauma/EMS system. However, time delays due to a lack of a surgical in-house team at the community hospital near a capable trauma center are unjustifiable. Also not justifiable are time losses due to extensive emergency department workups done prior to calling the trauma surgical team. Deaths and significant morbidity unfortunately result from the lack of a clear systems design with trauma treatment, triage, and operations protocols. These protocols are scientifically sound, technically appropriate, and effective only if they are utilized in an appropriate setting with a regional trauma/EMS system.

Developed in a uniform manner on a regional basis, these protocols provide effective trauma care. Such standardized trauma care can thereby be provided more effectively to a much larger number of critically injured patients. This was not possible in this country 5 or 10 years ago.

The real impact in trauma management is not in the importance of a single treatment but in the conceptualization and systematic implementation of an organized regional trauma/EMS system of care.

II. **Maryland's Trauma/Emergency Medical Services System** Maryland's Emergency Medical Services, based on a five-region system (Figure 3), evolved over a period of several years. Its roots go back to the mid-1950s when R Adams Cowley first began investigating the causes and treatment of shock. In 1973, an executive order of the governor of Maryland provided for the development and implementation of a statewide system. At the same time, the governor's order created the Maryland Institute for Emergency Medicine to concentrate on the study and treatment of shock and trauma. Both programs were directed by Dr. Cowley. Today they are continued within one institution—the Maryland Institute for Emergency Medical Services Systems, part of the University of Maryland at Baltimore.

A. **EMS Regional System** The EMS Division of MIEMSS is the field operations section and works to coordinate and improve treatment facilities, transportation and communications equipment, training of emergency medical personnel, and public education within each of the state's five EMS regions. Local EMS needs in each of these areas are determined by one or more professional regional coordinators and a volunteer EMS Advisory Council. Each Council is composed of consumers, providers, institutional personnel, government representatives, and EMS professionals.

The Appalachia Region (Region I) consists of Garrett and Allegany counties and also works in cooperation with the surrounding areas of southwestern Pennsylvania and West Virginia. The Mid-Maryland Region (Region II) consists of Frederick and Washington counties and also works in cooperation with southern Pennsylvania, West Virginia, and Virginia. The Metropolitan Baltimore Region (Region III) includes Baltimore City and Baltimore, Anne Arundel, Harford, Howard, and Carroll counties and also works in cooperation with the adjacent areas of southeast-

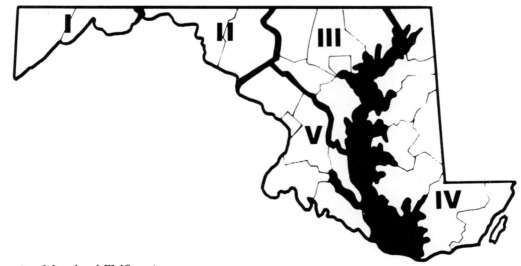

Figure 3. Maryland EMS regions.

ern Pennsylvania. The Eastern Shore Region (Region IV) consists of Cecil, Kent, Queen Anne's, Caroline, Talbot, Dorchester, Somerset, Wicomico, and Worcester counties and also works in cooperation with neighboring Delaware and Virginia. The Metropolitan Washington Region (Region V) includes Montgomery, Prince George's, Calvert, Charles, and St. Mary's counties and also works in cooperation with the adjacent District of Columbia and northern Virginia.

B. **Communications**   The Maryland EMS Communications System, the first state-wide system of its kind in the nation, ties the entire Maryland EMS system together. Ambulances, helicopters, hospitals, central alarms that dispatch emergency medical teams, all are linked with any EMS component in any region throughout the state. The Systems Communication Center (SYSCOM) is located at and operated by MIEMSS. It is manned 24 hr a day by trained communication dispatchers who are also emergency medical technicians. SYSCOM performs the following functions:

   —Dispatches emergency aid, including Med-Evac helicopters, to the scene of the emergency
   —Notifies the receiving hospital of the patient's estimated arrival time and probable injury so the hospital is prepared for the patient
   —Establishes cardiac and trauma consultations between physicians in hospitals and emergency medical teams in the field so that on-the-scene personnel can treat under physician direction
   —Transmits patient medical data from the field to the hospital through special telemetry units
   —Provides backup communications for national disasters involving mass casualties.

   A second communication facility operated by MIEMSS, the Emergency Medical Resource Center (EMRC), is located at Sinai Hospital in Baltimore. It is also manned by around-the-clock trained communications operators. Its function is to provide medical communications between ambulances and hospitals in the Metropolitan Baltimore Region. EMRC has a sophisticated radio-telephone switching system, and SYSCOM is connected through the EMRC to any hospital or ambulance in the Metropolitan Baltimore Region.

   The communications system plays an important role in EMS by ensuring that any accident or coronary patient in Maryland will receive life-sustaining care the minute that EMS personnel reach the patient and that the patient will be transported to a treatment facility prepared to manage the problem.

C. **Transportation**   Maryland's ambulance and rescue companies and the State Police Med-Evac helicopter system cooperate to provide extensive and rapid transport coverage in Maryland. At present, 240 paid and volunteer ambulance companies with well equipped vehicles serve Maryland. In addition, State Police Med-Evac helicopters are on 24-hr call to transport patients to specialty referral centers either from the scene of the accident or from other hospitals. Two U.S. Park Police and several U.S. Army Med-Evac helicopters supplement the State Police helicopter service.

D. **Maryland Specialty Referral System** Maryland has a unique system for the provision of highly specialized care for critically ill or injured persons who require sophisticated medical management. The system is called the Maryland Echelons of Trauma Care System (Figure 4). It consists of the specialty referral centers, the rapid transportation system, and the EMS communications system.

Specialty referral centers in Maryland have been established for adult trauma, pediatric trauma, burns, high-risk infants, upper and lower extremity amputations, poison control, eye trauma, and smoke inhalation. Each center is committed to accepting patients within the system unless their facility is full, in which case MIEMSS serves as a back-up. The centers and their criteria for admission are listed below:

1. **Maryland Institute for Emergency Medical Services Systems (MIEMSS)** Adults (age 14 and over) with one or more of the following problems are admitted: severe multiple injuries (two or more systems), cardiac and major vessel injuries, cardiogenic shock, multiple injuries with complications (e.g., shock, sepsis, respiratory failure, cardiac failure, alcohol and drug overdose, severe facial and eye injuries, burns), gas gangrene, poisoning, carbon monoxide intoxication, scuba accidents, drowning, and smoke inhalation.

MIEMSS also accepts patients in the following situations:
   a. Children (under the age of 14) when an adult family member is also a MIEMSS patient
   b. Children with spinal cord injuries
   c. An adult burn patient when the burn specialty referral centers are full
   d. Children requiring use of the hyperbaric chamber
   e. Head and spinal cord injuries.

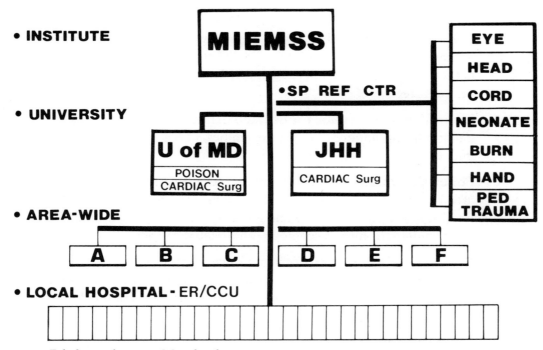

Figure 4. Echelons of care in Maryland.

2. **The Johns Hopkins Hospital Pediatric Trauma Center** Children (age 13 or younger) are admitted with one or more of the following: severe multiple injuries (two or more systems); head, cardiac, and major vessel injuries; cardiogenic shock; uncontrolled multiple injuries with complications (e.g., shock, sepsis, respiratory failure, cardiac failure, alcohol and drug overdose); severe facial and eye injuries, burns, drowning victims. The Children's Hospital in Washington, D.C., is utilized when the Hopkins Pediatric Center is full.

   The Johns Hopkins Hospital Pediatric Trauma Center also accepts children (age 13 or younger) having severe burns when the burn specialty referral center is full.

3. **Baltimore City Hospitals Burn Center** Patients meeting one or more of the following criteria are admitted:
   a. Age 60 or older having any burn injury
   b. Age 5 or younger having any burn injury
   c. Patients of any age having 30% or more of the body surface burned, regardless of degree of burn
   d. Patients of any age suffering respiratory system burns
   e. Patients of any age suffering burns of any degree on the hands, face, feet, or perineum.

4. **Maryland Intensive Care Neonatal Program** Five specialty referral centers cooperate to provide specialized care for high-risk infants. They are:
   a. Baltimore City Hospitals Neonatal Center
   b. University of Maryland Hospital Neonatal Center
   c. The Johns Hopkins Hospital Neonatal Center
   d. St. Agnes Hospital (as a back-up center when the other units are full)
   e. Sinai Hospital (as a back-up center when the other units are full).

   The program is managed by the Director of the Neonatal Program of the University of Maryland Hospital. Admission to all three institutions occurs on a rotational scheme, which is coordinated at the Baltimore City Hospital's Neonatal Center. The program accepts any neonates with serious illnesses or congenital defects.

5. **Union Memorial Hospital Curtis Hand Center** Patients of all ages having partial or full amputations of upper extremities, hands, or lower extremities are admitted.

6. **Poison Control Center** This center is a telephone referral service for the local area and throughout the state. It has three telephone lines plus two toll-free lines. It is staffed 24 hr a day and gives advice to physicians and the lay public concerning poisoning, toxicology, and related subjects.

7. **Eye Trauma Center** Any penetrating eye injury is transferred, using the statewide communications system, to the Wilmer Eye Clinic in the Johns Hopkins Hospital complex or the Georgetown University Eye Trauma Center.

8. **Smoke Inhalation Program** Smoke inhalation patients are assessed at the scene. They are transferred to MIEMSS if:
   a. There is a history of unconsciousness related to exposure to smoke

b. The carbon monoxide level at the scene is greater than 25%.
SYSCOM coordinates helicopter transfers to MIEMSS.

9. **Areawide Trauma Centers**   Within the City of Baltimore, four trauma centers have been designated (Figure 5). They are:
   —Baltimore City Hospital (BCH)
   —Johns Hopkins Hospital (JHH)
   —Sinai Hospital
   —University of Maryland Hospital (UM)
   Other trauma centers designated throughout the state (Figure 6) are:
   —Memorial Hospital, Cumberland
   —Washington County Hospital, Hagerstown
   —Peninsula General Hospital, Salisbury
   —Prince George's Hospital, Cheverly
   —Suburban Hospital, Bethesda
   Adults are admitted to these trauma centers with one of the following:
a. Trauma combinations (head, chest, abdomen, extremity)
b. Crush/blunt trauma (chest, abdomen, pelvis)
c. Penetrating chest wounds (gunshot wounds, stabbing, impaled objects)
d. Injury with severe hemorrhage (systolic blood pressure less than 80 mm Hg; MAST applied)

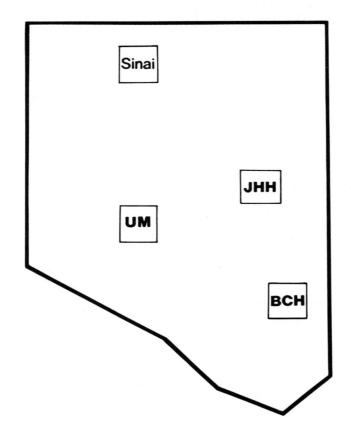

Figure 5.   Areawide trauma centers in Baltimore City.

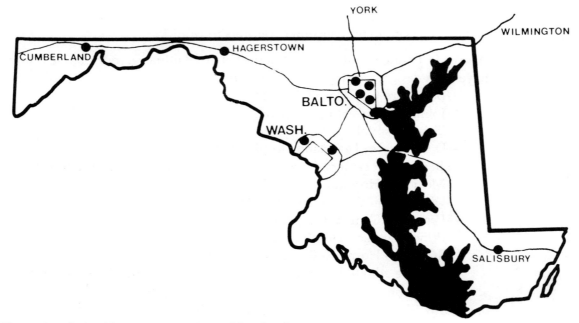

Figure 6. Areawide trauma centers in Maryland.

    e. One or more extremities paralyzed as a result of trauma

    f. Traumatic amputations (hand and foot cases are sent to Union Memorial Hospital).

E. **Training and Continuing Education** Training for medical personnel and lay citizens dealing with emergencies is offered through the cooperation of various agencies.

    1. Ambulance and helicopter crew members are trained to resuscitate and stabilize the patient at the scene of the accident and maintain that stable condition en route to the hospital. Most crew members are certified emergency medical technicians (EMT), and many are also certified cardiac rescue technicians (CRT). The CRT training instructs ambulance attendants to use telemetry equipment, to begin intravenous solutions and administer drugs ordered by a physician, and to utilize advanced life-support methods. EMTs and CRTs become an extension of the emergency room.

    2. Accredited nursing and physician programs provide an opportunity to update skills.

        a. For nurses, workshops are presented throughout the state on such topics as trauma, crisis intervention, child abuse, burns, cardiac emergencies, pediatric trauma, neonatal care, orthopedics, blood gases, diabetic emergencies, respiratory problems, mechanical ventilation, spinal cord injury, the nurse as a first responder, and principles of patient and family teaching.

        b. Various state and national seminars are presented on trauma and emergency medicine and intensive skills-oriented courses for emergency physicians.

3. CPR and first-aid courses are supported for the citizen. Through the cooperative efforts of the Maryland Institute for Emergency Medical Services, the Maryland chapters of the American Heart Association, and the regional school systems, CPR training has been introduced into all high school curriculums.

In summary, the EMS program in Maryland has evolved into a unique, comprehensive system and has proven that a system built on leadership, coordination, cooperation, education, and local participation works to provide the best emergency medical care possible and at the same time does what it was designed to do—save lives.

FAMILY SERVICES

I. **Family Services** is a multidisciplinary, ancillary team of professional behavioral scientists who work in concert with the medical and nursing teams to provide for the pyscho-social needs of the families of MIEMSS patients. Family services are available during the day and evening shifts and on-call for weekends. This team is comprised of:

A. **Director of Family Services** The Director takes responsibility for the managerial process of planning, organizing, staffing, coordinating, reporting, budgeting, educational programming, staff development, and research and evaluation and is responsible for the efficiency and effectiveness of the aforementioned operations. The Director also functions as a family counselor, as a liaison person for the local community agencies, and as an educator and consultant to the MIEMSS staff.

B. **Family Counselors** The Family Counselors are responsible for assessing the needs of families of MIEMSS patients and for the development and implementation of appropriate family treatment plans. Family Counselors provide service through direct casework, staff consultation, and community and staff education. Family Counselors perform program planning and assist in coordinating community resources for continued patient/family care.

C. **MIEMSS Chaplain** The Chaplain functions as a family counselor with special emphasis on the spiritual and religious needs of families. He also offers consultation and counseling to the MIEMSS staff.

D. **Alcoholism Counselor** The Alcoholism Counselor focuses on the problems alcohol abuse has created or poses for MIEMSS patients and their families. The Alcoholism Counselor works specifically with these patients and families and assists the Medical and Nursing staffs in assessing the needs of, and developing feasible treatment plans for, this patient population.

E. **Psychiatrist** The MIEMSS Psychiatrist functions in conjunction with Family Services and acts as consultant to the Division.

F. **Secretary** The professional staff is supported by a secretary whose function is to facilitate the work of the Family Services Branch.

G. **Graduate Student Counselors/Volunteers** Graduate students and volunteers in the disciplines of social work, psychology, pastoral counseling, and psychiatric nursing work with the Family Services team as student counselors in training.

II. **Services to Patients and their Families**
　　—Family psychosocial assessment
　　—Family treatment through individual and group counseling sessions
　　—Death and dying preparation and spiritual counseling for patients and their families
　　—Recommendations for appropriate posthospital placement and assistance with patient discharge plans
　　—Assistance in the coordination of community resources for patient rehabilitation
　　—Directing and facilitating the trauma patient recovery group
　　—Program planning and implementation to meet the needs of patient populations with specific problems

III. **Services to Staff**
　　—Individual and team consultation regarding psychosocial needs of patients and their families
　　—Individual personal counseling
　　—Classes, lectures, and workshops regarding the psychosocial dimension of patient/family care
　　—Staff development and in-service program planning and implementation
　　—Liaison between MIEMSS and community social service agencies and public health departments.

IV. **Community Involvement**　Areas of community involvement in which Family Services participates include:
　　—Assisting in MIEMSS community education programs
　　—Serving as liaison to community social service agencies and public health departments.

PSYCHIATRIC CONSULTATION
AND ABNORMAL BEHAVIOR

Psychiatric consultations in the trauma unit are common and cover a much broader spectrum than those required by other surgical or medical settings. Ten percent of all patients are seen by the psychiatrist, for a variety of reasons including severe agitation and confusion. Others are evaluated for psychosis, depression, or suicide potential, or because the patient requests a psychiatric consultation. Patients with a history of psychiatric illness or treatment and alcohol or other substance abuses need to be evaluated by the psychiatrist. Finally, the patient whose pain or other neurological symptoms are felt to represent a conversion disorder routinely receives psychiatric consultation. As in all settings, the usefulness of the consultation depends heavily on the surgeon's success at specifying which behaviors are to be evaluated and which questions are to be answered. Below is a brief discussion of common situations where psychiatric consultation is requested.

I. **Severe Agitation**   Severe agitation is a common sight in the trauma unit. Combative and disorganized behavior make history taking, physical examination, and diagnostic procedures more difficult than usual. Maintaining a venous line, cardiac monitor, and respiratory connections becomes an extremely difficult task.

    Rapid and accurate diagnosis is the key to appropriate management. In the trauma patient, the most common causes of severe agitation are hypoxia, sepsis, drug withdrawal or toxicity, pain, and head injury. Notably absent are schizophrenia, mania, and other psychiatric conditions; however, the psychiatric consultant's skillful interview can lead to useful information about pain or drug use. Sedation is often necessary to facilitate diagnosis and prevent injury to the patient and staff. Antipsychotic agents are the drugs of choice because of their effectiveness and low incidence of side effects. Haloperidol, 5 mg administered i.m. every 30 min, will reduce agitation to manageable proportions in many cases, but 6 to 10 doses (total dose of 30 to 50 mg) may be required. Hypoxia, sepsis, drug withdrawal or toxicity, head injury, and pain must be excluded as causes of agitation.

II. **The Confused or Organic Syndrome Patient**   Confusion is the rule rather than the exception in recently admitted trauma patients. Such patients are commonly agitated and, more generally, the causes of confusion are those mentioned in the section on the agitated patient. Management includes frequent reorientation, concise and repeated explanation of diagnostic and therapeutic procedures, and early removal from the excessive and unfamiliar stimulation of the critical care unit. Sedation routinely leads to a worsening of this condition. Accordingly, psychotropic medications are best left to the Psychiatrist or other physicians familiar with the use of these agents.

III. **Psychosis** Many confused or agitated patients are psychotic by most definitions. A group of psychotic patients that deserve emergency psychiatric evaluation are individuals who report or demonstrate persistent paranoid (unduly suspicious) thinking, auditory hallucinations (voices that talk to the patient or comment on the patient's behavior), or unusual thoughts, speech, or behavior. The latter signs depend purely on the physician's subjective impression but include such things as grandiose thoughts, articulate but illogical or incoherent speech, and bizarre gestures or postures. There are many nonpsychiatric causes of these phenomena, but they often respond, regardless of etiology, to antipsychotics. Failure to evaluate and, when appropriate, treat psychosis can lead directly to physical harm to the patient, other patients, or staff. A psychiatric consultation should be obtained if there is a question regarding psychotic behavior.

IV. **Depression** It is normal for the trauma patient to appear or report feeling sad or depressed. Those who report recurrent thoughts of low self-esteem or guilt and who report or demonstrate insomnia, diminished appetite, or a marked slowing of their thoughts may have a depressive illness. Diagnosis of this disorder can prevent unduly prolonged convalescence, suicide attempts, and other complications. Therefore, any patient suspected of being depressed should receive an elective psychiatric evaluation before discharge.

V. **The Suicidal Patient** Self-inflicted gunshot wounds, attempted hangings, jumps from bridges, and other suicide attempts are common causes of admissions. These patients are rarely a serious suicide risk while in the trauma unit; however, all such patients should receive a psychiatric evaluation before discharge. This evaluation will determine what type of psychiatric or other intervention is appropriate during the months after discharge when repeat attempts are not uncommon. Furthermore, any patient who acknowledges thoughts or plans of suicide or who attempts to harm himself/herself should receive an emergency psychiatric evaluation.

Numerous accidents, especially those involving a single automobile, may reflect disguised or unconscious suicide attempts. Patients with a previous history of suicide attempt, depression, or multiple accidents should have a psychiatric evaluation before discharge.

Confusion and psychosis represent two conditions where suicide may occur before or after discharge. The following **suicide precautions** are recommended:

—If any patient is thought to be actively suicidal in the hospital, then the Psychiatrist should be contacted to obtain an emergency evaluation for suicide precautions. Until such a patient is evaluated by the Psychiatrist, he is to be placed under one-to-one continuous observation. If such a patient is judged to be actively suicidal, then that patient will remain under continuous observation and the MIEMSS administration will be contacted immediately by the nursing staff so that they can make immediate arrangements for the patient's appropriate care. The Psychiatry Liaison Nurse and/or Psychiatrist will provide consultation to the staff and the private duty nurse as to choice of room, removal of dangerous objects, and so forth. Such patients will be reevaluated by psychiatry at least every 36 hr for removal of suicide precautions. In summary, an order for suicide precautions requires continuous one-to-one observation, a formal psychiatric evaluation, and reevaluation at least every 36 hr. In each case, the family spokesperson will be informed as to why such precautions are being followed and what they entail. Visiting privileges will be evaluated for each case.

—All patients admitted after a suicide attempt must be evaluated by the Psychiatry Liaison Nurse before discharge from the hospital. If any patient is felt to be actively suicidal, appropriate pre-cautions should be taken. Family Services will provide a formal family evaluation in all cases of suicide attemps.

—When a patient has been deemed suicidal by the above protocols, the following environmental precautions will be taken by the nursing staff:

Room designation (as indicated by the psychiatrist and approved by the administration)

The patient who is mobile will be escorted to, into, and from the bathroom under supervision.

Supervision by nursing staff or designated person to and from any area of the hospital (e.g., whirlpool, x-ray)

The following objects must be removed from the patient's immediate environment: needles, syringes, scalpels, scissors, razors, povidone-iodine (Betadine), peroxide, alcohol, any material made of glass, suture removal kits, and so on.

VI. The Patient Requesting Psychiatric Evaluation   All patients requesting a psychiatric evaluation should receive such an evaluation on a nonemergency basis unless the patient demonstrates a marked sense of urgency, in which case the request is treated as an emergency. The patient should not be merely reassured that his or her experiences are normal or that everything will be all right. Common reasons for these requests include thoughts of suicide, depression, an emerging psychosis or repetitive thoughts or flashbacks of the event that prompted admission.

VII. The Patient with a History of a Previous Psychiatric Disorder or Treatment   These patients should receive psychiatric evaluation, on an elective basis, because they may require psychiatric treatment during hospitalization or after discharge. This is especially true for those with a history of schizophrenia and those receiving antidepressants or antipsychotics at the time of admission. (Commonly used agents in these two classes are Elavil, Tofranil, Norpramine, Sinequan, Thorazine, Mellaril, Stelazine, Trilafon, Prolixin, Haldol, and Navane).

VIII. The Patient with a History of Alcohol or Drug Abuse   This group overlaps significantly with the above and, for the same reasons, should be evaluated by the psychiatrist or someone skilled in the treatment of those disorders. One way to screen for alcoholism is to refer all patients whose blood alcohol level at admission exceeds 150 mg %. Similarly, any patient having serum levels of benzodiazepines or other substances can be referred. The most reliable screening is done, however, by asking the patient and family members about alcohol and substance abuse (see p. 399).

IX. **The Patient Reporting Severe or Persistent Pain or Other Physical Symptoms Thought to Have a Psychiatric Basis (Conversion Symptoms)**   These patients require psychiatric evaluation. To enlist the patient's cooperation and thereby facilitate this evaluation, the patient should be told before the medical evaluation of the symptoms has been completed that all causes of the symptoms must be evaluated and that this will require a psychiatric consultation during or after the performance of other evaluations. Conversion symptoms often have a mixed organic/psychiatric cause. Evaluation and treatment generally require close collaboration between the primary physician and the psychiatric consultant.

> **Note**   **Emergency psychiatric consultation is available 24 hr a day.** Nonemergency psychiatric consultation may be obtained on weekdays by filing a consultation request.

REHABILITATION

At MIEMSS, rehabilitation is viewed as a process that contributes to a person's achievement of maximum functional potential and eventual return to the community. Consequently, it begins immediately following injury, continues throughout the critical care period, and includes the subsequent disposition of the patient. This is our concept of holistic care.

It is rare for trauma patients to be without some residual disability related to their injury. Therefore, the goal of the rehabilitative process during the acute care period consists mainly of preventing secondary disability and maintaining the existing function that the patient has. As the medical condition of the patient stabilizes and long-term needs become more apparent, the active restorative activities become more predominant and take place without unnecessary delay.

The rationale for a rehabilitation program in a trauma unit includes the following:

—Most trauma patients have residual disability of some type; in cases of neurotrauma and orthopedic trauma this may be severe, for example, tetraplegia or amputation.

—A system of care incorporating early rehabilitation activities has been shown to be cost-effective. The National Spinal Cord Injury Systems Data demonstrates decreased costs when a coordinated system of care is in place from the emergency care period through a completed rehabilitation program.

—A moral obligation to human life does not end when one saves a person; concern with quality of life for that individual is required.

I. **The Patient's Rehabilitative Needs**

   A.   The patient's ultimate success in rehabilitation and return to the community is expedited by an approach that considers the patient as a total individual. Physical, psychological, and sociocultural needs are present in everyone and need to be addressed. This holistic consideration transcends the narrow focus that concentrates only on specific medical problems.

   B.   Continuity of care is needed as the patient moves through the system. This means coordination and communication between each unit involved in care of the individual, whether it involves transfer between nursing units or transfer between facilities.

   C.   It is necessary to maintain an awareness that activities during the acute care period can have an effect on the patient's rehabilitation. For example, failure to employ preventive measures can result in complications, such as contractures or pressure sores, which interfere with readiness for active rehabilitation programs; or surgical location of a stoma can influence a person's ability to perform his or her own ostomy care.

   D.   Acknowledgment of the patient's inherent right to participate in decision making regarding factors that influence the patient's life needs to be part of the treatment philosophy.

II. **MIEMSS Rehabilitation Program**   To meet their rehabilitative needs, patients require a coordinated interdisciplinary team effort, no matter whether the location is an acute care facility or a rehabilitation center. In the trauma center, which achieves success by a protocol approach and has a staff of highly specialized physicians, nurses, and health care personnel, this is not an easy task. However, through a commitment to the rehabilitation process and the efforts of the staff, the following programs and services combine to meet rehabilitative needs.

A. **Primary nursing care system**   The nursing staff consists of professional registered nurses and is organized to deliver care as a primary nurse system. Under this method, each patient admitted to MIEMSS is assigned a Primary Nurse who is responsible for assessing nursing needs and developing an individualized plan of care. The Primary Nurse also is responsible for implementing that plan of care and seeing that it is carried out by other nursing team members. Incorporated within that plan of care are the practices basic to rehabilitation. These include positioning, turning, prevention of skin problems, attention to bowel and bladder needs, and communication with the patient's families or significant others. Responsibility for patient and family teaching rest with the Primary Nurse. This is planned teaching related to self-care needs; the resultant learning is integral to the rehabilitation process.

B. **Availability of clinical nurse specialists**   A neurotrauma nurse practitioner follows all neurotrauma patients through MIEMSS and is responsible for coordinating their care and supervising patient/family teaching and follow-up of these patients in the clinic to attend to their transitional needs. This type of specialist affords these patients regular contact with one individual and contributes to continuity. Another clinical specialist provides the same services for orthopedic patients. A Mental Health Clinical Nurse Specialist attends to the specific psychological needs of patients' response to trauma and also serves as a resource to the primary care nurses in this effort.

C. **Discharge coordinator**   Three discharge coordinators plan disposition for patients leaving the Institute. These persons are in contact with patients and families soon after admission and facilitate planning related to where the patient may be discharged. They are responsible for gaining necessary information from physicians, nurses, and other health care planners in order to furnish this information to the receiving institution. Disposition rounds are held on a regular basis so that a discharge status report on each patient is available. Information regarding rehabilitation facilities and other institutions is provided patients and families so they may participate in the discharge planning process. Such early planning decreases length of stay and eases some of the problems patients and families encounter when patients are transferred between institutions or return home.

D. **Rehabilitation rounds**   Twice weekly rehabilitation rounds are made by a cooperative team representing MIEMSS and the State Rehabilitation Center. This includes a psychiatrist, social worker, nurse, discharge coordinator, MIEMSS physician, and an administrative coordinator.

E. **Family Services Unit** This unit consists of family social workers, the Chaplain, and an alcohol rehabilitation counselor. They provide professional support, counseling, and direction to the trauma patients' families, who frequently find themselves in crisis due to the sudden disruption that trauma imposes on the family unit. This department collaborates with all other departments and focuses attention on the importance of the family unit to the rehabilitation success of patients.

F. **Psychiatrist** A full-time psychiatrist is a member of the MIEMSS staff and provides direct care and consultation regarding psychiatric problems that may occur in patients.

G. **Respiratory therapy** A respiratory therapy program is an inherent part of the Critical Care Medicine department and offers active chest physical therapy.

H. **Physical medicine and rehabilitation** Referrals to the Physical Medicine and Rehabilitation Department are made early upon admission of a patient with spinal cord or head injury so that consultation from psychiatrists, occupational therapists, and physical therapists may be obtained. While the patient is immobile, these services are provided at bedside; however, as soon as possible and when the patient is able to be moved, the patient is transported to the therapy department for necessary activities.

III. **Trauma recovery group** The trauma recovery group is an active organization that grew out of a need for former trauma patients to share common experiences. This support group, with guidance and participation of MIEMSS staff, focuses attention on the need for follow-up and continuity of care for trauma patients.

IV. **Center for Living** The Center for Living is designed as a nonmedical comprehensive "bridge" program to help trauma patients and their families readjust to their life situations following long-term acute and rehabilitation hospitalizations. It provides a place where professional counselors assist patients in sorting out and coping with the feelings generated by the traumatic injury. Individual, family, and group counseling and psychometric testing are available. As the program expands, there will be educational opportunities, job development, transportation, social reorientation, and respite care. This unique follow-up program addresses the special needs of the trauma population and functions as a primary resocialization agent for these persons.

Perspective
The cost of trauma is high and the cost of the resulting disability also is high. Early attention to rehabilitative needs of trauma patients is believed to contribute to lessened disability and decreased length of stay in institutions before persons return to the community. Enhancing that rehabilitation potential is an interdisciplinary team collaborating to meet the physical, psychological, and sociocultural needs of trauma patients.

TRAUMA REGISTRY

Quality assurance and evaluation programs are an integral part of the operation and continued evolution of a trauma center and trauma system. A major barrier to improving trauma care is a lack of cumulative knowledge and experience in the complex management of severely injured trauma patients. Medical records often are inadequate for evaluation of relevant data, and current methodology for abstracting pertinent information is usually tedious and often unrewarding.

MIEMSS has developed a computerized trauma registry with the following objectives:
—To facilitate and improve patient care by rapidly locating and reproducing significant amounts of clinical information
—To provide on-line clinical summaries of diagnostic and therapeutic methods
—To establish a data source for developing at-risk factors for accidental events
—To determine variables upon which patient morbidity and mortality depend
—To determine logistical and manpower requirements for trauma care in a given community
—To estimate costs and expenditures for certain injuries and their comprehensive care requirements
—To continuously monitor project planning for the care of the critically injured.

The following data sets are entered in a computerized registry:
—Patient demographic data
—Epidemiologic data
—Initial diagnostic data
—Patient care data
—Discharge diagnostic data
—Ancillary support service data
—Special procedure data
—Complication data
—Physician-nurse-paramedic field data
—Audit criteria data.

Demographic data capture includes such information as age, sex, race, occupation, home address, and so on. Epidemiologic data include information on time and location of accident, mechanism of injury, and so on. Initial patient care data captured covers the hospital management, including drugs that are given for medical support and procedures that are performed, the method and transportation time, and the standard of the institution to which the patient is transferred. Further data are entered into the patient file as the patient proceeds through the acute care unit. Laboratory, bacteriologic, and other data also are entered. They can be immediately accessed for the benefit of physicians and nurses and aid in the clinical management of the patient. Complication data such as incidence of atelectasis, septicemia, renal failure, and so forth also are entered during the hospital stay. In addition, there is a separate subfile that can be entered if the patient is in a particular clinical trial. Additional information concerning length of ventilator support, length of stay in the intensive care unit, number and type of physicians consulting on the patient, use of the ancillary services, and so on can also be recorded into the trauma data file.

At the time of discharge, the patient's cumulative inventory of information is sorted by the computer. This process will ensure that all relevant information has been collected. The computer abstracts portions of information for storage in the trauma registry. The entire patient file initially is stored on a disk for acute retrieval, and later is transferred to tape. Certain subprograms can be run against the data base in order to abstract relevant information to be used in the development of audit reports, mortality and morbidity review, utilization review, quality assurance reports, and other specific reports as required. In addition, the trauma registry can provide information and analyses of epidemiologic, demographic, clinical, financial, and societal impact of major trauma problems. This information can be used to satisfy local hospital, county, state, or federal requirements for data collection. These subprograms are in a state of development and will be used for developing injury severity scores based not only on anatomical data, but also on demographic and physiologic data which should provide useful information for optimal patient management. All of the reporting within the existing trauma registry data base is in standard format: International Classification of Diseases (ninth revision) Clinical Modification coding (ICD.9.CM) for disease entity, current procedural terminology (CPT) for procedures, and other information, allowing rapid and accurate recording for various agencies.

Design of the software package (in Fortran IV) follows a modular format that can be modified to fulfill any particular local requirement for analysis or data reporting.

TRIAGE

Triage implies the evaluation and classification of injuries for treatment and disposition. The decisions that must be made concern the need for resuscitation and emergency operations with the acceptance of the futility of surgery in certain lethal wounds. Triage also involves the establishment of care priorities.

In the Maryland EMS system, triage is performed at the scene of an accident and again on admission to a definitive care facility. Over 80% of the patients admitted to MIEMSS have life-threatening injuries, and are transported by the helicopter and ambulance systems from the entire state and surrounding states. The problem of triage is comparable to a military guerrilla situation, although admission criteria differ somewhat. The criteria for admission to MIEMSS are as follows:

—Severe multiple injuries (two or more systems)
—Head or spinal cord injuries
—Cardiac and major vessel injuries, generally of the chest and abdomen
—Multiple injuries with complications, e.g., shock, sepsis, respiratory failure
—Multiple injuries complicating previous illnesses, such as diabetes, liver cirrhosis, cardiac and pulmonary disease
—Severe facial and eye injuries (although generally not life-threatening in severity, these require immediate care if long periods of staged plastic surgery are to be prevented or if vision is to be saved)
—Scuba accidents, drownings, burns, gas gangrene, carbon monoxide intoxication, poisonings, alcoholism, drug overdose, and attempted suicides.

I. **Triage at the Scene** A direct pickup at the scene of the accident can occur in two ways: 1) The helicopter crew, while on patrol, may see an accident or be alerted by monitoring radio calls. In these instances, they would usually be the first paramedical assistance to arrive. 2) Alternatively, a civilian or a road policeman may call the jurisdictional county fire department for help, and they in turn will dispatch an ambulance with a simultaneous request for helicopter support.

The following criteria provide triage at the scene:
—Whoever arrives at the scene of an accident first assesses the injury. If the injury is serious, both helicopter and ambulance are summoned.
—If the ambulance arrives at the scene first, immediate first aid and resuscitation are given. If the injury is not life-threatening, the patient is transferred to the nearest hospital. If the injury is life-threatening, the ambulance crew continues resuscitation at the scene until the helicopter arrives. If the helicopter notifies those at the scene that undue delay would be encountered by waiting for arrival, or that the mission is not logistically possible, the ambulance crew will immediately proceed with the patient to the nearest hospital.
—If the helicopter crew arrives at the scene first, they in turn provide immediate first aid, resuscitation, and injury assessment. If the victim does not require

transport to a trauma center, they sustain the patient until the ambulance arrives for transport to the nearest hospital.

When flying to an accident scene, the helicopter crew radios an alert to the nearest trauma center to stand by for a possible admission. If, after triage, the patient is thought to need the facilities of such a center, a confirmation call is made and an estimated time of arrival is given. This call includes details as to the number of patients being transported, the types of injuries, and the condition of the patient(s).

II. **Triage at the Definitive Care Facility** Upon arrival at the helipad, the patient is met by a physician, admitting nurse, and anesthesiologist who provide immediate assessment and resuscitation if necessary. The patient is then met by an admitting team under the direction of a staff physician and team leader and initial resuscitative stabilization, diagnosis, and triage are continued according to established protocols.

In summary, our current philosophy is to attempt to save the lives of all patients, regardless of the injury or the duration of time between the initial insult and their admission. With this approach, we believe many patients survive who would die in more conventional medical systems. Thus, triage at the scene and on admission is a vital function necessary to carry out this goal.

III. **The Mass Casualty Incident: The MIEMSS Emergency Medical Response Team** A mass casualty incident (MCI) is defined as a medical emergency that overwhelms local capabilities and resources to deal with the situation. A minimum of 15 multiply injured persons is established for purposes of this definition. However, situations requiring lengthy extrication procedures may constitute exceptions to this rule.

Emergency surface evacuation becomes heavily burdened in a MCI, resulting in a loss of valuable time that increases the requirement for on-scene stabilization and resuscitation. In the pressure of a MCI there is an increased likelihood of error in the initial medical decisions that determine the patient's survival.

In their routine responses, emergency medical systems are structured to act with immediacy with resources adequate to the task. Personnel are trained to deal with individual specialized problems including fractures, lacerations, other trauma, heart attacks, and the like. However, in a MCI the emergency medical problems differ. The scene can create an environment of confusion, as medical radio communications are commonly overwhelmed and there may be a shortage of supplies and professional expertise. It is imperative that the elements of command, control, and communication be established promptly to ensure coordination of medical intervention with the efforts of police and fire departments.

As the lead agency for the statewide emergency medical services system, MIEMSS formed an Emergency Medical Response Team, referred to as the Go-Team, that is dispatched to the MCI to support on-scene emergency activities and establish an authority for medical control and supervision. The Go-Team is made up of the following MIEMSS personnel:

—One physician traumatologist

—One anesthesiologist

—One admitting area nurse

—One emergency medical systems communications operator.

At the operating base, the traumatologist is the physician in charge, with the anesthesiologist next in authority.

The Go-Team is activated by the Director of MIEMSS or his designated representative when help is requested through the Systems Communications Center (SYSCOM) by the local medical officer at the scene. On notification, the Go-Team assembles at the MIEMSS helipad for helicopter transportation to the MCI. In the event of inclement weather the team meets in the Emergency Room entrance of University Hospital. Transportation (both air and surface vehicles) of the Go-Team to the MCI is the responsibility of the State Police.

Initial medical and resuscitation supplies transported to the scene by the Go-Team are:

—State Police walkie-talkie kit

—Identification ensemble kit

—Stethoscopes

—Field dressings

—Sterile sheets

—Trauma blankets

—Pharyngeal airways

—Esophageal airways

—Endotracheal tubes

—Tracheostomy kits

—Cervical collars

—Plasma, crystalloids, and intravenous catheters

—Emergency and cardiac drugs

—Military Anti-Shock Trousers

—Elder valve units

—Ambu bags

—Flashlights.

Responsibility for resupply lies with the local medical groups.

The Go-Team's responsibilities at the MCI scene are to support the local medical officer in charge. The team:

—Establishes a predetermined command structure to minimize the potential for confusion at the scene

—Establishes expert triage for the most severely injured victims

—Provides early resuscitation and stabilization of the victims at the scene

—Provides a base for aeromedical evacuation

—Directs the transportation of the victims to the appropriate definitive care facility (specialty referral centers or areawide trauma center). The Go-Team possesses a thorough knowledge of regional hospital capabilities and capacities.

—Maintains the integrity of the emergency medical systems communications network

—Increases by its presence the confidence of the other medical and paramedical personnel at the scene.

In summary, the MIEMSS Go-Team provides an organized, preplanned response to the extraordinary circumstances presented by a MCI. It supports local emergency medical personnel by establishing an on-scene authority for triage, evacuation, and communication, and by coordinating the efforts of emergency personnel at the scene.

INDEX

Index

This index addresses itself primarily to those injuries and clinical problems that require urgent attention. Other listings have been omitted to prevent camouflaging those items which mandate a prompt response.

etiology, 349
management, 352
manifestations, 349
Renal insufficiency
diabetes insipidus, 356
SIADH, 355
see also Renal failure
Replantation, 274
Respiratory distress, 16, 313, 315, 326
Respiratory function
assessment, 16, 313, 315, 321
stabilization, 17, 314, 316
see also Endotracheal intubation; Pulmonary insufficiency; Tracheostomy
Resuscitative transfusion, 35
Retroperitoneal hematoma, 181
Rhinorrhea, 90, 94, 227, 422
Rib fractures, 24
first, 107
flail chest, 108
multiple, 107
simple, 106

Sacral fractures, 195
Scalp, 73
Scuba accidents, 512
Secretions, tracheobronchial, 323
Sepsis
bacteremia, 415
fever, 411
shock, 65
systemic stress, 414
Septic shock, 65
Sexual assault, 203
Shock, *see* Cardiogenic shock; Hypovolemic shock; Septic shock
SIADH, 355
Sinus fractures, 93
Sinusitis, 424
Skeletal injury
compartment syndrome, 246, 253
diagnosis, 241
ligamentous, 246
open fractures, 243, 248

radiography, 34, 242
splinting, 242
see also Fractures
Skull fractures, 21, 33, 75, 218, 220, 227
Skull x-rays, 33; *see also* Skull fractures
Small intestine
blunt trauma, 162
penetrating trauma, 161
Smoke inhalation, 289, 379, 508
Soft tissue
infection, *see* Infection management, wound infection
injury, 84, 260
Spine
cervical, 23, 233
initial management, 229
lumbar, 27, 235
medical treatment, 236
neurologic exam, 230
penetrating injury, 236
thoracic, 25, 235
see also Quadriplegia; X-rays
Spleen, 26, 151
Sternal fractures, 108
Stomach, 26
blunt trauma, 157
penetrating trauma, 156
Stress, systemic, 372, 414
Stress ulceration, 365
Subclavian vein catheterization, 470
Subcutaneous emphysema
barotrauma, 332
bronchial injury, 111
esophageal injury, 100, 119
laryngeal injury, *see* Larynx
tracheal injury, 117
Subdural hematoma, 221
Subglottic stenosis, 330
Sucking chest wound, 106
Suicidal behavior, 574

Tachycardia, 343, 345
Tachypnea, 17, 315
Tamponade, *see* Cardiac tamponade

Tension pneumothorax, 11, 19, 113, 333
Tetanus immunization, 429
Thoracic duct, 132
Thoracoabdominal wounds, 131
Thoracotomy, indications, 132; *see also* Reexploratory thoracotomy
Thrombocytopenia, 38, 414, 493
Trachea
injury, 25, 117
stenosis, 327
tube complications, 326
Tracheoesophageal fistula, 328
Tracheo-innominate artery fistula, 329
Tracheomalacia, 326
Tracheostomy
elective, 95, 481
emergency, 482
Transfusion
autotransfusion, 39
massive, 37
reactions, 41
resuscitative, 35

Ureter, 27, 179
Urethra, 27, 180
Urethrogram, 177
Urinary tract injuries
bladder, 180
kidney, 10, 27, 178, 182
ureter, 27, 179
urethra, 27, 180
Urinary tract infections, 424
Uterus
gravid, 206, 207
nongravid, 201

Vagina, 196, 200
Vascular prosthesis infections, 426
Vena cava, 181
Venous access, 9, 469
Ventilation, *see* Respiratory function

Ventilator support
    asynchrony, 315, 332
    indications, 314, 316
    initiation, 319
    weaning, 321
Ventriculitis, 422
Vocal cord injury, 99, 331

Von Willebrand's disease, 37
Vulva, 199, 200

X-rays
    chest, 4, 32, 33
    extremity, 34, 242

facial, 34, 83
pelvis, 32, 194
skull, *see* Skull fractures
spine, 31, 34, 232
see also specific injury

Zygoma, 89